My Body,
My Trauma, My I

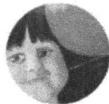

Green Balloon Publishing

Professor Dr Franz Ruppert, is Professor of Psychology at the University of Applied Sciences in Munich, Germany. He gained his PhD in Work and Organisational Psychology at the Technical University of Munich in 1985.

His publications in English include: *Trauma, Bonding & Family Constellations: Understanding and Healing Injuries of the Soul* (2008), *Splits in the Soul: Integrating Traumatic Experiences* (2011), *Symbiosis & Autonomy: Symbiotic Trauma and Love Beyond Entanglements* (2012), *Trauma, Fear and Love; How the Constellation of the Intention Supports Healthy Autonomy* (2014), *Early Trauma: Pregnancy, Birth and First Years of Life* (2016), all published in English by Green Balloon Publishing, Steyning, UK.

Ruppert teaches in Germany and many other countries including Brazil, Austria, Norway, Singapore, Switzerland, Britain, Ireland, Italy, Russia, Netherlands, Poland, Portugal, Romania, Turkey and Spain, furthering his insights into the deeper transgenerational effects of trauma in different cultures, and researching the methodology of constellations as a means of better understanding the effects and healing of trauma.

Dr. med. Harald Banzhaf is the Medical Head of the Healing Centre Zollernalb in Bisingen/Hohenzollern with his own practice for integrative medicine, and lecturer at Tübingen University. He works with the Identity-oriented Psychotrauma Therapy developed by Prof. Dr. Ruppert and is a trainer in mindfulness and an accredited MBSR teacher. His publications include: *Achtsamkeit und Mitgefühl in der Therapie* (2010) in Deutsche Heilpraktiker Zeitschrift, and *Meditieren heilt* (2015) with S. Schmidt published by Kreuz, Freiburg.

About this book

This book is a collection of essays on the topic of the connection between physical illness and early emotional and psychological trauma. The premise is that 'physical illnesses', whether structural problems, chronic illnesses, undefinable malaise or nameable diseases, are likely to have as their foundations some form of very early psychological traumatisation.

The book starts with an overview by Professor Ruppert from the perspective of IoPT theory, followed by a complementary essay by Dr Harald Banzhaf, Medical Head of the Healing Centre Zollernalb, Germany, considering how current scientific and medical developments support Ruppert's theories and thinking.

The other 23 essays are written by practitioners who work with IoPT theory and method, bringing their own particular interest and expertise to understanding the origins of a variety of physical complaints in early emotional traumas.

This book provides a further link in our understanding of ourselves as human beings, who we are, and why we suffer from the ailments that we do.

My Body, My Trauma, My I

Setting up intentions – Exiting Our Traumabiography

Franz Ruppert and Harold Banzhaf

Contributors:

Dagmar Strauss, Evelyn Hähnel,
Beate Herrmann, Ingrid Perg, Patrizia Manukian,
Aurora Wolf, Annemarie Denk, Marta Thorsheim,
Thomas R. Röll, Thilo Behla, Gerlinde Fischedick,
Martina Wittmann, Juliane von Krause, Catherine Xavier,
Isabella Gerstgrasser, Kate Collier, Nadja Palombo,
Bettina Schmalnauer, Ellen Kersten, Diana Lucia Vasile,
Stephan Konrad Niederwieser, Andrea Tietz,
Christina Freund

Translated by Julia Stuebs
with the assistance of Rick Hosburn

Edited for the English edition by Vivian Broughton

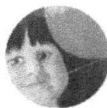

Green Balloon Publishing

First published in the United Kingdom in 2018
by Green Balloon Publishing

German edition first published under the title
Mein Körper, Mein Trauma, Mein Ich by Kösel Verlag,
Verlagsgruppe Random House

All case studies in this book are based on real events. In order to protect
the identity of those concerned, names and, where necessary,
personal details have been altered.

Green Balloon Publishing, Steyning
www.greenballoonbooks.co.uk

ISBN 978-0-9559683-8-9

Book production by The Choir Press, Gloucester
Set in Times

Contents

Contents

Preface

Doctors attempt to heal a patient's body without regard for the psyche. And psychologists treat the psyche without understanding what is happening in the body. The concept of psychotrauma forms a bridge between these worlds of the psyche and the physical, because in our experience psychotrauma is the source of many ailments that manifest in the body and in the psyche.

If we think about the traumas that we may experience in the very beginning moments of our life, we are able to understand better why our body and our psyche have developed as they have; we can see why many physical and psychological problems develop. If we can find a way of explaining these, mostly subconscious, correlations, we would then hold the key to healing the source of these physical and psychological afflictions. In this book we have collected many examples that support this claim. Our understanding of these causes also will help us to differentiate between medicinal and psychological treatments that are beneficial, and those that only address symptoms, and so only serve to support trauma survival strategies.

We would like to thank our colleagues for letting us include their practical experiences with the constellation of the intention in treating psychosomatic problems in this book, and we are grateful to those authors who have contributed reports based on their own personal experiences.

Our warm thanks go to Usha Swamy and Gerhard Plachta at Kösel publishing house for their helpful support in this joint project.

Munich, July 2017
Franz Ruppert and Harald Banzhaf

English Lanuage Editor's Foreword

As the editor of this English language version of Mein Korpe, Mein Trauma Mein Ich, I am very happy to present this book to you; another very important contribution to the growing bibliography of Professor Ruppert and his colleagues.

My thanks go to Julia Stuebs, the translator, for her excellent work. As a specialist subject editor for the English version, to be presented with a near perfect translation makes my job easy, and enjoyable. In addition my thanks to Rick Hosburn for his collaboration and support of Julia in her work.

I wish to acknowledge John McClean as our excellent proofreader, Miles Bailey and Rachel Woodman and their colleagues at Choir Press for the typesetting and technical work, John Mitchell of Green Balloon Publishing for his co-ordination and work toward publishing the end product, and several of my colleagues who assisted me with the editing.

I hope that English language readers find this exploration of the underlying causes of physical illness as fascinating as I have.

Vivian Broughton
English Language Editor

FRANZ RUPPERT

My body, my trauma, my I

From the viewpoint of Identity-oriented Psychotrauma Theory and Therapy (IoPT)

Physical Complaints – Fate or Psychotrauma?

Everybody has some sort of physical complaint. It's normal for different parts of our bodies to hurt from time to time. As we get older our bodies may be worn out by hard work, or by having children, or have permanent damage caused by accidents; that is part of human life. But why do children have all sorts of illnesses such as 'ADHD'[1], 'neurodermatitis', or 'asthma' that don't heal? Why do young people poison their bodies with drugs or starve themselves to death? Is the heart attack that is caused by stress a normal occupational hazard? Is 'cancer' unavoidable, and what about 'dementia' in old age? Do we have to put up with illnesses such as 'diabetes', 'rheumatism' or 'stomach ulcers' and just accept symptomatic treatments?

My therapeutic work has frequently shown that 'illnesses' are not the consequence of fate or 'bad genes', or even age. When we look more closely, we find they are caused by life experiences that we have been unable to process. 'Illnesses' are the result of psychotraumas that have to express themselves physically. This is demonstrated again and again in the therapeutic groups in which I work with the intention method and the constellation process:

---

[1] As the term 'illness' is frequently used as a trauma survival strategy and names of 'illnesses' are often simply verbal fantasies with no content-related message, I usually use quotation marks to make this background clear. The same applies to other terms in quotation marks, such as 'sexual abuse'.

- 'I want to know why I'm ill.' That was the intention expressed by a seminar participant who was on dialysis. Her constellation pointed to sexual abuse in early childhood. Even now, she is unable to express the pain and tears associated with this. The little child within her still has to pretend to her original family that nothing bad happened to her and that everything is fine.
- 'I want to be rid of the pain in my jaw.' This was another woman's intention. A constellation process brought to light that the removal of one of her wisdom teeth had triggered a psychotrauma from a long way back: the pain from an abortion she once had.
- 'I want to have my lungs back.' That was another participant's intention. She is a heavy smoker. Her constellation brought to light that she had suffered because her mother smoked while she was pregnant with her. Even before she was born this participant had a dilemma: not being able to stay in the womb, nor wanting to leave, where the smoking ordeal would continue. With every cigarette, she re-stages the psychotrauma that began before she was born, because her mother hadn't wanted to have her and didn't take care of her.

In my experience it is always worth facing up to the existence of psychotrauma and its far-reaching consequences for the human body and the human psyche. To do this we need to know:

- how the human psyche works;
- how psychotraumas arise and develop;
- the way they manifest in the body;
- how psychotraumas can be channelled into a healing process.

Living human organism (LHO)

The living human organism is the starting point for all illness and attempts at therapeutic healing. It is the interaction between matter, energy and information.

Matter – this refers to cells, organs, muscles, bones, blood, lymph, nerves and the genes with all their substructures. Both the male and female body are centred around the sexual and reproductive organs. Below the reproductive system is the primary means of locomotion: the legs and feet. Above it lies the food digestion system; above that the respiratory system, and above that again the head as our system of orientation. On each side of the trunk is an arm functioning as an instrument of action. The body is covered by skin that is permeable for what is allowed to move from inside the body to outside and vice versa.

Energy is produced by the living organism through its own activity at the motoric level. It is increased and decreased by biochemical reactions: for example, the intake, metabolism and elimination of food, neurotransmitters and hormones. It is created by electro-magnetic vibrations at the cellular level, and is structurally developed in the organs (e.g. the heart), and in the brain as electro-magnetic fields.

If we go by the observations of modern physics, matter is simply highly compressed energy (Laszlo, 1995). Where there is matter and energy, *information* is created. A great deal of information is needed in the living human organism, so that

- cells can inform each other of their state and requirements;
- organs can coordinate their actions with one another;
- behavioural patterns can be refined;
- the internal and external world can be understood on the basis of the individual's needs.

A living organism must continuously communicate with itself and its environment; it has to resonate with the environment; it is both a sender and a receiver. This happens verbally and consciously, but also to a greater extent unconsciously and non-verbally. Unconscious stimulus-response processes (e.g. breathing), hormonal behavioural impulses (e.g. the urge for sexual satisfaction), and actions based on emotions (such as searching for a loved one), often precede conscious perceptions and thoughts. The structure of the human brain – the brain stem, the diencephalon and the two hemispheres of the cerebrum – conveys a rough impression of the extent to which physical processes can become conscious. The connections run in both directions: unconscious processes in the body give rise to conscious decisions, and conscious decisions influence unconsciously regulated physical functions (Damasio, 2006; Siegel, 2010). Consciousness is a special feature of the human 'psyche' and is sometimes referred to as 'mind'. I will explain later in more detail what else is part of the human psyche.

The living human organism (LHO) as a modular system

We know that single cell organisms evolved into complex multicellular organisms through different single cell organisms learning to live in symbiosis with one another. The different qualities of the single cell organisms thus gave rise to the new qualities of a multi-cellular organism. The mitochondria, for example, which are responsible for the energy resources in a cell, were originally independent entities. And to a certain extent in the merged cells they are still separate. Fungi and bacteria form symbiotic communities to their mutual benefit. Countless fungi and bacteria that carry out useful functions for the whole organism settle in various places in the LHO, in the mouth, the stomach, the intestines or on the mucous membranes of the penis and vagina. In return they enjoy a secure existence under the protection of a powerful host. At the same time, studies of bacterial strains have shown how they keep each other's growth in check, thereby protecting their host from damage (Enders, 2014).

It is interesting to note the frequent occurrence of pairs in the LHO: legs and feet, arms and hands, lungs, kidneys, nostrils, eyes, ears, testicles, ovaries and the cerebrum. This is not only in case one of the systems should fail; it can also lead to further specialisation. The right and left halves of the body can have different abilities because they are directed by different brain structures. One obvious example of this is whether someone is right-handed or left-handed.

The modular structure of the LHO, consisting of many individual parts, is the reason its reactions are specific and do not always affect the whole organism. Sometimes, however, certain causes do affect the whole body: a virus, for example, which spreads throughout the LHO.

Since every human being is either a man or a woman – although there are also forms of intersexuality – every human body is also gender-specific. Men and women not only differ anatomically, they also go through different psychological processes of development and maturing. Male and female physical experiences can be very different. It is only a woman who can experience feeling a male penis inside her vagina, being pregnant, giving birth or breastfeeding. A male will usually experience some form of competition with other males, and many will carry mental and energy traces from this for the rest of their lives. Some men have become 'warriors' in the course of their lives. Others have become 'dealers', 'thinkers' or 'philosophers'.

Stages of Development of the LHO

Every human organism develops in a maternal body. During its formation it passes through a sequence of developmental steps: penetration of the egg cell by the sperm, initial cell division, implantation in the uterus, development of placenta and amniotic sac, development of organs, bones, muscles, nerves and brain, and finally emergence from the maternal body, birth and the cutting of the cord.

What then follows is subject to a far greater degree of variance than the events inside the maternal body. Some babies remain with their mother, are nourished from her breasts and experience her love, care and support. Other babies are removed from their mother immediately after birth, transferred to an incubator, not breastfed and have no eye or skin contact. Yet others are immediately given to an adoptive mother, or are passed from their 'surrogate' mother to the woman or couple who have paid for her to carry the child.

5

The paternal genes have a significant influence on the child's physical formation and his development; however, the importance of the father is usually overestimated, and that of the mother usually underestimated. Children are physically, energetically and informationally much more dependent on their mother than their father, and they only make more effort to bond with their father if their mother is not available.

To summarise: everything an LHO experiences from conception onwards is reflected in a combination of matter, energy and information, making him into his unique self. We may not consciously remember our early years, but they shape the foundation of our body and our psyche.

What is the meaning of 'being alive'?

Human life is breathing, moving, eating, drinking, excreting, growing, being active, resting, opening up as well as protecting oneself, being injured and healing, playing, working, having sexual intercourse, conceiving and giving birth, giving children a start in life ... and finally, dying. Being alive can be described with words such as intense, dynamic, gentle, flowing, in contact. By contrast, expressions such as blocked, petrified, hardened, turned to stone, frozen, calcified, ossified, wooden, rigid, over-controlled, or isolated indicate that an organism shows little liveliness. Liveliness is reflected in friendliness towards oneself and other beings. Lifelessness is expressed in a lack of concern, lack of feeling, indifference to the point of open hostility. It is purely based on their lifelessness that human beings start wars, carry out acts of terror, and make life difficult for one another. A person, who is filled with liveliness, loves life.

To be properly alive, a human being needs a supportive environment – according to his developmental phase. This includes clean air, clean water, good food, protection from heat and cold, sufficient room to move, relationships that are supportive and promote autonomy, and above all other people who develop constructive social systems. People who are alive create a healthy environment. People who have frozen their liveliness destroy their environment without any thought and, in their fight to survive mode, make the earth uninhabitable.

What is the meaning of 'my body'?

Is my body something independent and separate from me? Is my body at my disposal? Or am I supposed to serve my body? Am I my body? We treat our body differently according to how we view it:

- Some people regard their body as a tool to enable them to achieve their goals (for example professional athletes). They are often disappointed by it and angry when it does not do what they ask of it.
- Many men and women use their body to impress others. They do bodybuilding, go on diets, wear make-up, have cosmetic surgery, and squeeze themselves into tight clothing and uncomfortable shoes.
- Others, however, neglect their body. They scarcely wash or look after it, they poison it with cigarettes, alcohol and poor food. They do little exercise or sport, become lazy and allow their body to become fatter.
- On the other hand, there are people who appreciate their body and look after it. They experience their body as the source of their vitality. It is their greatest life resource and their friend.

Our bodies give out signals

An itchy scalp, stinging eyes, runny nose, ringing in the ears, split lips, sore throat, racing pulse, stomach ache, painful knees, inflamed genitals, swollen feet – there are many sensations attributable to our bodies. Some of these are temporary; they last for minutes, sometimes days or weeks, and then suddenly disappear again. Others are more permanent and stay with us our whole lives. Sometimes they bother us more, sometimes less. Sometimes they can be unbearable and rob us of our quality of life.

For some physical reactions there is a straightforward explanation: the itchy scalp may be caused by a drying shampoo. Stinging eyes can be attributed to sitting in front of an open fire. A runny nose maybe the result of a bacterial infection. Ringing in the ears maybe due to spending time in a loud discotheque. We have a split lip because someone has punched us. The sore throat is due to singing too loudly. Racing up four flights of stairs has led to a racing pulse. The stomachache is caused by having eaten too much. The knees are hurting following an exhausting trek in the hills. A fungal infection following sexual intercourse has caused the inflamed genitals. The feet are swollen from standing for a long time in a queue.

The more we understand the connection between our body's reactions and the cause, the better we can ensure that we feel well again. We can also adjust our behaviour to prevent such cause and effect correlations. However, if we do not understand the cause, we may take the wrong steps. For example, if we treat a runny nose, which is simply getting rid of dead cells and bacteria that have been rendered harmless, with sprays that suppress it, we undermine the useful work of our immune system. If we ignore other causes by continuing to lift heavy objects even though our back already hurts, we force our body to react ever more strongly. If we continue eating although our stomach cannot take any more, our body can only react with nausea and vomiting.

In order to treat the body well, we need to understand causal relationships, to gain experience with effective methods of healing, and be prepared to listen to the signals of our body. It is vital that we are not indifferent towards our own body, or regard it as an opponent or even an enemy whose aim is to hurt us. It is our friend, doing its best for us if we take care of its basic needs.

The human psyche

The human psyche is there to allow us access to reality, both inside and outside of our bodies. As *reality per se* is multi-faceted, so the human psyche also must be multi-faceted.

It fulfils its task of creating *my subjective reality out of the objective world* in the following ways:

- by sensory perception in the form of smelling, tasting, hearing, touching and seeing.
- by experiencing and feeling emotions such as fear, anger, love, joy, grief, pain, shame, pride, disgust or desire.
- by imagining and re-connecting perceptions and feelings.
- by analytical thinking.
- by making decisions consciously.
- by the transformation of consciousness into spoken words.
- by transforming perceptions, feelings, imagination and thoughts into actions.
- by retaining and dealing with memories.
- by self-reference and the formation of the personal self.

The modular structure of the human psyche requires the individual psychological components to be integrated: seeing for example has to be reconciled with feelings, imagination, thoughts, words and actions. That is most easily achieved in a friendly and supportive social environment. Under conditions of stress, the focus is restricted to coping with the danger. Action is then taken with no consideration of the consequences. Above all, the long-term results of our actions require deeper reflection including the functions of the 'I' and of the will.

The human psyche serves the preservation of the individual and the species. Its functions do not just relate to the natural environment a person is born into (such as a dry, sandy desert or snow-covered mountains). Above all, the psyche of a person is geared towards other people close to them, and getting into contact with them. It is designed to comprehend other people in detail: what they are like, what their intentions are, whether they like the individual or not, whether they are open to sexual relations, whether they are a threat, etc. The human psyche is aimed at ensuring and keeping the person's place in a society, which is necessary for survival. For this reason the individual's own interests are often deferred if membership of a group is at risk.

The psyche of a new human being grows together with his body. A human being is not first just a body, into which at some point a psyche or even a 'soul' enters. Right from the beginning it is a joint growth process of material, energetic and psychological aspects.

We will never be able to comprehend with our psyche all the aspects of the particular reality in which we find ourselves. This becomes apparent when comparing the human psyche with that of other creatures that are able to perceive colours, sounds or smells that we humans cannot. Therefore the human psyche is always selective in how it observes reality. It adapts itself to the respective circumstances, and it is also creative and can discover and develop new things.

One significant characteristic of the human psyche is its ability to create its own world, which can be completely independent of the external reality. This is not a problem so long as the person can differentiate between his psychological world and the real reality. However, it can cause huge problems if the psychological world created is confused with reality. A large amount of energy is then expended trying to bring this fabricated world into reality, with people devoting their whole lives to this task. Other people may then be regarded as enemies if they do not believe in this created reality, this make-believe world, and do not take part in its realisation. 'Germany above all' (*Deutschland über alles*) and an 'empire lasting 1000 years' (*1000-jähriges Reich*) was the unreal plan of a maniac that collapsed in ashes and rubble after 12 years. Unfortunately the experiences of history do not prevent others from striving to do the same.

Being a subject

From the very beginning, a human being is a subject, not an object. He develops from inside and reacts with his unique nature specifically to the external world. The growing child within his mother's womb, if developing healthily, will seek a suitable position in the uterine wall in an immunologically fine-tuning with his mother. He will anchor himself there and allow

10

the placenta, the umbilical cord and the amniotic sac to develop, within which he has the required symbiotic connection with the maternal environment as well as the necessary autonomy. This is why I do not refer to an unborn child as an 'embryo' or 'foetus', because this represents a way of thinking of the child as a non-specific 'something', only becoming a person at a later date (Ruppert, 2014).

A person's whole development is subjective: our breathing, our perception, our emotions, our feelings, our needs, our thoughts and our actions. Development takes place in the interaction with the environment. For this reason even identical twins are also individual subjects. They react in their own ways to their mother, their family or their teachers. Our suffering also is always subjective and every psychological or physical 'illness' is an expression of our subjectivity. There are no objective illnesses. Wherever possible, we should stop other people attempting to reduce us to objects, as often happens, when they diagnose us.

The I-function in the human psyche

"Who am I?" This is the most fundamental question human beings can ask themselves. No other creature on earth can pose such a question, let alone answer it. As humans we are therefore in the privileged position of being able to develop a conscious awareness of ourselves. At the same time we are in the dilemma of possibly having to say: "Who am I and what do I want from my life? As yet I haven't found an answer to these questions!"

From the perspective of evolution theory, one could say that the purpose of the human body is to procreate, and that all physical and psychological structures are subordinate to this basic purpose. However, a specific feature of human life is not exhausting itself in reproduction, as happens in many animal species. There are many people who do not want to, or are unable to reproduce, and who do not see that as their purpose in life. As humans we seem to have the fundamental task of finding a constructive relationship between the body and the 'I', so that the physical processes leave space for individual decisions and the psyche does not abuse its own body. If, for instance, a woman thinks she has to become a mother at all costs before her biological clock runs out, it will not benefit her or her child.

If a person is not in touch with himself, he has no inner focus on which to base all his psychological experiences. His 'I', feelings, will, realisations and actions do not form a cohesive entity. They each follow their own impulses. Put another way: without an 'I' there is no captain steering the ship. In a storm all the passengers race around frantically and aimlessly, giving each other different and contradictory instructions and advice. Sometimes there is even a small, overwhelmed child at the wheel of an adult ship (Langlotz, 2015). If there is no one on the bridge or the person is unable to take command, the ship will soon be in distress.

Only a healthy 'I' is usefully able to connect all the psychological dimensions and choose the appropriate action for the body. All psychological and physical capacities are then at the disposal of this 'I' and know what they can aim for. The person's 'I' is the inner authority that determines what is important and what their life is all about.

I-existence and I-consciousness

From the very beginning I-existence is in the nature of human beings. Becoming aware of one's 'I', on the other hand, is a question of time. It takes two to three years for a child consciously to realise and reflect on who he is, what he is experiencing and doing. This I-consciousness helps the person become more and more the subject of his life. He can thus improve his understanding of his own perceptions, feelings, expectations, thoughts and memories, and his own actions can be directed more purposefully.

This I-development seems to have a clear connection with the differentiation of the prefrontal cortex. It is not until the child's second year that his orientation towards his environment and his mother can be replaced by a sufficiently stable self-direction (Bauer, 2015). To have a clear awareness of 'I' a person has to learn first and foremost to differentiate himself from his mother. The more clearly the mother has developed her own sense of her 'I', the more likely this is to succeed. It is much more difficult for a mother's children to differentiate themselves from her and develop their own 'I' if she is not clear in her own 'I'.

Human self-awareness is a wonderful evolutionary development. It increases the possibilities of options in life. However, it also shows a darker side when we have to become consciously aware of something that places too great a burden on our psychological processing ability. This can happen in two ways:

- Something is done to us that we can't bear emotionally, because it causes us too much fear, pain or shame.
- We ourselves do something terrible that excludes us from social communities, and we are unable to bear the consequences emotionally and whilst fully self-aware.

The will and healthy desire

Besides the I-function, the function of the will is the second significant component in the human psyche. This is immediately evident in therapeutic practice. No therapeutic method can have any effect if a person wants to neither look at his problems, nor change anything in himself. It is therefore a crucial criterion for my psychotherapeutic work that a client is prepared to formulate his own intention. I believe that it is not possible to help someone who has no intention of his or her own. On the other hand, formulating an intention displays a person's determination to attempt to change. The more an intention is thought about, the better it is for the ensuing process of change.

Wanting something in a healthy way is realistic, and an assessment of what is possible and what is not. Many people learn only in therapy to have patience with themselves, and not take on too much. In the beginning people often want to do everything at once and achieve their goal immediately. The more they realise the extent and depth of the harm they have suffered, the less they put themselves under pressure and the more they can appreciate modest progress and be proud of themselves.

I, You and We

Every 'I' develops in relationship to their objective reality, thereby learning something about the objects in their environment. The 'I' makes discoveries about their ability to deal with objects in a focused and meaningful way. The 'I' also develops in relation to other subjects, thereby learning to understand what subjectivity is and how relationships function. In addressing a discussion with a 'You' I can understand more clearly who I am.

The interrelationship between the 'I' and 'You' perspectives results in the new psychological category of 'We'. 'We' and 'I' develop in parallel and are linked to one another. The 'We' is experienced, felt or thought in the same way as the 'I'. Concrete forms of 'We' are partnerships, family relationships, groups of friends and clubs, as well as larger social units such as towns, districts or nations.

But such a 'We' can be possibly no more than a meaningless postulation, purely a thought construction. No constructive social relationships can develop if the 'We' construction is confused; instead such a 'We' disguises the reality of envy, ill will, violence, exploitation and oppression.

Identity and identity development

What is a human being as a whole? What is his 'identity'? The word 'identity' comes from the Latin and means 'the same', the quality of being identical with oneself. How does a person stay 'the same' if his body and his psyche are constantly changing?

Interest in the subject of identity recently seems to be increasing again in psychotherapeutic circles (Ammon and Fabian, 2014; Waltz-Pawlita, Unruh and Janta, 2015). There are a number of identity theories, the best known being the psychoanalytical stage theory of Erik H. Erikson (1902-1994). Erikson has linked the concept of identity with the stages of development in a person's life cycle. He regards the age of youth as the phase during which a person is either successful in developing his own identity or fails to do so (Erikson, 1976).

In my opinion the development of identity begins at the moment of conception, with the fusion of egg and sperm, in whose genetic code the whole heritage of the history of mankind is contained. Thus a new person is created who is entirely unique. Although our life comes from our parents, it is not identical with their lives. Our life holds within itself its own life force and its own will to live.

At any point in a person's life he is the result of his development from the beginning up until that moment. Everything he has experienced forms part of his being. Nothing can be ignored, disregarded or edited out. A person's identity is therefore the aggregate of all his life experiences.

Identity and the mother

The first touchstone for every person's identity development is his mother. From the moment of his conception she represents his first experience of a relationship; she is his environment. Even before he is born she is his immediate counterpart, the first 'You'. She is the basis for the formation of the first 'We'. Every child has to deal first of all with his mother. In his relationship with her his 'I' and his will have to assert themselves.

This is easy if the mother welcomes her child, accepts him lovingly, nourishes and looks after him during pregnancy, enjoying his presence and his development. After his birth, the child can then feel himself reflected in the eyes of his mother and feel that he is loved (Strauss, 2014). Through this he gains a sense of basic trust in himself, in his life and his relationships. On this basis he can effortlessly live out the basic formula of a healthy identity: 'I' = 'I'. Then nothing is added to this equation that does not belong there.

Attributions

If, on the other hand, a mother rejects her child, does not want to have the child, misuses the child for her own purposes, or projects her own trauma survival strategies onto the child, then it is extremely difficult for the child to perceive himself in his identity. The child cannot feel and experience who he is beyond the maternal rejection experience or maternal expectations. He cannot distinguish clearly what belongs to him and what doesn't. It is impossible for him not to apply his mother's attributions towards him to himself and so, identify with them. Attributions such as

- "You're too much"
- "You arrived at the wrong time"
- "You're the wrong sex"
- "You're too restless and you make too much noise"
- "You're too slow"
- "It's your fault", etc.

The danger is that his identity will consist of nothing but these maternal attributions, hostile rejection and expectations he cannot fulfil. In a case like this, a child has to put aside his own perceptions, feelings and needs in order to escape his mother's rejection and excessive demands, and behave the way he thinks his mother wants him to. He is ashamed of himself, in other words ashamed of the fact that he is there in the first place, and suppresses his own characteristics. The paradoxical logic behind this is: "Only if *I* weren't here would my mother be satisfied *with me*! If I can succeed in not being here, I can be here." As time goes on, such attributions may also come from the father, older siblings or relatives and there may be new expectations and demands, which prevent the child from being himself.

However, such attributions say more about the person making them than they do about the child. Attributions as mental constructs are superimposed onto reality. Medical diagnoses, for example, often say more about the doctor than the patient. Attributions may continue in kindergarten, school and in the child's or adolescent's circle of friends without him being able to retaliate or distance himself from them. School grades, for example, are nothing more than attributions of a competitive school system on students (Kohn 1986). It is a mark of 'total institutions' (Goffmann, 1973) that they mercilessly subsume people to their attributions.

It is bad luck for someone if they live their whole life in a society and culture that only recognises attributions with which the person has to identify, and which leave him no room to develop his own identity. There are social groups in which everything is regulated and an individual has to behave and do things in a certain way: the circumstances of his birth, the religion he belongs to, his progress at school, his choice of partner and starting a family, his work and his death. The basic formula of such a life states: *You = Me = Us.* You should be, and have to be, the way I need you and the way 'we' need you to be. Such collectivism stifles the merest attempt at individuality. 'We' know best which direction your life should take! What 'we' want from you should be and has to be what you want for yourself! In a fascist dictatorship, the basic formula then states: The nation is everything and you are nothing! We can only gain our own identity if we have the chance and the freedom to question and reject the attributions laid upon us.

Identifications

In the course of forming our identity we not only have to watch out for attributions, we also have to ask ourselves whether what we identify ourselves with is good for us. The basic formula for identifications states: *I = You.*

Identifications are not *per se* negative. Identifications with other people can accelerate learning processes, such as when a child learns his first language by imitating the language of his mother. Identification processes can also motivate a person to be as good as his admired role model. But they can also prevent him from perceiving for himself, feeling and thinking for himself, and cause him to identify with something that harms him.

17

If an individual is not able to form his own 'I' in a robust manner, he will have difficulty in freeing himself from his parents, his family, his relations, his origins or even from a religion, and in creating sufficient distance to allow his own development. His whole life long, 'others' will remain the reference point for his own existence. There can then be no perceived and definite distinction between what he has experienced himself and what others have experienced. For this reason many people are symbiotically entangled in the traumas of their parents, siblings, ancestors or compatriots, which they perceive as though they were their own. In a collective that does not promote the formation of identity, the 'fate' of each member of the collective will become the 'fate' of all the others. There is then no clear distinction between collective pain and individual pain. Whole collectives can then sink further and further into the pain of their 'ancestors' and the resulting perpetrator-victim dynamics. They all disappear together into the abyss of their past, and a new future becomes impossible.

We cannot achieve an identity for ourselves from identifications, in other words from the formula $I = You$ or $I = Us$. To achieve our own identity we have to measure by our own yardstick what we assume from others. What does it mean for *me* if I learn to do what my role model can already do? Why do *I* need it? Why is it important to *me*? We then often realise that the reason something is important to us can be very different from the reason it is important to the person we took it from.

Even if we love another person, how far do we have to identify with his perceptions, feelings and thoughts, or how far can we demand that he identifies with ours? $I = You = Us$ is a symbiotic relationship formula from which nothing new can emerge. If, on the other hand, we think and practise $We = Me + You$, the 'We' has added value and becomes something unique, something that neither the 'I' nor the 'You' alone could achieve. Only such a 'We' is worth the trouble of coordinating the different needs of those involved. It makes no sense to invest time and energy in the repetition of old patterns.

Separateness

While in collective cultures separateness is seen as betrayal of family, religion or culture, in individualistic cultures we are told, not infrequently, that we should separate ourselves better or protect our boundaries more clearly from external attacks. This sounds well meant, but we will not achieve our own identity by just separating ourselves from others. Saying what I do not want, what I am against, and from whom and what I differentiate myself, may be a first step in seeking my own identity. However, it does not constitute a personal identity. On the contrary, it can even indicate a lack of identity if I continually refer to others, finding fault with them or rejecting them. 'I never want to be like my mother' or 'I want to free myself from the entanglement with my mother': such thoughts continue to centre on the mother and direct the person's eyes and energy onto her and not onto oneself. Hidden beneath this is the unrequited childish longing for the mother's love.

Healthy identity

We talk of a healthy identity when the unity of our psyche is assured and we do not have to split in order to do something or to have a relationship with other people. Then a healthy Identity means ...

- having one's own will,
- own perceptions,
- own feelings,
- own thoughts,
- own memories,
- own actions
- in the individual's own body,
- in relationships chosen by the individual

and one can interact simultaneously.

A healthy identity proves itself first and foremost in our relationships. In a healthy identity there is no identification with perpetrators and their attributions put on us. We can then enter into and shape relationships that are of mutual benefit, with a balance of give and take, and that create win-win situations for all concerned. We are then easily able to free ourselves from relationships that are not good for us and make us ill in the long term, relationships that in other words are win-lose or even lose-lose situations.

As Jesper Juul so aptly puts it: 'Love is the art of transferring the emotions of love into loving behaviour without the need to give up oneself.' (Juul, 2013, p. 76) Love that asks a person to give himself or herself up cannot be healthy love. If an individual sacrifices himself for his family, his people, his country or his god in order to think himself loved, he should ask himself how his life has come to that. Why have I become like that? What have other people done to me, and what have I allowed them to do, for self-sacrifice to seem the only way I think I can find happiness? Particularly since, for someone with such a sense of victimisation, 'family', 'people', 'country' or 'god' are simply general constructs, in other words attributions to reality that have little or nothing to do with the variety and differentiation of real life. They often originate from fantasies of violence.

I and self

'Self' is a special term in connection with the question of identity. It appears in different variations, such as "I want to do it myself", "I have to protect myself" or "I have low self-esteem". 'Self' is a reference word when talking *about* the personal 'I'. In healthy psychological structures, there is no contradiction between I and Self, when 'Self' means the same as "Identity'. To be Self also means to be grounded in one's own body and psyche. However, if trauma survival strategies gain the upper hand in a person's psyche, the term 'Self' could instead be used to name a dissociated survival state. It will then function as the idea of an ideal-self, separate from the real characteristics of a person. As the term 'higher Self' for example, it might be used as a construct by traumatized individuals to seek to connect with something that seemingly exists outside the reality of trauma.

Self love or egoism?

Spiritual teachings, and moral and religious dogmas often deliver the message that wanting to be 'I' is 'egoism', 'selfishness' or 'self-love':

> "Man lives by his ego that always hungers for power. Every 'I want' is an expression of this claim to power. The 'I' puffs itself up and finds a way using new and sophisticated disguises to force the person into its service. The 'I' thrives on separation and is afraid of giving itself, of love, and of becoming one. The 'I' differentiates and develops a pole and blames the shadow that arises on the external, on the 'You', on the environment." (Dethlefsen and Dahlke, 2008, p. 83)

In my experience, if a person consciously places himself at the centre of his life it is in no way socially damaging. On the contrary:

- The healthy 'I' as the centre of the person's own identity does not have to cling onto other people or interfere in their lives.
- It has no need to gain power and control over others because its desire is to be aware of itself and not divert attention from its own real suffering or identify with the suffering of others.
- The healthy 'I' needs no compensation strategies such as accumulating possessions, consuming drugs or other forms of compulsive behaviour in order to escape from itself and cover up its existential and abandonment fears, or its pain.
- A healthy 'I' wants to be alive in the here and now and wants to develop. It can develop further because it accepts itself with its biography and its own history of suffering.
- It is self-sufficient because it has recognised that it has enough to do in feeling its own experiences and integrating them within itself.

What is possibly being denounced here as 'ego' is in my opinion a trauma survival strategy. Someone who has lost contact with his healthy 'I' through trauma, replaces this with a pseudo-I as a trauma survival 'I'. This can be inflated and behave as listed in the diagnosis criteria for a 'narcissistic personality disorder' (ICD 10, F60.8 and DSM IV, 301.81).

This pseudo-'I' has an overstated understanding of its own importance; exaggerates its abilities and talents; expects to be recognised as superior without proof; is absorbed by fantasies of limitless success, power, brilliance, beauty or idealised love; believes itself to be 'special' and unique and only understood by, or having to associate with, other special or highly-regarded people or institutions; needs to be admired to excess; displays a sense of entitlement; has exaggerated expectations of special treatment or automatic recognition of own expectations; exploits others in relationships, in other words, uses others in order to achieve goals; lacks empathy; is not prepared to recognise the feelings or needs of others; is frequently jealous of others, or believes others are jealous of it; displays arrogant, supercilious behaviour or views.

A pseudo-'I' could also be the opposite: full of self-doubt and feelings of guilt and shame. Traumatised people often develop both versions of a pseudo-'I', and the external situation determines which pseudo-'I' is shown. For example a man might feel invincible in competition with other men, but become a picture of misery in bed with a woman.

Since 'spiritual concepts' are not normally based on an understanding of trauma, it is easy to throw the baby out with the bathwater. In this kind of thinking the way to overcome a pseudo-'I' is to give up the 'I' altogether. My experience with 'spiritual' people has shown that they use their spirituality as a way of detaching themselves from their painful experiences and from their body, which suffers the consequences of severe trauma. They conclude that only their 'spirit' counts and that their body and feelings are incidental. In the end they believe their spirit has created their body. I think this is another far-reaching trauma survival strategy. In my work I experience these

'purely spiritual parts' as only in the mind, and continually activating endless reflections. By doing this they ignore the body's
distress as the traumatising experiences are suppressed. They
talk incessantly without feelings; they impress others with the
intellectualism they have developed; they immunise themselves
against any possible improvement in their life. Afraid of their
true feelings, they retreat into their thoughts.

Individuality and loss of the whole

As long as a person can develop healthily, he remains an 'indi-
viduum'. He is something that is not split, that seeks to broaden
and perfect his form and retain it as a unit. It is only if he experiences something totally overwhelming that he has to give up
this unity in order to survive, and body and psyche are forced to
split. The unity of body and psyche, of 'I', of wanting, perceiving, sensing, feeling, thinking and doing is lost. What remains is
the false impression that there is a body without a 'spirit' and a
'spirit' without a body.

The fact that individual components within the body (such as
the human psyche) can break down without the whole system
collapsing, allows a survival strategy in the case of a trauma
emergency reaction:

- If there is insufficient nourishment, oxygen, or functioning
  temperature regulation for the whole body, what is
  available will be concentrated on the essential organs
  (heart, brain).
- If even breathing is too dangerous it can be reduced to a
  minimum.
- If movement might be fatally dangerous, it can be frozen.
- If the perception of what is actually happening is unbearable, the function of the senses can be reduced or
  completely stopped.
- If we have no freedom to make decisions, we can switch
  over to reflex actions.
- If a person is unable to bear the flood of feelings, these

feelings can be suppressed, numbed and switched off.
- If the person's thoughts are unbearable, the thoughts can be moulded and altered until they are bearable.
- If memories are too distressing they can be suppressed, glossed over and forgotten.
- If the person's own will does not function any more, an outside will can be assumed and experienced as the person's own.
- If we as human beings feel we do not matter any more, if our personal needs and values no longer count, before we wear ourselves out in futile resistance, we can experience the 'I' of another person as our own. In this way we are still able to function even in the worst circumstances. In dictatorships the suppressed are still able to identify with 'their' dictator.

Psychotrauma and splits

A psychotrauma is an event that a person, with his psychological capacities, is unable to deal with. Even the stress reactions that are usually helpful in warding off a threat become a danger to the person in a trauma situation. These stress reactions have to be stifled so as to avoid further provoking an attacker or becoming over-heated for the system. During a stress reaction the body goes into overdrive, and the trauma emergency mechanism slams on the brakes. Figuratively speaking, we have one foot on the gas pedal and one on the brake. Relinquishing the unity of body and psyche is the immediate solution to this dilemma; the unity disintegrates into fragments and is only sustained by the process of splitting the whole.

The following diagram shows the disintegration of the human body and the human psyche through the experience of trauma (Figure 1):

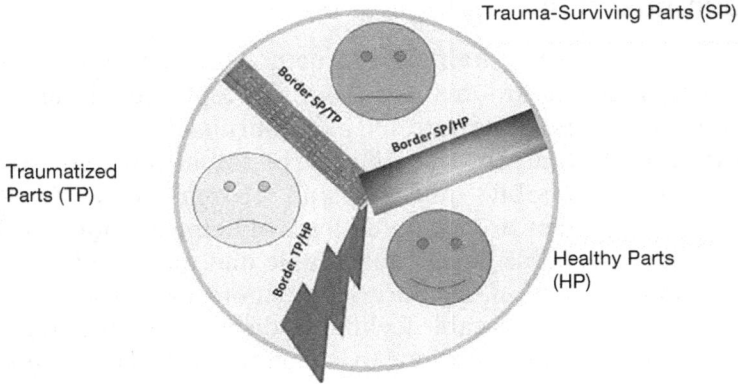

Figure 1: Basic model of the psychological split caused by the experience of trauma

Healthy psychological parts

The human psyche is innately healthy. Overwhelming experiences force it to adopt special survival programs that enable it to continue living. In figurative terms, it is when lightning strikes the human organism that it is forced to split.

After the traumatisation there is still an area of healthy physical reactions and healthy psychological structures. These are still able to react adequately to reality, to process it and to comprehend it in its complexity. The healthy psychological structures are still interested in reality as it is. They can express feelings if the occasion demands it. They assist in entering into interpersonal attachments and close relationships, and in withdrawing from them if the relationship pattern becomes increasingly destructive rather than constructive. They enable us to experience sexual desire in a responsible way. They can reflect our own actions self-critically. In difficult times they allow us to hope that we will find suitable solutions to our problems. They can persist in continuing to find a way out of the split.

Traumatised psychological parts

I call the second psychological structure formed by a trauma lightning strike the traumatised parts. On a physical level these are different forms of unbearable pain (burning, stabbing), regulatory circuits that are out of control (breathing, digestion, movement), immobile muscles and frozen body. On an emotional level they are terrifying fears of being abandoned and dying, uncontrollable anger, unbearable and never-ending pain of loss and desolation, all born in the moment of the trauma. They can also be unbearable feelings of disgust, shame and guilt.

Traumatised parts continue to live, perceive, feel and think as they did in the original trauma situation. They come to a standstill at the moment of the trauma. Stimuli can easily trigger the images, feelings and thoughts from the trauma situation, and then they swamp the individual, flooding him and re-triggering the original emergency response again. Thus intense pain, inflammation, rashes or panic attacks can suddenly appear seemingly out of nowhere.

Trauma survival strategies

The third structure in Figure 1 I have termed trauma survival parts. In a trauma situation these parts have to prevent the worst from happening: psychological disintegration and physical death. They allow the individual to survive the trauma situation by splitting. They block the manifestation of the traumatised parts by stripping them down into their individual components, removing the emotion, distancing them from the 'I' and banning the experiences from consciousness. The person can only continue to function because those parts of the body that were particularly involved in the trauma are numbed, blood flow to them is decreased, or they remain in a frozen state of tension. Trauma feelings are parcelled away by the survival mechanisms into certain regions of the body and suppressed. The survival parts work hard at undoing the whole trauma experience for the individual's consciousness. The survival parts see no alternative but to carry the traumatised body, or parts of it, like a heavy burden through life. They develop various basic approaches:

- They avoid memories of the original trauma.
- They tell themselves that it wasn't so bad, and still isn't.
- They devise a new reality, for example a world full of mysterious 'forces of fate' and 'illnesses' in which the trauma doesn't feature.
- They control themselves, and everyone else in their environment to ensure that the trauma does not surface.
- They numb themselves, if necessary, with alcohol or drugs, or by using sedatives, sleeping pills or painkillers provided by the pharmaceutical industry.
- They distract themselves with all kinds of activities, such as burying themselves in work.
- They keep coming up with new strategies if the old ones are not enough to keep the inner onslaught of the traumatised parts at bay.
- They are extremely grateful for any offers of support by others that help them to block out the trauma, and those who show them ways to get by without dealing with their trauma. They invest a lot of time, money and effort in this.
- They visit doctors and healers, showing them their body as if it is not really theirs but an annoying thing that someone else can look after.
- Without any emotional engagement, they may allow operations to remove parts of their body.
- They undergo painful medical treatments in the hope of having some peace within their body, which through inflammation and pain, is actually signalling that something isn't right.

To survive a trauma the human psyche uses its abilities to create a psychological life that is separate from reality. It is important for the psychological trauma survival strategy that the healthy 'I' has to disappear. The 'I' is then replaced by a different 'I'-construct that in the end believes itself to be the real 'I'. That can be a role into which the individual flees (e.g. the mother role or a professional role), or it can be an identification with a religion, nationality or regionalism. The 'We' then becomes more important for a traumatized person than the 'I', and usually causes the person to become extremely aggressive if others throw such survival 'I' forms into doubt. The rampant hate-filled tirades on the internet and in social media show the large number of people worldwide who are traumatised and can only cope with their fears by becoming aggressive.

In the same way as the 'I', 'wanting' also is defined by trauma experiences. It is a clear sign of a trauma survival strategy if a person tries very hard to

- heroically bear something that is actually unbearable,
- block something out that needs to be looked at,
- distract themselves by talking non-stop and constantly doing things,
- obsessively help others,
- fight against something at all costs,
- force something impossible to happen.

Other trauma survival strategies are the will

- that completely capitulates,
- that submits to authority and obeys orders unconditionally,
- that would like to disappear completely.

Many people have grown up in families where their will has been broken; or they have spent their childhood and adolescence in authoritarian regimes or dictatorships in which it was dangerous even to express an opinion, let alone have a will of their own. Or they have lived in a partner relationship in which they had to submit to their partner's will. Then they have to realise that having a will of their own is not dangerous, and will not necessarily result in rejection, criticism, punishment or violence, and that presupposes that they can leave relationships, families and social systems that function to suppress their will.

In accordance with the finding that survival strategies can neither question nor recognise themselves (Ruppert 2007 p. 30), in a 'We' some perspectives and approaches might be seen as healthy that are actually extremely damaging for all concerned. One example of this is the high percentage of caesarean sections taking place in many countries, which traumatise mothers and child alike and lead to psychological splits. The election successes of despotic presidents show that the majority of voters do not recognise who is a perpetrator, and so out of their trauma survival strategies they become their victims.

Boundaries between the psychological parts

In principle there are six boundaries between the different psychological parts (see figure 1):

- the boundary between HP and SP and the boundary between HP and TP,
- the boundary between SP and HP and the boundary between SP and TP,
- the boundary between TP and HP and the boundary between TP and SP.

Although the healthy parts (HP) are able to learn what the survival parts (SP) are, they cannot deliberately override them as long as the traumatised parts (TP) still exist. They might also have an idea that the traumatised parts are behind the 'lightning strike' but they have no conscious access to them. They can only identify the reality of their trauma when they approach their traumatised parts emotionally, getting in touch with their own traumatised feelings.

The survival parts differentiate themselves from the healthy parts in that they maintain it to be impossible, illusory and dangerous to address the trauma, if indeed they acknowledge that the trauma actually exists. They stick to a strategy of resisting coming into contact with the horror that the person has experienced. The stronger the emotional pressure from the traumatised parts becomes, the more the survival parts experience stress, become overactive and confused and escape into dissociation, fog and incomprehension. They dissociate more and more, fleeing from reality and from the body, and adopt the perspective of an observer. In extreme cases they end up in a completely dissociated state as if they were not there at all.

The traumatised parts feel let down by the healthy parts and the survival parts. They oscillate between resignation and angry rebellion. They are open for a sympathetic approach, but their own experiences with interpersonal relations have been extremely bad and so they hesitate to expose themselves to more such contacts, and so any approach to them has to be slow, cautious and gentle. If the healthy and traumatised parts get so close that the boundaries between them start to dissolve, strong feelings and life energies are released, and physical tension drains away, and muscular tensions that serve as a protective barrier can be relinquished. Body tissues that have suffered from inactivity and lack of blood flow and been kept in survival mode can then be reactivated and brought back to life. This is immediately noticeable in the case of hands and feet that were previously icy cold becoming warmer, eyes shining once more and the face taking on a rosy hue.

A structural model of psychotrauma

As not all psychotrauma is the same, so we have to differentiate. Experts make a classic differentiation between a monotrauma – a single event such as a serious car accident – and continually traumatising situations, such as years of imprisonment and torture.

They also discuss the term 'complex traumatisation', which is used to describe children in ongoing abusive familial relationships. In this context mention is also made of 'development trauma' (Garbe 2015; Heller and Lapierre 2013).

Several years ago I developed a classification that groups together the many possible reasons for traumatisation into the following categories (Ruppert 2002, 2005, 2007, 2010, 2012):

- *Existential trauma*: This is a matter of life and death, for example when a mother attempts to abort the child growing inside her. In such a case it is important for the surviving child to split and suppress his mortal fear and become numb and inert so that he does not die from this state of over-excitation.
- *The trauma of loss of a loved person*: If a child dies, for example, his death traumatises his parents. In the same way the early loss of his parents will traumatise a child. The worst trauma feeling here is the pain of loss that continually flares up and is difficult to subdue. The psyche may then, for example, develop the illusion of a reunification with the loved one in the 'afterlife'.
- *The trauma of love*: Every human being is dependent on the loving contact and care of his mother, and it is therefore psychologically unbearable for a child if this quality is missing. A father too, if he does not love his child, causes a trauma of love. In a trauma of love, my experience has shown that the person make use of six different survival strategies:
  - They fight their whole life for the parental love they have not experienced.
  - They idealise their parents.
  - They identify with their parents' trauma survival strategies and attributions.
  - They attempt to help and save their parents.
  - They connect with their parents' trauma feelings.
  - They ignore their own psychotrauma.
- *The trauma of sexuality:* If a person is sexually stimulated against their will and forced to take part in sexual acts, this is such a major invasion of their whole identity that the feelings of pain, of betrayal and humiliation, the unbearable sensations of fear, anger, shame and disgust have to be split off from their consciousness (Rhodes 2014). In most cases the 'I'-function is almost completely split from all physical sensations. The phenomenon of so-called 'anorexia' is one instance where this is most clearly seen.

Those affected would like to be rid of their body because their need for physical contact is through the body, a need that is then exploited by perpetrators. The separation of body and 'I' means that, even after years of therapy, those affected are still not sure whether they experienced sexual abuse or not. Even if countless indicators point to sexual traumatisation in childhood, they may not really believe it happened. One loophole is often the idea that feelings of sexual abuse might have been 'assumed' from the mother, in other words they might have identified unconsciously with her feelings from her abuse. The shame of sexual traumatisation is so immense that even with obvious physical symptoms such as inflammation of the genitals, abdominal pain during sexual intercourse, severe pain in the anal area, etc. the person may not admit to sexual traumatisation in their biography.

- *The bonding system trauma:* In such a case, an individual is stuck in a society that consists mainly of perpetrator-victim relationships. This could be his family of origin, the village he is growing up in, his place of work, or the whole country of which he is a citizen. Whoever lives in a society like that is either a victim or perpetrator of violence, and in most cases both at the same time. In systems like that even young children become perpetrators of violence towards their siblings or playmates. On a psychological level this produces a large number of victim and perpetrator attitudes. Those concerned will often make use of many new forms of survival strategies in order to suppress the truth of being a victim and perpetrator, and avoid feeling the consequences of the violence. They deny acts of violence, defining their reality in whatever way they choose, and pretending that there is harmony between victims and perpetrators. This is the basis for every possible ideological construct, whether racist, nationalist, sexist, religious or economic. One survival strategy frequently chosen is to seek refuge in the concept of 'illness'. Obvious perpetrators and victims are termed 'psychopaths' or 'psychologically ill'. The physical consequences of violence are given names such as 'cancer', 'auto immune disease' or 'trigeminal neuralgia' (a form of facial pain), in which their traumatic origins are no longer recognisable. Relationship tragedies based on violence thus become supposed scientific problems requiring a technical solution. All involved in such a system avoid realizing the causes of victimhood and perpetrations and are only looking at the symptoms.

'Early trauma'

If we look at the possibilities of becoming traumatised from the perspective of a person's biography, we can see events at the very beginning of a life that I have termed 'early psychotrauma' (Ruppert 2014). Some examples of these are abortion attempts (Hoppe 2014, Evertz 2015), lack of contact and violence experienced in the mother's womb, trauma during the birth by caesarean section, forceps or ventouse, separation from the mother immediately after birth and being transferred to an incubator following a premature birth.

The 'early trauma' is particularly relevant for the consequences of traumas that manifest themselves in the body, because body and psyche have to form a stable relationship in this early phase of development. These events cause them to become easily separated from each other:

- In order to survive, the living organism has to switch from the development program to an emergency program at the very beginning of its life. The basic material-energetic functions have to be maintained; otherwise, early death would be the outcome. It is a question primarily of surviving the damaging effects on the organism and enduring the emergency situation. There is no room for subjective happiness or the search for contentment.
- In these adverse circumstances, the consciousness of having a body, sensing and feeling it, has to be reduced

or completely abandoned. Thus dualism is created early on: here is my psychological being and there is my body that is thrown on the mercy of the world like an object. In order to survive, I have to distance myself from my aching body and regard it as a foreign object that has nothing to do with me.

In early psychotraumas the first developing 'I' of an unborn or a newborn child is strongly under the influence of the maternal psyche, and thus the trauma feelings of the mother often overlay the child's feelings and his 'I'. However, because the child has to seek close emotional contact with his mother, that results in his not being able to differentiate clearly between himself and his mother. What does belong to me, and what belongs to her? Where do I end and where does my mother begin? What are her feelings and what are mine? What did I experience during my birth and what did she?

Traumatised mothers are unable to help their children differentiate between his experience and her experience. On the contrary: there are some mothers who are glad to be able to hold onto the child because they themselves have no firm psychological basis of their own, and no healthy 'I' of their own. They use the child's problems to distract themselves from their own traumas, preferring to occupy themselves with their child's 'problems' rather than their own. Thus the child becomes the doll for the maternal survival strategies.

A mother should really be the source of nourishment, protection, care, love and happiness for the child, but with an early trauma she becomes the source of illness, stress, aversion and even death. The child is then frightened of contact, of touch and nourishment and this manifests itself in 'childhood illnesses' such as 'tummy ache', 'bed-wetting', 'asthma', 'neurodermatitis', or 'food allergies'. A child who has to live with a mother who rejects him will become psychologically and physically ill.

With the extent of early trauma that usually affects whole generations, it seems not surprising to me that we jointly submit to an economy that is similar to a dysfunctional mother: we can only have nourishment if we accept self-abandonment, submission and the necessity to work extremely hard. We have to serve 'the economy', and not the other way round. We 'live to work', and we do not work to live. We have to feel guilty for even existing, and pay the debt with a life of hardship and toil. Our own value is measured in externals: in money and in debt (Graeber 2014).

The trauma biography: From 'trauma of identity'...

'Early trauma' is a chronological category, and I have now termed the logical first form of psychotrauma as the 'trauma of identity'. This basically calls into question the individual's very existence, his own being. Why? Because a person in this situation should really not be there at all, since his mother did not want him. Very often his father did not want him either. This means that the child has to stand his ground against a mother who rejects him and who is either hostile towards him or, at best, indifferent. The child is literally fighting for his right to exist from the very beginnings of his life. In most cases of early trauma, the union of egg and sperm cell is already part of a perpetrator-victim dynamic, because the woman has become pregnant against her will. The father of the child might have been a one-night stand, who disappears the next morning, or a husband who insists on his right to have sex regularly, or a rapist who simply takes what he wants.

From the moment of conception the new life has to find his or her place in a uterus that does not welcome him. Implantation in the uterus wall becomes the first obstacle he has to overcome, because the maternal organism does not want to create space for him. If the child does succeed in finding a place where his mother's immune system does not identify him as a foreign object that must be destroyed, he then has to fight for his nourishment because his mother is reluctant to provide it.

Weeks may well then pass for the child under a Sword of Damocles while the mother considers whether to abort him or not, or wishes not to have him. There may even be attempts at abortion, which he has to survive. In some cases that I have seen in my practice the mother even believes an abortion has been successful because one of a pair of twins has been killed, although the other child has survived.

Even if, later on in the pregnancy, the danger of being killed is no longer a threat and the mother has come to terms with the inevitability of her pregnancy, the child still receives little consideration. His mother may drink alcohol or continue smoking, might not eat healthily, might do hard physical work or live in a noisy and cold environment. The whole pregnancy is an ordeal for the child to survive. He feels unprotected, not cared for, and left completely alone. His mother ignores or rejects all his attempts at making contact with her.

For such a child the aim is to hold on until the birth, which itself in such circumstances is usually unpleasant, because the child and mother do not cooperate. For a mother who does not want her child, the birth can be a final opportunity to give birth to a stillborn child. The child might stop moving down the birth canal, which in emergency obstetrics requires the use of ventouse, forceps, or result in a birth by caesarean section. Sometimes the birth is very fast ('precipitate birth') which could be the mother ridding herself of the unwanted child quickly. The birth then becomes a trauma experience for the unwanted child.

For these children the unloving experience continues after their birth: there is no warm skin connection with the mother, no eyes looking lovingly at them, no loving breastfeeding and no care and protection. The child is held by cold, hard hands, looked at by empty, hate-filled eyes, and cleaned, dressed and fed purely mechanically. Most of the time the child is left alone without being spoken to. He is left to cry until he exhausts himself. The child cannot trust anyone in his environment. He has to be permanently on his guard from psychological and physical attacks when he makes his needs known. A child who needs to be loved holds his hands out to his mother and father. After a few failed attempts at seeking contact, an unwanted child will leave his arms hanging by his sides.

Existing, when your existence is not wanted by your mother, is unbearable and affects the person's whole life. A human being needs to have his own life, to be himself, and this has to be given up in order to fit into an environment of rejection. Instead of being himself, being 'I', the person has to fit in with the rules of a hostile and indifferent environment in order to survive. How can the pain of rejection be endured, the horror of being alone? How can he survive with the little that is left to him? And this leads to the crucial question: how can he adjust sufficiently to the needs of others so that he is at least able to survive? His own joy and vitality, his own will, trust in his own resources, his own 'I' – all this has to be given up in order to stay in relationship with a hostile environment, and that prevents his own healthy development.

When I formulated the intention 'Why must I work so much?' in a constellation for myself, I became painfully aware that until then I had identified with my mother's strong work ethos: "Someone who doesn't work doesn't need to eat!" Underneath this lay my shame of being an unwanted child who was always in the way. I was ashamed of my existence because I was a burden to my parents. As a result I wanted to do everything myself as soon as I could: no longer needing nappies, tying my own shoelaces, needing no attention and making myself as useful as I could for my parents. I encouraged my younger siblings to do the same. I wanted them to be able to do everything for themselves as soon as they could so that they were not a burden to our parents. I despised my childish needs. From the age of twelve I didn't ask my parents for money, but 'earned' enough for my modest wants by helping out my grandmother and a wealthy uncle. Later, although I had achieved a lot in my professional life, the shame of not being good enough, being incapable and not worth anything, stayed with me until this and some other subsequent constellations.

An important variant of this identity trauma is gender: if a mother or father does not want a child because in their eyes it is the 'wrong gender'. In patriarchal societies this particularly affects girls, because having a boy represents a higher 'value' for the family. This is linked with the idea that the son will carry on the father's name, will continue to lead the family/clan, and take over the father's farm or business. Some marriage practices exacerbate this idea if a dowry has to be paid if a daughter marries, while a dowry is received if a son marries. In India, for instance, families sink deeper and deeper into debt because they have to take out loans in order to marry off their daughters (Kakar 2015).

The rejection of the child's gender can also spring directly from the mother, because it triggers her own trauma. For an expectant mother who has suffered violence at the hands of men it may be a shock to realise – consciously or unconsciously – that she is carrying a male child. Part of her may resist this growing boy, reject him or fight him. The boy she is carrying receives the unconscious message: 'You are not right being a male, you should not become a man'. On the other hand, a survival part of the mother might see a boy child as a potential saviour, someone who can protect her from male violence in the future. The unborn child is then unconsciously given the job of becoming a 'superman', a protector of his mother... but he may also not be allowed to be sexual, so that his mother is not threatened by his sexuality. As a result he becomes unsure, ashamed and confused, which may continue throughout his life in his relationships with women. For fear of his mother's rejection, he may experience his own masculinity and sexuality as a threat and may be burdened with feelings of guilt.

Mothers may also show pre-natal trauma reactions when they realise they are expecting a girl child, because they connect their own experiences of powerlessness, suffering and victimisation as a girl. Then the unborn girl may also feel that it is wrong to be what she is. As far as her mother is concerned she will never be right, no matter how hard she tries. As long as her mother projects her own trauma onto her daughter, she blocks her daughter's future as a woman with her own worries and distress.

With an identity trauma, the basic survival strategy is striving for non-identity. That means that a person in his shame struggles to hide the fact that he was not wanted and is not right in the way he is. He therefore does not develop any empathy for himself. He refuses to acknowledge the reality of his childhood and instead makes out that it was wonderful; he is determined not to look at his blind spots, identifying uncritically with the opinions, attitudes and beliefs of others. In the course of his life he may increasingly immerse himself in external things at the expense of exploring his inner world. He willingly accepts attributions from others because he feels hollow inside, and tries to put some order into his life with such attributions.

So the trauma of identity is the basis by which a person identifies uncritically with his family, his religion, nation, culture, political party or anything else that is available within their environment. This does not get noticed in an environment in which identity is always equated with identification. On the contrary, identifying himself with external groupings becomes a demand that the person has to comply with in order not to be excluded from these trauma-survival communities. Gratitude for being allowed to live, feelings of guilt of being a burden to others, and making sacrifices without complaint for these groups are the required attitudes of living.

The idea of having an individual 'I' is experienced as threatening, because wanting this provokes the perpetrator's aggression, and any connection to the traumatised parents would have to be relinquished. Thus trauma survival strategies will mean pushing aside the person's own 'I' completely. Instead the person must identify with the perpetrator, who cannot be recognised and named as such. Of all the writers I know, Arno Gruen has made this point most clearly. He says that under such conditions we have a sense of our own 'I' as a stranger within us, and so, continually betray ourselves (Gruen, 2000, 2014, 2015).

A young man I worked with in therapy stated it as follows: "I don't want a personal 'I'. A personal 'I' is betrayal, failure and abandonment." He had been an unwanted child, and his mother had used him and manipulated him as it suited her for her survival strategy purposes. In such circumstances, just existing for their mother or father becomes the person's *raison d'être*. He has no idea what it might be like being alive without being completely at the disposal of his parents. He believes himself incapable of life without his parents.

Instead of wanting something for his own life from his mother, such a person needs his mother so much that she becomes the replacement for his own identity, and vice versa, because such a mother needs the child without his 'I' as a replacement for her identity. She herself suffers from a 'trauma of identity' and acts out her 'trauma of love' with her child.

... to the 'trauma of love' ...

From the 'trauma of identity' immediately arises what I have termed the 'trauma of love'. Split off from his own healthy 'I', the person's needs now become subordinate to the needs of the person from whom he expects love, his mother. From here illusory ideas of happiness and love are created:

- "I'm happy when you're happy!"
- "If you're not happy I'm responsible for making you happy again."
- "I have to put everything I've got into saving you from your suffering."
- "I am not important myself; the main thing is that you feel better."
- "My task in life is making sure everyone around me feels good."
- "As far as I'm concerned, the most happiness anyone can have on earth is to make others happy!"
- "That's why I'm will become a nurse, doctor, psychotherapist or pastor, entrepreneur or politician."

The child's love that is not reciprocated by the parents is then transferred onto an object (such as a teddy bear) or another living creature (such as a pet dog or cat). If later in childhood or early adolescence this love is transferred to a sports club for example, it often ends in blind allegiance and fanaticism. If it is projected in adolescence onto 'the Fatherland' or a 'nation' ('Germany above all!', 'America first!') the original childish innocence is gone, and the originally projected images of trying to save the traumatised parents from their suffering then lead to 'patriotism', 'nationalism', 'racism', and from there to antagonism towards other nations and peoples, and finally to a readiness for war. As history has shown, this eventually can draw the whole world into the trauma-abyss of an 'emperor', 'Führer' or 'president'.

The 'trauma of love' as a survival strategy from the trauma of identity sucks the person into another's trauma, because this is the only way they can feel an emotional attachment to the other. If the person also reacts unconsciously to the split trauma in the other person, both are likely to feel as if they are 'soulmates', and may take that as the basis for a long-term partnership and marriage. Both people's survival parts then keep searching longingly and obsessively for emotional contact at the trauma level, because this is the only possibility of providing a heart connection. This dynamic can also be seen in people who originally were a twin if the other twin, due to a lack of life resources or an abortion, died (Bourquin and Cortés 2016).

... to the 'trauma of sexuality' ...

The 'trauma of love' in turn is the fertile soil, which gives rise to the 'trauma of sexuality'. The rejection and unrequited childish longing for closeness and physical contact make the perpetrator, who is stuck in an identity trauma and trauma of love, greedy and unscrupulous. At the same time, the victim, who is usually lonely and neglected, is receptive to his approaches and his attention. Once the barriers are down and healthy feelings of shame no longer prevent inappropriate sexual contact, abuse and violence in parent-child, child-child and man-woman relationships can become a 'normal' matter of course. The sexual contact cannot be halted, even if it is experienced as disgusting and guilt-laden. "I preferred having any form of contact to having none, so I just went along with everything!" This was said by a woman whose father had sexually traumatised her as a child.

It is depressing to see the sexual traumatisations brought to light in therapy:

- For years, the father has sexual intercourse with his daughter and the mother pretends to know nothing about it. When the daughter becomes pregnant, the mother arranges the abortions.
- Parents sell their children to wealthy 'friends' for sexual perversions.
- From early puberty, mothers regularly seduce their sons to have sexual intercourse.
- For years, brothers have oral, anal and vaginal sex with their sisters with their parents' knowledge.

In such familial systems sexuality has the function of a trauma survival strategy in many different variations: to manipulate another person, so that they are always available for physical contact and sex; to take revenge by proxy on the other sex; to satisfy an addiction to orgasmic feelings; as a distraction in situations that are actually unbearable. Behind this is the profound loneliness of all concerned who, through their sexual practices, succumb to the illusion of being lonely no longer, and instead feel powerful rather than powerless. Sexual orgasms make them somehow feel alive, at least briefly. Illusions of sexuality, which have nothing to do with the reality of sexuality, serve as survival strategies in a 'trauma of sexuality' in the same way as illusions of love in a 'trauma of love' are a survival strategy for that trauma. Putting such strategies into practice comes at a high price, psychologically and physically.

... to the 'trauma of own perpetration'

All forms of traumatisation lead, to a greater or lesser extent, to perpetration against the individual himself and against others. The basis for this is that those internal parts that identify with the original perpetrators, especially their own mother and father and are therefore 'perpetrator-loyal' (Huber 2013). This is because as a child they were completely dependent on the parents, so they have to suppress themselves and avoid showing their anger and aggression towards their perpetrator parents. They therefore turn these in on themselves. This might take the form of continually ignoring their own traumatised parts (that for example make themselves noticeable through physical symptoms), or even directly harming themselves. They, for example, might misuse medication or drugs, cut or burn themselves, or even attempt suicide.

Their suppressed anger is then directed at others, either openly or covertly, who happen to be in their environment. This might take the form of hurtful remarks or a hand that 'slips out' to hit their own child. Therefore, if I have traumatised other people by what I have either done or not done, and harmed them irreparably, then I have myself become a perpetrator. I have not only traumatised my victim, but I have also traumatised myself by my own actions, or by not offering the necessary assistance, which is my responsibility to do. I then have to force from my consciousness my fear of social condemnation, my shame for my actions, my feelings of guilt and my remorse. I have to behave as if nothing had happened, as if it was not my actions that had traumatised another person.

What chiefly links being a victim and being a perpetrator is the shame that makes this unspoken, thereby creating permanent inner stress of no longer being able to show themselves to others, and having to be self-denying.

Victims are ashamed

- because they exist, although they were not wanted,
- because according to their begetters they are the wrong gender,
- because they do not feel loved,
- because they are humiliated by physical violence,
- because they are sexually humiliated,
- because they are referred to as useless,
- because they are allegedly 'sick'.

Perpetrators are ashamed

- because they know they have done wrong,
- because they fear they will be ostracised from society,
- because they will be openly accused if their actions become known.

In concealing their actions and their responsibility, perpetrators have to carry out further perpetrations. They have to deny their own identity, thereby becoming more and more alien to themselves. Above all, perpetrators fear the truth, so they lie, suppressing the truth in any way they can. For them the extent of their power defines the truth. In addition, they silence any accessories to the perpetration. They pretend to be the very picture of innocence, passing on their responsibility to others. They blame the victims and pass them off as the real perpetrators. They are appalled at others' behaviour, and they depict themselves as victims and feel immediately insulted and as if their honour has been violated if anything is said against them. Increasingly violence to others becomes their preferred trauma survival strategy, attracting other perpetrators and entangling them in power struggles until, in the most extreme case, someone is killed.

Through their excesses of violence, perpetrators revert to an animalistic state. Their body tries to discharge the inner tension through acts of violence that often ends in the destruction of another creature. Their increasing lack of contact and relationship is transformed into a permanent willingness to fight, and those people around them only feel fear and are constantly prepared for violence. In order to do this they have to make their body emotionless, to harden it. For the perpetrator who is prepared to kill, his body is ideally just a machine that he can use for his aggressive impulses. His whole life becomes a theatre of war. It is not only in wars that the full picture of this perpetrator-victim dynamic comes to the surface. In times of peace as well, people who are prepared to resort to violence spend their time looking for opportunities to fight and escalate violence. They become real 'violence freaks' (Buford, 2010).

As a result, no rational sense can be expected from perpetrators. They can only allow themselves to become conscious of what they have done and are doing when they feel their own victimisation. That is the reason they have become perpetrators, in order to avoid those feelings. This victimisation often lies a long way back in their childhood and is hidden deep within them.

The risk of becoming stuck in a perpetrator-victim dynamic is very great, because if the parents are stuck in it they will also draw their children into the dynamic with them. Thus, perpetrator-victim dynamics spread further from generation to generation until they take over whole communities. If we look at the Earth more closely, we will see that there is hardly a country that is not entangled in countless perpetrator-victim dynamics – both within the country but also involving their neighbouring countries. In a community that is permeated by perpetrator-victim dynamics, couples and families do not have much chance of escaping. If it is possible, they seek out niches in society where they can be untouched by the perpetrator-victim dynamic. Instead of succumbing to the illusion of wanting to 'save the world', it seems to be more realistic to try to save oneself *from* the world that is ruled by perpetrators.

Many societies are more 'perpetrator-loyal' than 'victim-loyal'. It is more of a taboo to talk about the traumatising perpetrators than to talk about the traumatised victims. Those who oppose war are quickly classed as idealistic dreamers and receive less publicity than those deciding on the deployment of tanks, rockets and machine guns. It is the rule rather than the exception for communities to be controlled and governed by perpetrators: royalty, rulers and democratically-elected presidents are loved by their subjects because these subjects see them as their supposed saviours in times of emergency, even if they are actually the cause of the people's distress, and have created the 'enemies' from which they now are saying they are protecting their people. Particularly in emergencies, it would be far more useful for as many people as possible to take part in political decision-making processes, rather than giving all rights and powers to a single person, leaving them to decide on whether to wage war or peace. How is a single person supposed to deal emotionally and mentally with the complexities of social, economic and political facts and interests? The 'strong man' or 'strong woman' is an archaic myth and a collective illusion of the trauma survival parts of people. In other words, this means that a community wants to be prepared for violence and ruthless. History has shown that the concentration of power in one person (for example Alexander the Great, Genghis Khan, Caesar, Napoleon, Hitler, Stalin, Saddam Hussein, George Bush, etc.) leads sooner or later to that community's demise.

The further on someone is in his or her trauma biography, having become a perpetrator themselves, the more difficult it is for them to escape. This is often the case with politicians who, once they have achieved power, increasingly become perpetrators and then, in order to conceal and justify their actions, turn into dictators and, using every means available to them, forbid society to see them as perpetrators.

If a trauma biography is not consciously interrupted, it develops further in the individual and passes from one generation to the next by means of parenthood and the assumption of positions of power within society. Might it not be a sensible idea to check the trauma biography of those seeking power and 'responsibility'? Instead of them having to make their financial affairs public, they ought to disclose anything they found particularly painful in their childhood and how they have learned not to transform this pain into their own perpetration.

I have summarised my development model of psychotrauma in Figure 2 which shows how the other forms of trauma follow on logically from the 'trauma of identity'. Many people I work with therapeutically have a trauma triad: Not wanted! Not loved! Not protected! They usually end up in the trauma of their own perpetration. This, and all previous traumas, can only be overcome if the 'trauma of identity' has been worked on therapeutically.

Possible Trauma Biography

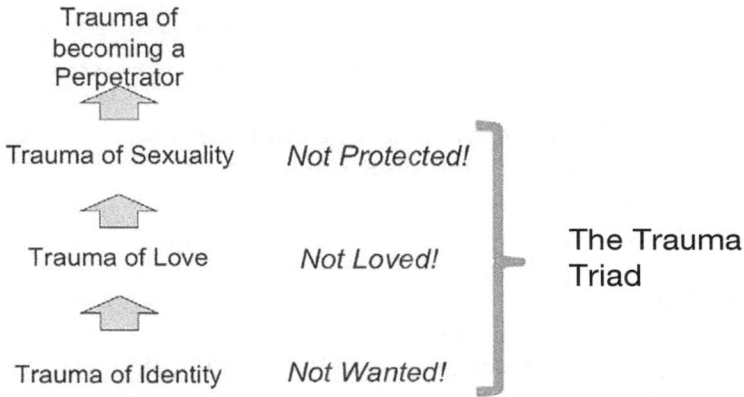

Trauma of
becoming a
Perpetrator

Trauma of Sexuality   *Not Protected!*

Trauma of Love   *Not Loved!*   **The Trauma Triad**

Trauma of Identity   *Not Wanted!*

Figure 2: Possible stages in a trauma biography

Psychotrauma as a source of physical distress

A psychotrauma can be driven from a person's consciousness. Nothing seems simpler than switching off the light of consciousness when reality becomes too much to bear. However, we are unable to rid ourselves of our traumatised bodies. The actual experiences of a trauma remain in the body even when emotional pain, fear, anger, disgust or shame no longer force their way into the consciousness as a result of emotional numbing and psychological splitting. Similarly, it is illusory to think that the body does not experience a trauma from a medical operation just because an anaesthetic switches consciousness off. Moreover, even that is questionable because there are instances of people, while anaesthetised, remembering conversations the operating team had during the operation. We can therefore state, the truth concerning our experiences is stored in our body. The body does not lie!

If, because of traumatisation, the individual's consciousness has withdrawn so that it only functions from the cerebrum, the body below is subject to conflicting forces, which use the body for their own purposes. The body becomes a complicated puzzle of different structures into which the traumatised parts are forced, for example an inflamed toe that does not heal. The different survival strategies of the person fight for their right to make use of the whole body.

People caught in their trauma biography live their lives under extreme stress. The amount some people can physically endure in these circumstances is often nothing short of miraculous. Nevertheless, this endurance comes at a price:

- Heart and circulatory system are permanently under extreme pressure and may collapse.
- Skeletal and muscular systems cause pain and buckle under the increasing burden of adjusting to traumatising relationships.
- Teeth are ground down to stumps if the traumatising situations keep re-appearing during sleep.
- The digestive system has no reliable criteria for distinguishing what is nourishing for the body and what is not, nor what should be excreted and what should be retained for further use.
- Under toxic stress, the organs gradually cease to function.
- The immune system is no longer able to distinguish between what is foreign and what is part of the body, and starts to attack the person's body.
- The whole nervous system can collapse under the permanent stress, and even the brain can gradually cease to function, leading to dementia.
- The body is increasingly poisoned with poor food, medication and drugs.

The more deeply a person is trapped in their trauma biography, the more physical symptoms can appear. There are some specific forms of suffering that point to a direct connection with a trauma situation (for example inflammation of the genital area often indicates sexual trauma). Others are non-specific and appear in different parts of the body as physical warning signals (if, for instance, physical violence in childhood was ignored or glossed over). In every physical symptom, there is a piece of personal history. 'Illnesses' are symptoms and usually just the tip of the iceberg.

The ACE study

It has long been scientifically investigated and known that traumas make people physically ill (Maté, 2011). For example in one study Vincent Felitti, Robert Anda et al investigated the health of 17,500 mainly white, well-educated patients in an obesity clinic. At the same time, they asked them about events in their childhood, Adverse Childhood Experiences (ACE)[2]. This included physical, emotional or sexual abuse, neglect, parents with psychological illnesses, drug dependency or prison sentences, parental separation and divorce, and domestic violence.

The results were unequivocal: the more ACEs a person had in their past, the worse their physical constitution. Of those asked, 67% had experienced at least one ACE and 12.6% had had more than four. The risk of lung cancer was three times higher in someone with more than seven ACEs in their childhood, and their risk of suffering a heart attack was 3.5 times higher. Even if the individual had no further risk factors such as smoking, poor eating habits and lack of physical exercise (which in themselves are actually trauma survival strategies), their risk of developing an illness was greatly increased. It was the 'toxic stress', according to the authors of this study, that destroyed the health of these people (Felitti, Anda et al, 1998).

Further investigations have confirmed these findings: childhood traumatisation leads to an increased risk of psychological disorders and physical illnesses, and lower the life expectancy. The body is unable to forget the violence it has suffered. The childhood traumas remain stored in it. Time does

---

[2] http://acestoohigh.com/2012/10/03/the-adverse-childhood-experiences-study-the-largest-most-important-public-health-study-you-never-heard-of-began-in-an-obesity-clinic

not heal trauma wounds; on the contrary, the older we get, the less able we are to push these issues aside and the more our survival strategies prove futile and the more our old wounds reappear.

A long-term Harvard University study that has been looking at American white-collar and blue-collar men for 75 years has shown that it is secure and supportive relationships that lead to a physically and psychologically healthy old age more than cholesterol values. Living alone and isolated, on the other hand, leads to illness.[3]

"I don't feel traumatised!"

One of the characteristics of psychotrauma is denial on a personal and societal level (Broughton, 2013). The following example illustrates this:

Maria M. (22 years old) goes to see a doctor because of a bladder infection. The doctor asks her whether she has experienced a trauma. Maria M. initially denies any trauma experience, but after having spoken to her foster mother, she tells the doctor that she was given to her foster parents when she was two. Her mother had a heroin addiction and had used drugs during the pregnancy. The doctor advises her to consult a psychotherapist.

The therapist Ms M. consults tells her not to worry, and says she is a healthy young woman and not in the slightest traumatised. Although she is relieved to hear that, she is uneasy and asks me what I make of the situation. When she tells me that her weight at birth was very low I congratulate her on having managed to survive despite having suffered, in my opinion, massive traumatisation in her mother's womb. Even after the birth she did not receive any love or care and was likely to be completely overwhelmed by this situation. She says: "But I don't feel traumatised!" She has sorted out her bladder problems with antibiotics.

---

[3] https://www.youtube.com/watch?v=vmIEnstv0-c&app=desktop

I reply that it is entirely up to her whether she wants to deal with her early history, in other words with issues such as a possible abortion attempt, lack of nourishment, poisoning during pregnancy, lack of maternal love and being left alone as an infant. But that it might be sensible to look at these issues more closely before she becomes a mother herself. This seems to convince Ms M. because she has a friend who, just like her, was given to foster parents early in life. This friend had become pregnant and had a baby and these experiences had been a huge disaster for her.

Everything I have experienced and experiences I observe in people I work with therapeutically lead me to the conclusion that psychotraumas keep being restaged until they are understood, felt and thereby resolved.

'Illness' – cause, condition or consequence?

My wife recently set off on a mountain hike in good spirits. She came home two days later feeling miserable and ill. The first symptoms had appeared on the descent from the summit: nausea and physical weakness. Later on she had diarrhoea, felt very cold, and had a temperature. We quickly decided the cause was a lukewarm potato soup she had eaten in a mountain lodge, in other words, a possible bacterial infection.

Therefore, what exactly is her 'illness'? Is it the physical symptoms? If we assume that poor hygiene in the mountain lodge, or food that had gone bad meant that toxic substances had entered her body, then the symptoms are not the cause but the consequences. And even though having diarrhoea and a temperature and feeling very cold are not pleasant, they are *not* the signs of an 'illness', but the information that her body is fighting the toxic invasion. Her body is trying to get rid of the toxins as quickly as possible. It slows down the metabolic processes in those places reached by the toxic intruders (the abdomen in particular). By raising the temperature, it stimulates the immune system to attack the harmful bacteria. Even the loss of appetite and aversion to food on the following day were unpleasant for my wife, but they were sensible, preventing her from possibly consuming further toxic substances while her body was still fighting the previous invasion.

So what is the cause of an 'illness', what are the consequences, and what are the conditions under which a cause can lead to consequences that might even be very serious? We humans suffer not only the immediate effects of harm to our body, such as the pain of a burn, but we also suffer the consequences of our body fighting the damage done to it and attempting to heal itself. We therefore use the term 'illness' for both of these. We are usually unable to distinguish one from the other and we confuse causes, conditions and consequences. As a result, we might take measures that negate the body's defences and prevent it from healing itself. For instance we might have a hot bath, although the body is lowering its temperature on purpose; or we might try to get our temperature down even though a high temperature is essential for the immune system to function successfully. 'Illnesses' can even become chronic if we continually sabotage the body's attempts to heal itself by well-meaning treatment. This frequently happens if we hope for a quick recovery because, for example, we do not want to miss an important appointment, so we take antibiotics in the hope of speeding the process up. Eventually we will pay dearly for that.

'Illnesses' – objective or subjective phenomena

In addition to the inconsistency connected with the term for illness, a further difficulty arises which makes its use problematic:

Is there really such a thing as 'the illness', for instance 'the cancer', 'the allergy', 'the migraine', independent of the person who has the symptoms? Are the physical symptoms objective facts that can be tackled with objective measures and standardised forms of treatment? Alternatively, can we only really understand their appearance and development if we look at the individual sick person as a subjective whole? We would then be better able to explain why not all people become 'ill' despite carrying the same viruses and bacteria within them, because these viruses and bacteria are also a part of their subjectivity and we cannot simply disregard them.

Thinking of and classifying 'illnesses' as something objective, independent and separate from the human subject, is a basic paradigm in scientifically oriented medicine. Science-influenced medicine regards the human body as an object that allegedly functions purely according to the biological, physical and chemical laws of nature. According to this viewpoint, even the human psyche is nothing more than the result of the workings of a complex brain machine. The spirit, the will, the consciousness are regarded as being determined by material bodily processes and thus reduced to physics, chemistry and biology. From which the question arises as to why people even need their own 'I', their own will, feelings, thoughts etc. for their existence.

'Conventional medicine'[4] implements this reduced paradigm with the claim of scientific accuracy by categorising the possible expressions of 'illnesses' according to the 'symptoms'[5] and giving them each a name. This might be the name of the person who discovered a 'clinical picture' (for instance Bekhterev's disease). Frequently the term is taken from the Latin or Greek, for example 'migraine' which comes from the Greek word meaning 'half skull'. These names can be difficult to understand and pronounce, making their use impressive to non-medics and distancing the sufferer further from their own body.

This sort of medicine is not concerned with the concrete living conditions of the 'ill' person. Possible political, economic or interpersonal causes for 'illnesses' are hardly ever considered. For that reason, conventional medicine often assumes the illness is 'genetically' caused: the cause of a person's illness must lie in their genes and therefore within them, and since not much can be done about 'the genes' in the body, the treatment of the illness is usually confined to treating the symptoms. The treatment then

---

[4]   This has become standard terminology for this type of medicine.

[5]   'Symptom' stands for that which 'coincides' with each illness.

consists of attempting to separate the ill person from their illness. This means, amongst other things, that in order for the person to be healed, parts of their physical body are destroyed by, for example, medication, radiation or an operation.

The consequences of such a way of thinking became clear to me when working with a woman whose intention was: "I would like to inactivate my herpes simplex virus". The virus turned out not only to be a childish part of her but also to be her mother, who had tried to control her and to put her under constant surveillance. Her healing consisted therefore not of deactivating herself, but of activating the split off traumatised part of herself and allowing it to live. That is the only way she can quieten her perpetrator mother within her. She cannot win an inner battle against her mother and it would only lead to further stress.

In conventional medicine, someone is defined as 'healed' if he is free from symptoms that, often more or less by chance, have become the focus of medical measures. As this is frequently not successful, the goal of medical treatment is to reduce the symptoms to a minimum, with the danger of the 'side' effects of the treatment leading to new symptoms and thus no end to the treatment. This is no way to make a person healthy. It simply supports, to a greater or lesser degree, the person's ability to function and survive from day to day – despite the unresolved trauma in his organism. This sort of medicine is itself a trauma-survival strategy.

Discourse: Positivism and dualism

Since coming into existence as a modern science in the mid-19th century, medicine has committed itself to the paradigm of 'positivism', which arose at the same time. Auguste Comte, mathematician, philosopher and critic of religion, who lived in France from 1798 to 1857, supported the idea that in science metaphysical assumptions made no sense and were therefore unnecessary. One should refer more to the factual, the observable and measurable, leaving aside speculation and questions of faith (for example concerning the existence of God) (Chalmers,

2001, p.7). For medicine, which for centuries had been impeded in its research through religious objections and controls, positivism was a convenient idea. It was able elegantly to dissociate itself from doctrines of faith and metaphysics. From then on physicians delegated responsibility for the 'soul' to religion and philosophy. In exchange, they claimed responsibility for the body cleansed of the soul. The split of 'naked body' on one side and 'pure soul' on the other is one of the origins of modern medicine and is even today regarded as one of its important traditions. According to its orthodox advocates, medicine is a strict science that must not be mixed with metaphysical ideas.

The discussion of philosophy in the western world cites René Descartes (1596-1650) as the father of the idea of the dualism of body and soul. Descartes's *Discourse on the Method of Rightly Conducting One's Reason and of Seeking Truth in the Sciences* containing the famous phrase "I think, therefore I am", is seen as proof that it is possible for there to be a mind without a body and that the body is also imaginable without a mind. "From that I knew that I was a substance, the whole essence or nature of which is to think, and that for its existence there is no need of any place, nor does it depend on any material thing; so that this 'me', that is to say, the soul by which I am what I am, is entirely distinct from body and is even more easy to know than is the latter; and even if body were not, the soul would not cease to be what it is." (Descartes 1961, p. 31ff, quoted from Damasio 2006, p. 330)

In my opinion, this dualism is itself a consequence of trauma. Traumatised people lose connection with the body and escape into the head and, finally, no longer even sensing its attachment to the body, they experience it as 'soul', that can exist free from constraints of time and place.

The success story of conventional medicine

For secularised societies at the beginning of the 19th century, the findings of medicine, freed from ultimate religious supervision, were very convincing. The medical illness paradigm gained an increasing number of followers from all levels of society, particularly as it mostly refrained from criticising social relationships. Medicine had released many people from the belief that their complaints were caused by their sinfulness or godlessness. They were now allowed to be physically ill without having to suffer intimate questions as to their lifestyle. Instead of going on a pilgrimage, they could now go to a doctor who looked at their physical complaints and did not question their personal life.

At the start of the 20th century medicine was even able to show that severe forms of 'madness' and 'insanity' could be caused by bacteria entering the body, for instance in the case of syphilis. As a result, the medical paradigm of illness was immediately applied to the suffering of the soul as well (Davison and Neale, 1979, p. 17ff.) Thus, psychiatry was established as a branch within medicine and it claimed medical responsibility for all forms of psychological anomalies. 'Psychological illnesses' were deemed illnesses just like all others. They were said to originate from irregularities in physical processes and could therefore, like other physical illnesses, be treated by physical applications, medication or surgical operations (Schneider 1992). Sedating emotionally imbalanced people became one of the main societal tasks of psychiatry. Even if this does not enable them to function again, it means at least that they no longer cause a public disturbance. The reasons for these people being unable to control their impulses, feelings and thoughts are of no interest. Even knowing that their patients are traumatised does not stop psychiatrists from giving them medication.

Imposing an idea on reality – in this case the concept of 'physical illness' on people with psychological anomalies – is an ideological action and the opposite of science. Serious science obtains its concepts and terms from investigating reality. It explains reality and does not subordinate this reality to economic, social or political interests. Real science therefore does not have to insist dogmatically on its concepts. If it has gained new insights, it can confidently forget the old ones.

'Experts' and 'patients'

Physicians who pursue a positivist and dualist worldview learn during their studies to treat the human body like a machine from which, according to the rules of their art, they can remove old things and into which they can insert new things. They can drill, cut, hammer, saw and laser the human body as though it were simply an object to be worked on. Liquids and chemicals are pumped through the vessels as though lymph and blood vessels were nothing but tubes inside a rather complicated technical appliance. 'Health' and 'illness' thus become simply a question of technical feasibility and scientific progress. Conventional medicine scarcely takes into consideration the fact that such treatment methods

- do not alter the cause of the physical ailment in any way (for instance in the case of a heart attack),
- can further traumatise the person receiving the treatment (for instance in the case of an operation such as a caesarean section, or by the use of aggressive radiation therapy and chemotherapy).
- can even trigger trauma reactions in traumatised people (for instance in the case of medical procedures on previously traumatised body orifices).

In a profit-oriented medical system, the tendency is also to keep the patients in a chronically ill state, needing elaborate intervention measures for the rest of their lives.

This model of medicine thus creates two defined roles: 'experts' (from the Latin meaning 'specialist' or 'authority') and 'patients' (from the Latin meaning 'the suffering'). The 'experts' are thereby defined a priori, at least psychologically, as healthy. They put pressure on themselves to know as much as they can about an 'illness', while 'the patient' must be passive and assent to the experts' treatment without protest.

Many people accept their role as 'patient' uncomplainingly and are happy that doctors are looking after them and their affliction. There are 'patients' who gain a 'secondary gain' from apparently being cared for comprehensively within the medical system. Such people can become very demanding in this attitude and make unrealistic demands of the 'experts', causing them to try even harder to demonstrate their medical skills. Some doctors may then really start to feel that they are demigods.

A further aspect of this extreme division of roles in scientifically oriented medicine is the experts' fear of making mistakes and being taken to court by the 'patients'. The relationship between doctor and patient, instead of being one of trust, can quickly turn sour and become one of fear and mistrust, combined with the associated power gap and authoritative and submissive attitudes on both sides.

I suspect the following: the more severe the perpetrator-victim dynamic that leads to the physical consequences diagnosed by conventional medicine as, say, 'cancer', 'autoimmune disease', 'psychosis', 'anorexia' etc., the greater the danger of such perpetrator-victim relationships being replicated by the technical-scientific treatment. This happens without the doctors and 'patients' involved being aware of it.

Is this the end of conventional medicine?

Doctors perform almost miraculous acts in emergency medicine to save people's lives. They are able to keep many people alive who without their help would definitely have died. Many doctors have a high level of personal commitment in their efforts to relieve other people's physical distress. Even so, there is increasing doubt in the population concerning the sense of the medical illness paradigm, not least because the optimistic medical aim of being able to conquer all illnesses by medical actions and the use of an increasing amount of technical and pharmaceutical products has turned out to be incorrect. The advertisement disclaimer "consult your doctor or pharmacist about any risks or side effects" is asking for trouble, because it is palpably obvious that the pharmaceutical industry is seeking commercial gain and does not stop at the manipulation and bribery of doctors and politicians.

In my opinion, the blatant failure of the medical paradigm becomes most apparent in the 'fight against cancer', amongst other causes, where no great progress has been reported despite massive financial investment. Also with so-called 'psychological illnesses', the wide use of psychiatric medicines simply means that the symptoms become chronic, and does not restore health to those concerned. I believe that conventional medicine desperately needs new concepts and approach if it wants to do more than protect and promote trauma survival strategies.

Psychosomatics and stress concept

An alternative to conventional medicine that has been around for some time is psychosomatic medicine, which attempts to identify the correlation between body and psyche (Adler i.a., 2017; von Uexküll, 1976, Wirsching, 1996). 'Psychosomatic illnesses' point to a causal relationship between a person's physical and psychological states and their social conditions. This leads to the conclusion that in the case of many symptoms such as circulatory problems, back pain or obesity, treating the body on its own will not lead to success and the psychological and social causes need treatment as well.

In the 1970s the stress concept was developed in physiology and was then taken over and adapted by psychology. It states that the stress reaction in a person's body is a functional way of mobilising additional energy quickly to cope with a situation that is acutely dangerous. If the danger passes, the body can begin to recover and regenerate. However, if the stress reaction does not subside because the external danger is still present or still having a psychological impact, then the organism lacks the periods of rest that it needs. In the long run this causes damage to the organs, the vascular system, the muscles and joints. Immune reactions will also stay at too low a level, thus increasing the danger of catching an infectious illness.

The stress concept is still one of the most important explanatory models of psychosomatics. It has entered into the thinking of the medicinal nonprofessional. "Too much stress" has become a popular line of reasoning when symptoms such as a heart attack, high blood pressure or stomach ulcers appear. The panacea for such physical ailments has become 'rest', 'relaxation', 'meditation' and 'recuperation'. However, experience has shown that physical and psychological symptoms increase during such periods of rest, and that some people can enter a trauma state if they have to meditate in a psychosomatic clinic, which refutes this concept. When doing breathing exercises personally I found myself becoming either tired very quickly or getting into a state of over-excitation and unconsciousness. The reason for this was the experience I had as an infant, when I was almost killed by my father who attacked me violently. It was only when I dealt with this traumatisation that my breathing permanently changed for the better.

Psychosomatics is still based largely on depth psychology or behaviour therapy (Ermann, 2007). For instance, one of the standard explanations states that suppressed feelings 'somatise' into physical illnesses. Suppressed anger is supposed, for example, to lead to pressure in the stomach, and in the long term to stomach ulcers, and the recommended solution to this problem is the 'release' of feelings, supported with therapeutic methods (for example beating cushions with a wooden stick).

However, my experience has shown that acting out feelings in this way does not have the desired cathartic effect. On the contrary, the feeling of helplessness following such an explosion of anger is often even more profound than before. Or feelings of guilt increase towards the people the anger was directed at. Why? Because as a rule these feelings were suppressed within the mother- or father-relationship that the person concerned was unable to leave. He is still trapped in his longing to receive his parents' love, or having to save and comfort them. Acting out feelings of anger can deepen the split in a person even more, as I have frequently seen in constellations. The person will only stop suppressing his feelings

- when his conscious I wants to escape and succeeds in escaping completely from the relationship with a perpetrator,

- when he loves and esteems himself,
- and when he feels the pain of his own victimisation.

Psycho-neuro-immuno-endocrinology and powers of self healing

A further step in the direction of the holistic view of physical phenomena is psycho-neuro-immuno-endocrinology (Schubert, 2011). Here knowledge is focused on the psyche, nervous system, immune system and hormone system all being connected with each other via the same information carriers and neurotransmitters (Pert, 2001). Thus, words alone can influence a person's psyche to such an extent that hormones are released, which in turn activate the immune system and send neurotransmitters through the whole body (Bauer, 2015). This explains amongst other things the placebo and nocebo effects. If 'patients' expect an improvement in their health from a certain medication or operation, they feel better even if they are given a tablet with no effective ingredients or the operation has not taken place. On the other hand, a doctor's diagnosis such as: "Your life expectancy with this type of cancer is only six months" can lead to the patient giving up and dying according to the timescale of the prognosis.

Psycho-neuro-immuno-endocrinology sharpens our eye for the human organism's self-healing powers, which we need to support. At the least, these self-healing powers should not be interrupted or halted by external measures. We therefore have to ask: what promotes a person's self-healing powers and what impedes them? It seems to me that thinking in categories of illness tends to weaken them rather than strengthening them.

'Illness' as a trauma survival strategy

For a long time, thinking in terms of illness categories was something I took for granted, and so to begin with in my own theories I tried to put a psychotraumatological interpretation and explanation on medical diagnoses such as 'panic attacks', 'depression', 'borderline personality disorder', 'schizophrenia' or 'psychosis' (Ruppert, 2002, 2005). I hoped that explaining the causes would also be of interest to conventional medicine, particularly psychiatry. I now realise that the use of the category 'illness' – whether purely physical or referring to psychological phenomena – can constitute a trauma-survival strategy for both experts and laymen.

Calling oneself or someone else 'ill' can mean not looking further into the person's current personal circumstances and seeking the deeper causes in their life history, or examining critically their situation within society. The use of illness categories can be an implicit agreement between doctors and 'patients', to avoid looking more closely at the possible causes, immediately initiating a course of treatment to fight the symptoms. As a 'patient' I am then not responsible for my 'illnesses' myself. It seems to be easier to say: "I've got an illness" than to think: "I am my physical affliction". The opposite attitude would be: "My physical affliction is my own and no one can know myself and my life better than I do. And thus it is only I who can know, feel and sense the possible causes of my affliction."

Discourse: 'Depression' as a result of trauma

Illness diagnoses in current psychiatry do not as a rule offer explanations; on the contrary, they cover up reality. 'Depression' as an 'illness' is today largely an accepted diagnosis, and millions of people in the world are supposed to have this mysterious 'illness'. Whether a person shows depressive symptoms such as

- being chronically exhausted,
- being unable to sleep properly,
- thinking everything is pointless,
- not having any future perspective or any joie de vivre

because

- his job has completely worn him out,
- his partner has just left him,
- a hurricane has demolished his house,

- he is trapped in a victim attitude following childhood neglect,
- he is trapped and powerless in a societal system, or
- he feels the political situation worldwide is hopeless,

is irrelevant when adding up the individual cases to millions of depression 'illnesses'.

If we look more closely at the list of symptoms in the case of 'depression', its psychotraumatological background becomes obvious. If we define the psychotrauma as a phenomenon

- where a person gets into a state of powerlessness and help-lessness,
- where all his attempts to liberate himself only make the situation worse,
- and the best solution is for him to take no outward action and
- to try to reach a place of safety internally and save himself,

then it is clear: the symptoms of a 'depression' can be freely explained by the fact that:

- people are in a traumatising situation, or
- their current experience makes them revert to an earlier trauma situation
- they feel helpless and incapable of acting in the situation and protect themselves by retreating internally and giving up their efforts
- they can thus remain in relationships from which they cannot and do not want to disentangle themselves.

A person calling himself 'depressed' without taking the causal situation into consideration I term a trauma survival strategy. Even thoughts of suicide that often accompany depression are a trauma survival strategy inasmuch as they are a means of avoiding dealing with the trauma situation and persistently trau-matising relationships.

Identity-oriented Psychotrauma Therapy (IoPT)

There are several different theories about trauma, and different therapeutic approaches (Reddemann, 2008; Levine, 2010; Seidler, Freyberger and Maercker, 2011; Heller and Lapierre, 2013; van der Kolk, 2015). The therapeutic approach must correspond with the theoretical understanding of trauma, and where the emphasis is placed on different forms of trauma.

My basic trauma model is the split model (see Fig. 1). For me, therefore, the therapy of a psychotrauma consists of the following steps:

- A person's healthy parts have to be activated. They have to be developed further and stabilised. Above all the healthy 'I' has to be developed and strengthened. The person's own will has to be present and doing its part to overcome the splits.
- Becoming aware of personal trauma-survival strategies is the primary cause of an increase in healthy structures. The better survival strategies are recognised for what they are, and the more clearly their negative consequences for the person's life are understood, the more they lose their credibility, powers of persuasion and lack of any alternative.
- Recognising that I am in survival mode is the basis for accepting that I have a psychotrauma of my own and that I might be living in a trauma biography.
- Encountering the traumatised parts only becomes possible when the person is in stable contact with their healthy parts. That means that the person is then able to give up his survival strategies, disengage himself from his physical, emotional and spiritual numbness and feel the suppressed emotions in his body that have been incarcerated by the split. The survival strategies then become superfluous. The traumatised body is able to develop further.

In psychotrauma therapy, the various possibilities of failure are because:

- Trauma situations are re-stimulated without sufficient healthy parts, resulting in the person becoming re-traumatised and sinking even more deeply into trauma feelings.
- Reinforcing existing survival strategies, or learning new ones, is incorrectly claimed as overcoming the trauma.
- Attention is focused on eliminating the symptoms, and not on seeing the person and their way of life as a whole.

I believe psychotrauma therapy is not possible without referring to the reality, the facts and the truth concerning what has happened and is continuing to happen. Since most people are entangled in massive victim-perpetrator dynamics, this is no easy task. It requires therapists who are clear in themselves about their own trauma; they cannot allow themselves to be drawn into the perpetrator-victim entanglements of other people, and have to be prepared to address their own perpetrator-victim structures therapeutically. If a therapist still lives in his own illusions, he will recommend them to others in trauma therapy as a supposed solution. In my opinion, the quick fix sought by conventional medicine and spiritual healers does not make any sense when faced with a trauma biography.

Constellations

My preferred method of therapy is the use of constellations. Since 1994, I have been gathering experience with this approach. I originally became familiar with 'constellations' by attending events with Bert Hellinger who popularised them in the form of so-called 'family constellations' from 1990 in Germany and later worldwide (Weber, 1995). I have set out my critical analysis of family constellations in various publications (Ruppert, 2005, pp. 204–214; 2012, p. 179ff.). With my current insights, I have identified the danger in family and systemic constellations of distracting the person from their own traumatisations and instead seeking a supposedly appropriate place in the 'system'.

The principle of the method of constellations consists of people being set up as 'representatives' in order to make a person's external relationship structure as well as his inner psychological state visible as a 'constellation of people'. People who speak and move function in this method as mirrors and seismographs for the psychological-physical state of other people. These 'representatives' do not have to know each other or anything about the life history of the person they are representing. This seems to be unbelievable. How can someone who is a stranger to me know what is going on inside me? How can he have access to my physical state, my feelings and even my hidden thoughts?

On the other hand, we could ask ourselves: What could be better suited, other than another person, to grasp the complexity and specificity of psychological-physical conditions so that they immediately make sense to the person concerned? What diagnostic method, technical apparatus, brain scan or elaborate questionnaire could do this better than another human being with similarly complex structures could?

Intention and Intention Method

I have known for some time that meaningful therapeutic work with people is only possible if they themselves want to achieve clarity about themselves. To do this they have to have an intention that they have explicitly formulated. I therefore developed the following technique: the person seeking my therapeutic support states his intention and then chooses a representative for his intention from the other people in the therapy group, and stands opposite this representative. This led very quickly to an intensive exchange that could go very deep (for concrete examples see Ruppert, 2012 and 2014). Using this method that I called 'the constellation of the intention' between 2009 and 2014, I could ensure that a person's intention was not lost sight of during the therapy process. Even if, following a suggestion of mine, further representatives for the person's inner life were called for, the focus remained on his intention. That was important to me, because this person ought to receive what he was asking support for – no more and no less. That way he was able to take responsibility himself for his own inner steps, and as his therapeutic support, I was in less danger of wanting something different from or for my client.

Words and Sentence of the Intention

A fundamental innovation for this therapeutic process came about early in 2015 when I thought about setting up a representative for each word of the intention, which was usually in the form of a sentence, instead of one representative for the whole intention. If the intention states: "I want to perceive and allow my needs", these are eight words that can be portrayed by separate people. In addition, there is the full stop at the end of the sentence that can also contain an important message about this person's intention. I have discovered that the punctuation mark at the end of a sentence of intention, whether it is a full stop, a question mark or an exclamation mark, can provide crucial information about the underlying psychological dynamic of an intention. Indeed, if a punctuation mark is missing, that is also a message, because the people who write their intention down leave it out consciously or unconsciously.

Representatives for words – does that work?

First, I had to convince myself that representatives could resonate with individual words in a sentence and that this makes sense to the person whose intention it is. Just a short while later I had gained so much experience confirming this that today I am in no doubt the method works! The representatives resonate with individual words in a clear and defined way; and not only with the words that appear more important, the nouns and verbs, but also with the definite and indefinite articles, pronouns and also with an 'and' or a 'to'. The meaningfulness of the representative's reflection is confirmed when the person whose intention it is, recognises himself in it. In addition, I have noticed that this happens almost without exception.

It is even more remarkable for me to experience that this technique does not require any prior information. The person writes down his sentence of intention and the process can begin. Everything that is important in the context of the sentence of intention appears during the process – whether it is a prenatal trauma, a life-threatening situation following the birth, the symbiotic entanglement with the parents, sexual traumatisation or experiencing violence during childhood, etc. The representatives need not have heard anything about this beforehand. They are still able, through the resonance process with the individual words, to access a reality that the client until then had split off inside himself and suppressed.

Once, during a two-day seminar, I was intrigued when every participant except one immediately wrote their sentence of intention on the board and began their constellation process straightaway. The one female participant who insisted on telling her detailed history was the one who, by describing a tragedy in her family, distracted attention from the real focus, which was that after her birth, a nurse had almost killed her.

The resonance phenomenon

My term for people willing to act as representatives is 'resonators', because we resonate with a word from the client's sentence, therefore with information that is transferred consciously and unconsciously. We attune ourselves with this word and become certain of its content within the sentence of intention via the feedback received from him and the other resonators. There is always something wonderful when this person who is now dealing with his intention, finally feels recognised and understood.

These resonance processes are often breathtakingly precise. During a resonance, I once had the feeling that my fingers were being crushed and I needed to call for help. Whereupon the client, whose father I was representing, said that during the potato harvest her father had once trapped his fingers in the harvest machinery and she had witnessed it. Apart from the horror of having seen it, she had also felt a certain amount of malicious joy because her father had hit her with that hand shortly before.

Procedure

I believe a procedure consisting of seven phases is the most effective in the Intention Method:

1. The client writes or draws his intention on a whiteboard. He must not be influenced in any way in finding his intention.
2. He chooses resonators for all the words or elements of the drawing. He then gives the starting signal and all resonators leave their seats and begin to interact with one another. (Since this process is new, the constellations in this book are described using an earlier procedure, in which the representatives are chosen one after another.)
3. In the non-verbal phase the resonators do not speak. They can move about and use gestures, body language or sounds to express what they are experiencing.
4. The client stays close to the whiteboard. He can choose to react emotionally or, depending on his intention, retain his exploratory attitude.
5. In accordance with the client the therapist ends the nonverbal phase after one or two minutes.
6. The client decides in which order he is going to ask the resonators for their input. They talk about it in concentrated form. The client matches their accounts with his biographical experiences. As therapist, I support the client in clarifying his intention by my questions and comments. I help him kick-start a crucial inner change. This is particularly the case when the client gets further into his feelings and he is able to assign his feelings to the original trauma situations in his biography.

7. The client dismisses the representatives, during which they can still say something to him that is necessary for them to be fully released as resonators. This also can have an emotional impact on the client, thereby leading to further clarification of his intention.

In most cases the sentence of intention comes from a mixture of the healthy, traumatised and survival parts. If an intention mainly consists of survival strategies, the facilitator has to have a particular skill in making it clear to the client in a sympathetic way how his survival strategies are again building up stress inside him, and causing him to resort to activity. For example, by conveying in clear words to the client how a perpetrator-victim dynamic has unfolded in the work as a continued excluding of the split trauma feelings. The client should be made aware that his survival strategies were previously necessary in order for him to be here today, but that he still has to pay a high price as a result and that his quality of life is suffering as a result.

Bringing a survival strategy to the fore through a sentence of intention does not mean that the therapy has failed, because all survival strategies that are re-staged in a therapeutic situation, and consciously recognised and understood, then do not have to be repeated unconsciously in everyday life. It is important that the client not only recognises these survival strategies in his head, but feels them: what happens when I dissociate, become confused, give up contact with my body, split within my body, give up contact with my 'I' and then act? On the other hand, I have found that there is a healthy part in every intention that has to be emphasised during the constellation process. Sometimes it is the full stop at the end of the sentence that carries an important message.

As a facilitator, I encourage the client to feel and sense during every phase of the constellation process. If necessary, the whole process is halted or slowed down. Sometimes not all words in the sentence are explored, especially if the client comes into contact with his trauma feelings. What has occurred might be enough for the client at that moment. As therapeutic support, I should not force him to express his feelings and nor should I block them. I encourage him with sympathetic words and gestures and respect his boundaries.

Native language or learnt language?

Which language should I use to formulate my intention? The language I first learnt as a child, in other words my 'mother tongue'? Alternatively, in a second or third language I have learnt later? When this question arises, I let the client decide for himself. Both alternatives have advantages and disadvantages.

I encountered an interesting example in my work with a Chinese woman. The seminar took place in English. The intention she formulated in English was: "I want to divorce my husband". She then had the idea of putting this intention into her native language, Chinese, and the intention translated then read: "I want leave marriage" (see Fig. 3.).

These are definitely two different matters: wanting to divorce one's husband or to leave the institution of marriage. The constellation established that it was the latter that was more important to the woman. Her main reason for getting married was because her parents had pushed her into it, and in her social environment, it was expected of her. So first and foremost this was about her social status and not about her wish to be in a partnership and enjoy sexuality and having her own children with a loved person.

She had studied at university and was happy with her professional progress. Her traumatic childhood experiences had also made her feel that she had not wanted to get married. Her parents' marriage had also been more of a deterrent for her. She treated her marriage more as a friendly alliance of convenience that, over time, she found more restricting than fulfilling.

The single-child policy in China that meant that girls were regarded as inferior, and suffered a trauma of identity because they were the 'wrong' sex, also became apparent during this work.

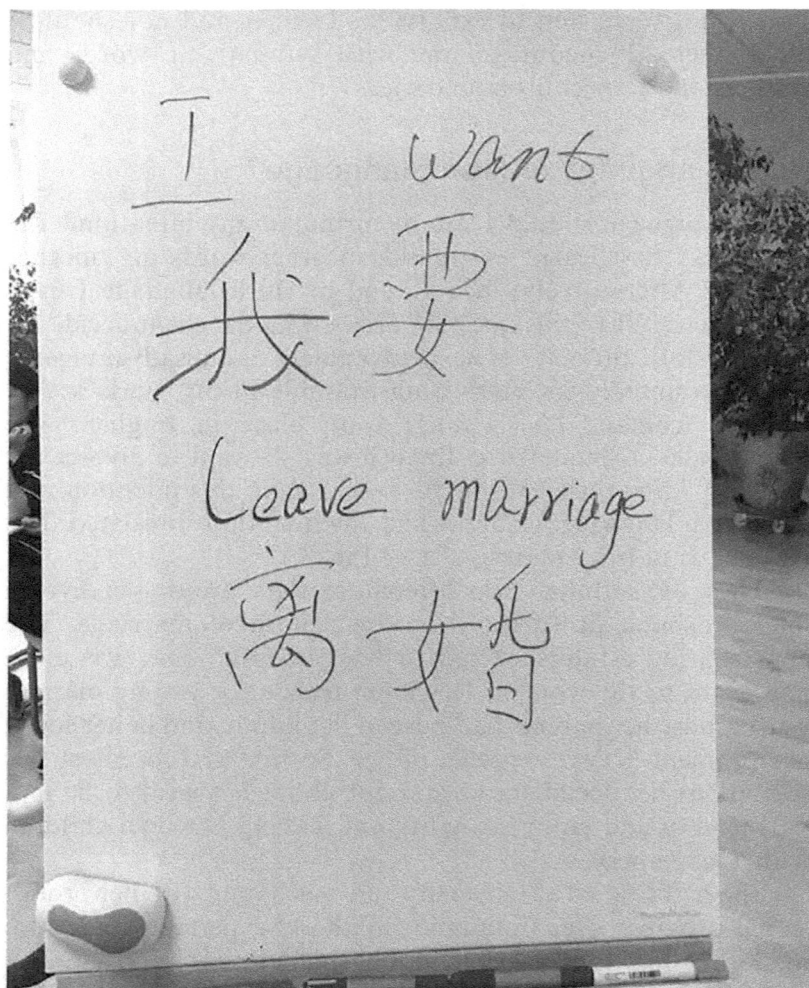

Figure 3: Intention of a native Chinese speaker

How does the resonance phenomenon work?

There have been some attempts to interpret the resonance phenomenon, which is the basis for constellations, scientifically. For example referencing the mirroring neurons in the brain (Bauer, 2005) or 'morphogenetic' or 'knowing' fields (Sheldrake, 1998) or quantum physics assumptions. In fact, there is not yet any scientific explanation for this phenomenon, although it can be reproduced at any time and anywhere. In my opinion, it is not necessary for the practical work, which has its basis in the humanities and social sciences, because anyone wanting to convince himself of this method has only to be a representative a few times and experience the effects himself. From one moment to the next, he can have the most varied experiences in a role. He can:

- suddenly be full of stress and fear,
- feel extreme anger or shame,
- feel pain in exactly those parts of his body which are the same as those of the client,
- become tired or even faint,
- be flooded with a wave of sadness and begin to cry,
- receive specific images,
- feel that there is something else in the room that is not yet represented,
- feel nothing, because that also corresponds with the role.

What would it add to such personal experiences if we knew what energy waves and exactly which parts of the brain and body are involved? It is enough for me to know that we humans have a very high capacity for empathy that connects us with other people at a deep level, and this has a life-sustaining function within the mother-child attachment in particular. I have noticed that people, who have suffered a great deal with traumatic attachment experiences, have developed a pronounced ability to perceive the feelings, moods and thoughts of other people. However, in principle everyone can resonate with other people and take on the role of representative in this therapeutic work. The important thing is for him to do it gladly and willingly. As resonators, we can open ourselves during the constellation process to the deepest feelings of another person, and afterwards close the open sensors relatively easily.

The human psyche – an open book

As therapist and observer of constellations, I can understand the in-depth structure of an intention when using the intention method. I therefore become aware of how a person's psyche is presented in its basic elements in a sentence of intention, that is, in ...

- its function of the 'I',
- the function of the will (expressed as for example want, would like, must, should, may),
- the different forms of cognition (see, hear, sense, feel, know, understand),
- the different forms of acting (for instance, healing, letting go, developing),
- its state (for instance was, am, be, become), and
- in the words for personal attribution (my, me, mine, self).

The intention method makes one vividly aware of the psyche's modular structure as well as its workings and it becomes possible to read a person's psyche like an open book.

The healthy 'I' in therapy

The healthy 'I' has to be re-activated in identity-oriented psychotrauma therapy. It has to free itself gradually of having a traumatised mother, a traumatising father or a perpetrator superimposed on it. It has to start being able once again to take over its steering function and responsibility for the whole person. Only a healthy 'I' is capable of properly coordinating all psycho-logical functions and fine-tuning them. Only the healthy 'I' has the ability to take appropriate decisions in the interests of the whole organism.

When it is ready once again to take up its task as leader, the healthy 'I' experiences the trauma survival parts, which tried to replace the 'I'-function in the original traumatising situation, as adversaries, which are not easily persuaded to hand the reins over, even if the immediate danger to life has passed. They keep intervening when something reminds them of the original trauma situation. It is therefore difficult for the healthy 'I' to develop after a trauma experience, and grow with its responsibilities. It often fades into the background.

Sentences of intention and everyday psychology

Most sentences of intention sound plausible. Below are some examples:

"I can trust my powers of healing." (1)
"I want to have relationships and still be able to remain in my power."(2)
"I want to be able to deal with money."(3)
"I want to disentangle myself from my terrible family."(4)

During the constellation process, it transpired that:

- the client still trusts in her mother ('healing') and father ('strength') who seriously harmed her during her childhood; (1)
- 'relationships' are still relationships with perpetrators because the client still idealises the original perpetrator from his childhood; (2)
- 'money' is the word unconsciously used for the perpetrator, whom the child was unable to deal with; (3)
- the word 'terrible' trivialises the violence, sexual traumatisation and even murder in the family of origin.

In the face of trauma, everyday psychology fails. It neither recognises the extent of trauma, nor does it know how to really help. It glosses over things and believes it has overcome the old horrors. The intention method can put such sentences of intention, and with that our everyday psychology, under continuous review. This method has the potential to allow people to recognise and resolve their 'blind spots'.

When I set up constellations for myself, the representatives help me to notice my own splits. My ability to self-reflect is limited – I am no different from anyone else in that respect – even though I have learnt a lot about trauma. Under the precondition of psychotrauma, a person's ability to self-reflect is fundamentally restricted because forcing the experiences into unconsciousness helps to survive a trauma. Part of the character of a psychotrauma is also the denial of this reality and being blind to traumas.

'Identity constellations'

Since this form of therapeutic work is concentrated on a person's identity development, this process can also be termed 'identity constellations'. Identity constellations are not simply exercises in self-awareness but psychotherapeutic processes based on Identity-oriented Psychotrauma Therapy (IoPT). My understanding is that every identity constellation reveals a person's healthy psychological structures and allows them to strengthen and grow. One of the ways this happens is by vividly experiencing our trauma survival strategies; because it is only then that we recognise that unconsciously they preserve our splits. Some people are shocked at the extent of the activity of their survival parts, and the way in which they act. However, as a rule this beneficial shock motivates the person to change their situation.

In order to integrate a person's traumas, in other words to remove the psychological splits, feelings that were suppressed in the original trauma must be allowed to be experienced in the therapy. However, in this process the original unbearable experience must not be a repetition. Instead, a healing pain should be experienced, that then recreates the connection with the person's 'I' that was split off in the original trauma situation. The focus should be on the person developing good feelings towards himself, and a self-acceptance that includes all the bad experiences that he has had. Therefore, it is not so much about trauma 'confrontation' – which is an aggressive term anyhow – as about developing empathy and self-love. It is the accessing of his original joie de vivre, the enjoyment of his own existence, curiosity for his life and trust in his own life forces. It is about being 'I' in the fullest sense of one's own possibilities. More and more I have realized that the trauma of identity takes centre stage in all steps towards change.

Constellations and the body

The whole organism is involved in the constellation, not just the psyche. There is movement, touch (for instance holding hands), embracing, and occasionally aggressive contact, which in the process of the work can only be stated but not enacted. Therefore, constellations always contain elements of physical therapy. Physical blocks can be experienced and there is a physical discharge of tension when we shake, cry or scream or even exhale deeply and physically relax. That is why constellations are a suitable method for healing physical phenomena. After a constellations process physical symptoms sometimes completely disappear, as I found for myself in the case of gum disease, reflux problems and a permanent tickle in my throat.

Healing

The literal meaning of the word 'healing' is 'becoming whole', and the healing of a psychotrauma can only take place from the inside of the person. Medication, surgical procedures or external treatments can have no effect if they do not activate a person's own healing powers. Since the experience of a psychotrauma makes people into objects, the healing of trauma must begin with making them into the subject again, calling into action their own 'I' and their own will, developing and stabilising them.

In terms of setting one's intention, since every person can only begin the process of change from his own inner place at that particular time, there can be no wrong intention. Since our survival strategies always aim to resist our belief in the reality of our splits, and our recognition that psyche and body live in two different realities, those intentions that enable our trauma survival strategies to be experienced and touched are very helpful for our further healthy identity development. These trauma survival parts tenaciously maintain that they know the only true and sensible escape route: splitting off and suppressing the traumatising reality and projecting it to the outside. For instance, in constellations a client often interprets one of the words represented as follows: "That is my mother!" In reality, however, it is a part of the client that has been split off and made external.

Lara: "I want to learn to live"

Lara sits down on the chair next to me. Her head is completely empty, she says, as she waits for me to ask her something. I do not say anything, knowing that by doing so I would be supporting her in her survival strategy of orienting herself according to the outside world. I wait for her to continue. She begins to talk about her overactive thyroid gland. Doctors have discovered a lump and advised her to have an operation, but she is unable to make a decision.

She then continues talking about where her last therapeutic work had finished. This had been about her birth. She says she had to stay in hospital after she was born because there was something wrong with her blood, probably something to do with incompatible rhesus factors of her mother and father. She stayed in hospital for two months. She does not know what was done to her; she might have had a blood transfusion. She bears a scar on her right shoulder from this time. Her mother went back to work shortly after she came home from the hospital. At eight months old she was given to her grandparents during the week and only saw her parents at the weekend.

Finally Lara finds her sentence of intention: "*Ich will lernen zu leben*" ("I want to learn to live"). As the first word in this sentence she chooses 'I'. Instead of choosing a person as a resonator (apart from me there were three other people in the therapy room) she takes a red meditation cushion for this 'I' and places it in the middle of the room. She then runs away from the cushion and hides behind an empty chair. After a while, she leaves her hiding place and stands on the six-inch high cushion. She complains that it is pulling her further and further upwards and she is hardly able to think and feel any more.

I ask Lara to choose a representative for another word from her sentence of intention. She gets down from her 'I'-cushion and chooses one of the women present to resonate for the word 'will' (want). To begin with this woman is at a loss, then she is drawn to the 'I'-cushion. She puts her feet under the cushion, raises it a little and begins to push it along in front of her using both her feet, as king penguins do with their eggs. This resonator for 'want' then says: "This 'I' is completely lifeless. I would like to crawl inside this 'I' as if it were a toy that I could then move from the inside so that the 'I' appears to be alive. It could then do everything, above all, it could move. But it can't feel." Lara stands at the side and watches with interest what the 'want' is doing with the 'I'.

For the next word from her sentence of intention Lara chooses '*lernen*' (learn) and again chooses one of the women present. She walks up and down a small corridor made by the pattern of the carpet in the therapy room; she says her head feels empty and she would like other people to come and tell her what to do. She has no connection with 'I' and 'want'. The resonator for 'want' confirms this. Lara says "that's true!" She sometimes feels as if she lives in parallel worlds.

Lara then chooses the last word in her intention: '*leben*' (to live). She chooses me and places me under the 2-metre tall tree in a corner of the therapy room. My head gradually disappears inside the branches of this plant. To begin with, I think the plant is alive, because plants produce oxygen to breathe. However, as a resonator, my breathing gets more and more difficult, and I notice that I cannot move away from the tree. I feel more and more as if I am in prison. I realise that I cannot live properly here, nor can I die. I panic and start to call for help, sometimes louder and more demanding and sometimes more quietly with a pleading note.

While I gradually get into my role, Lara has hidden behind the flip chart and starts to cry. After a while she comes out of her hiding place and goes to the resonator for 'learn'.

Again, I cry for help, but none of the others comes to me. On the contrary, they block their ears. In addition, when Lara begins to take a step towards me, the representative for 'learn' stands in her way. As 'to live', I have no hope that anyone is going to come and rescue me.

At this point, I leave my position as resonator and take up my position as facilitator again, and suggest interrupting the constellation. I ask Lara if she wants to hear how I understand the constellation process so far. She answers yes. I give her the following interpretation:

- When she had to stay in hospital after she was born, she found being alone so unbearable that she had split psychologically and give up her 'I'-function. That had become clear to me both from her reaction when standing on the 'I'-cushion and by what I experienced in resonance under the tree. Her child 'I' is traumatised and in great distress and mortal danger.
- She also suppresses her feelings, not crying in front of others (just a brief moment of crying behind the flip chart). After coming out of hospital, she became a 'good child' and was easy to look after.
- From then she moved through her life not with a natural healthy will but a strong survival will. Externally she tried to appear 'normal', which was exhausting for her. That may be the cause of her thyroid problems. She had to expend an enormous amount of energy to keep her frozen body alive

and moving. That would lead over time to complete exhaustion and the potential failure of her thyroid.

- Since the representative for 'to learn' seemed detached from her 'I' and her 'want' in the constellation, what she 'learns' may also not be helpful for her. Therefore, the function of this idea of 'learning' is a survival strategy that distracts her attention from contact with the traumatised child in her that is calling out for help. Learning in this way makes her dependent on what other people say; thus, she cannot come into her autonomy.

Lara agrees with my interpretations and adds that she has only cried twice in front of her husband during her marriage, and both times he severely criticised her for it. I offer her the following on the topic of love: there is a false concept of love that she has been following, "be good, don't cry, then you will be loved". A more real love would be to allow her own feelings, because then she would be more in contact with herself, and feel empathy for her own distress. The resonator for 'want' confirms that this feels right; she only felt some connection with Lara when Lara cried behind the flip chart.

I encourage Lara to look again at the 'I'-cushion and at the 'want' resonator. She does so, and after a while, she walks over to them. She touches the cushion and is pleased to hear it rustle (it is filled with grains of wheat). She then pokes her index finger into the cushion. This prompts 'want' to say to her that she should be more careful with the 'I' because it is only a little child. I add: "That's probably how you were treated as a baby. You were pricked with needles and that was painful for you."

Lara becomes gentler and strokes the cushion carefully. 'want' joins in and together both gently touch the 'I'. Lara is much moved and begins to cry. After a while we end this constellation.

This case study is a classic example of the 'trauma of identity'. Because of an early traumatisation the healthy 'I' disappears. It splits off and drifts into nothingness leaving the body without authority. That is why survival strategies, such as endurance and purely cognitive processes ('learn') have to continue on their own. However, they are not in contact with the client's real life, which is still stuck in an early trauma that turns into a trauma of love because the parents are not emotionally available to her.

Anne: "I want to be I"

Anne has been having individual therapy with me for some time. She also sometimes works in groups with constellations on her topics. On this occasion only I am there and after the preliminary conversation, Anne formulates her sentence of intention: *"Ich will ich sein"* "I want to be I".

In the individual session, when there are no other people to resonate for the client, the facilitator can take this function along with the use of floor markers.

Anne first asks me to resonate with the first 'I' in her sentence of intention. She takes hold of my hands but then quickly wants to pull her hands away from mine. But as the 'I', I hold on to her hands, which are ice-cold, for a while, and I am shocked at how much Anne appears to be just skin and bones with a layer of clothes hanging on her. She pulls her hand away, and when I tell her my thoughts, she confirms them. Yes, that is often the way she sees herself. Suddenly she realises what this "I want to be I" really means for her: "I want to be 'I' without a body."

This idea makes me shudder in my resonance, and I think of Greek mythology, the underworld, Hades, where the shadows reside, spirits without bodies that only exist because they can think. I tell Anne my thoughts and feelings and that it makes me feel very sad: as the word 'I', I want to be alive even if I only half feel my body now. But I am convinced that I can develop further and acquire more vitality.

Anne's intention then becomes even clearer to her: up until this moment, because of the massive traumatisations she experienced from a very early age, her solution has been not to feel her body. Her mother tried to kill her several times and her father traumatised her sexually for many years. Her parents' actions drove her out of her body and she had to flee into the idea of a bodiless form of existence. Anne now realises that experiencing her body means feeling all the violence she experienced from her mother and father as realities rather than merely cognitive facts. She recognises where her fear of her own body comes from, and how she had blocked her physical development.

In further identity constellations Anne has increasingly succeeded in saying 'Yes' to herself, in accepting her own body, sensing her feelings, understanding her extremely cognitive survival strategies and internally no longer needing her relationship to her traumatised perpetrator parents.

Words and pictures

Images or drawings can also depict an intention, as well as a combination of words and image elements. Drawings are particularly suitable for expressing unconscious and pre-speech experiences. Fig. 4 depicts the intention drawing of a man who wanted to address his chronic stomach pains. The constellation showed that these stomach pains pointed to an abortion attempt by his mother that he had survived.

With drawing intentions the client and therapist consider together which individual elements of the drawing need to be separately represented. In the case of Fig. 4, there were four representations:

- for the man lying down, who it transpired was an unborn child,
- for the (red) arrow which turned out to be an abortion attempt with a sharp object,
- for the (brown) line in the unborn child's stomach, that showed the abortion trauma,
- for the question mark that expressed the client's unwillingness to believe that his mother could have done something like that.

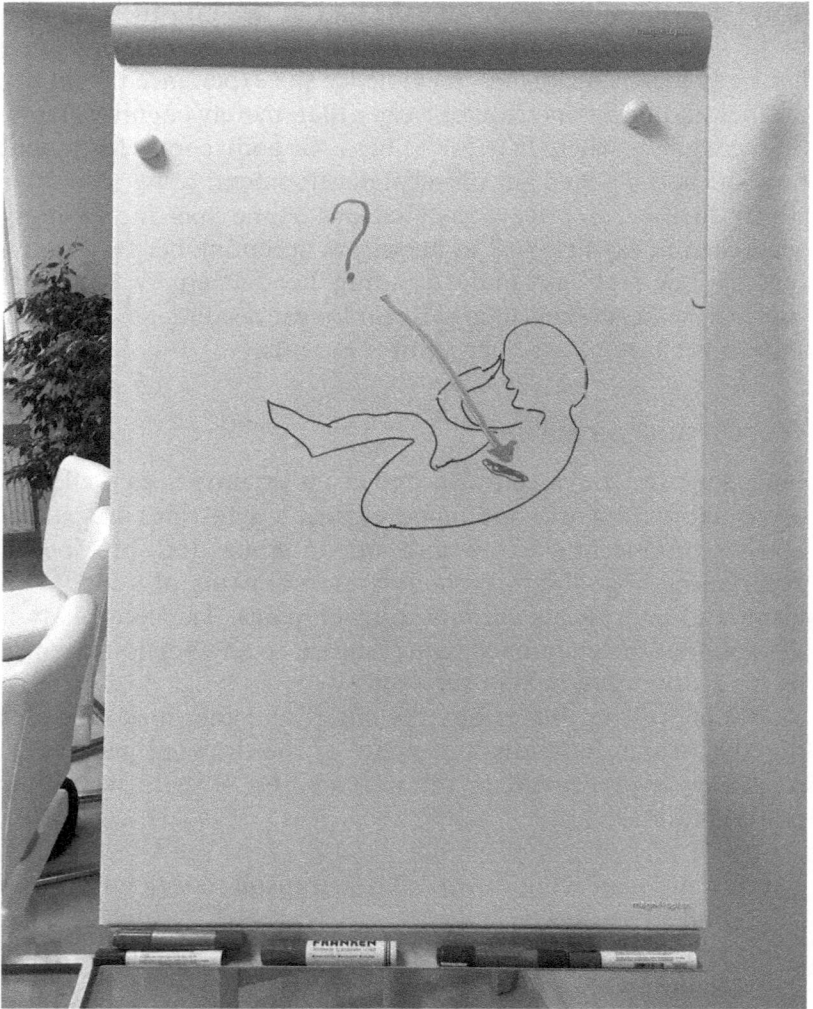

Figure 4: Intention drawing of a man with chronic stomach pains

The following case (Fig. 5) shows an intention of my own. I wanted to find out why I have a small skin growth under my left eye. Instead of several words ("the skin growth under my left eye"), I chose to depict it as a drawing. This can be a good way to avoid packing too much information into an intention. The amount of cognitive information that can be absorbed by the client during the constellation process is limited. It is a case of 'less is more'. Longer sentences of intention are frequently a sign of dominant survival strategies that distract from clarity and feelings; a lot of talk and reflection prevents feelings from surfacing.

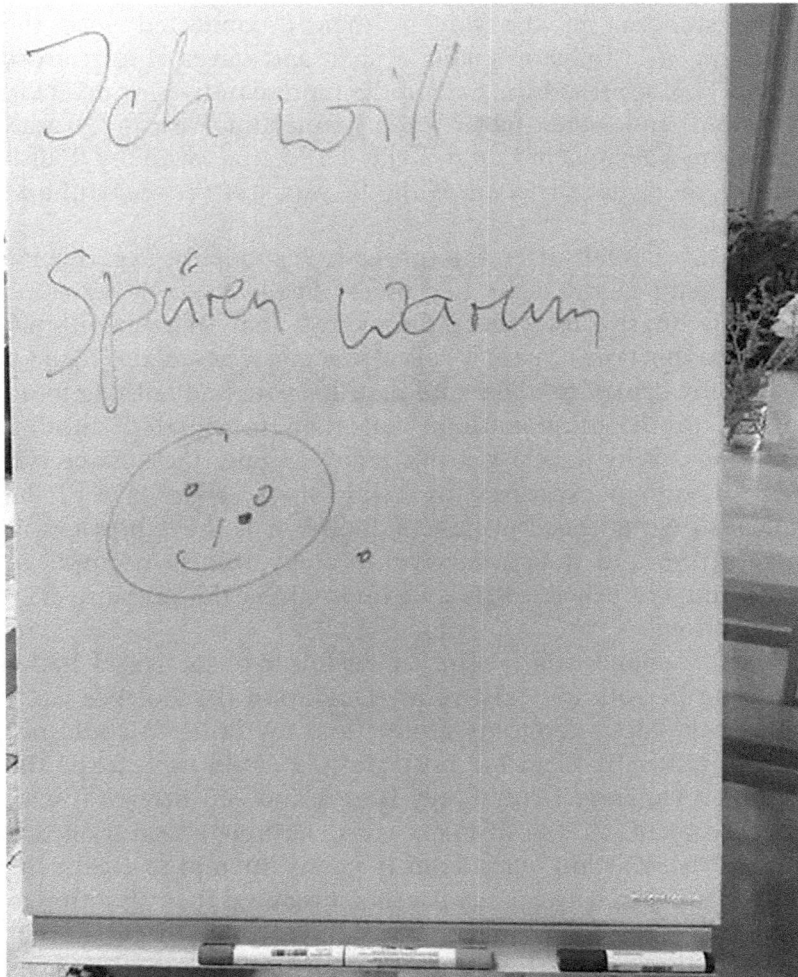

Figure 5: "I want to feel why (the skin growth under my left eye)."

In my case it turned out that the representative for the *'hautsymptom'* ('skin symptom') was full of anger and hate. My 'I' drew back in fear and my 'want' took on a submissive posture. I could attribute that to the extreme violence I had experienced from my mother during my childhood. *'spüren'* ('to feel') rolled around on the floor in despair and felt that it was totally unseen. *'warum'* ('why') said bluntly: "You got it because you happened to be standing in the way". When I connected with the *'schlusspunkt'* ('full stop') pain, despair and waves of tears arose in me. This appeased the hate in the representative for my 'skin symptom' and I then felt a better connection with my 'want', which was able to stand up straight. The contact with my 'I' also became more intense, even if the 'I' was still very fearful and cautious.

About a week after this process, I suddenly experienced violent pain in the right side of my head. After doing some research on the internet I discovered that in conventional medicine this type of pain is called trigeminal neuralgia. I paid a visit to my dentist to make sure that this pain had nothing to do with a tooth inflammation, and then formulated another intention: "Why have I got this pain?" Again, the answer was clear: The pain expresses my helplessness in the face of the violence I experienced in my childhood. It is the expression of dissociation and thus a survival strategy, which attempts to block out the perpetrators and internalises the pressure they have exerted.

In this connection it also became clear to me why I had a whistling in both my ears: in my childhood the violence came from both sides – from my mother and my father. I could not turn to either of them for protection. I could not escape the continual violence; I could only bear it and get through it with clenched teeth. In one of many constellations I set up on this subject, the whistling turned out to be my attempt to escape the daily arguments between my parents; I reduced their shouting to a thin whistling sound and tried to do everything right so that perhaps they might love me. Even before my birth, I was subjected to the infernal racket of masonry saws because right up to the seventh month of her pregnancy, my mother worked in a marble factory. In a further constellation on my 'tinnitus' I realised how, even as an unborn child, I was unable to escape this sound and my physical development was affected by my tendency to curl myself up into a ball to try and counter the sound and my fear. For a long time I puzzled over the fact that this 'tinnitus' only appeared when I was 35 years old. Today I realise it was triggered by a professional situation where, in a similar way to the start of my life, I felt rejected and unwelcome and was very afraid. Often 'parallel situations' to the original trauma will trigger physical symptoms.

The violence I experienced as a child had also become firmly lodged in me as a 'dry cough' in my throat and chest. If I was getting over a 'cold' this dry cough remained for some time after. This symptom disappeared following a constellation during which I clearly recognised, and felt, that as an infant I had only just survived a physical attack by my father. For the first time in my life, I had the feeling that I did not need to worry about what might happen next. I felt fully in the here and now.

Physical signals contain important messages

It is a major error to regard the manifestation of pain, inflammation, degeneration or injuries as the actual problem, because these phenomena are actually warning signs that something is at work that needs attention and has to be sorted out. It is a serious error if the physically discernible manifestations of psycho-trauma are simply 'removed', suppressed or repaired. Focus is then not placed on the essential issue, which can then not be brought into a healing process, but remains in the person's body as an unsolved problem. Traumas then are not worked through and the body does not become more alive, but, at best, is only temporarily able to function better. It is then likely to become more of a prison, even a real personal enemy. This is why new physical signals then appear which are usually more severe than the original ones. Thus, an escape from the trauma biography cannot take place without addressing and working through the trauma.

Survival strategies do not heal, they cause further splits

The earlier in his development that a human organism experiences trauma, the deeper, more diverse and more permanent the consequences are. If in the prenatal phase a child is harmed by toxins, incorrect diet, inter-human conflicts or violence, this leaves traces on those organs and body parts that were in development at the time of the trauma. Because we are unaware of these early injuries stored in our bodies, we orientate ourselves later towards what appears to be consciously understandable, and we search in vain for healing from our suffering where it cannot be found (Evertz, Janus and Lindner, 2015; van der Kolk, 2015; Sauer and Emmerich, 2017).

A lot of time has usually passed before we experience our distress at the physical level, time during which we have put an increasing strain on our bodies. This results in increasing signs of wear on joints, damage to the mucous membranes, inappropriate stress on sensory organs, or in complete organ failure. This time was also occupied with suppression, denial and appeasement of our traumatisation. Usually no one in our environment alerts us to the fact that these physical pains, deficiencies, or degenerations could be based on a psychotrauma. We might have tried various healing treatments, and some of the symptoms of our supposed illnesses might have been alleviated. However, this is unable to resolve the underlying trauma. On the contrary, we have only strengthened the splits within us. In my practice, I can clearly see the damaging effects of the well-meant survival strategies put to clients within the framework of conventional medicine, as well as by conventional psychotherapy.

Visualising 'self-mothering' for example, is not beneficial, because it unconsciously re-activates the real mother, who was a perpetrator to the child. Instead, we must feel the painful reality that there was no loving mother for us, because she herself was traumatised and still has a small, needy child inside her. Otherwise we will stay in a victim attitude and in our inner fragmentations.

How big is our self-healing potential?

Ultimately, it is all about communicating lovingly with our own body, looking after its needs and taking the signals it shows seriously. It also means that we do not continue to allow others to have our body at their disposal and to abuse it for their own trauma survival strategies. We must also learn to withstand any temptation to exercise power over someone else's body in order to transfer our traumatic experiences onto them.

This painful process engenders fear. Pain and fear can have different functions:

- There are pain and fear that separate our body and our psyche further from one another, deepening the splits. Preoccupation with these feelings serves as a distraction from our traumatisations.
- There are pain and fear that are beneficial. If we feel them deeply, they connect our body and our psyche with one another again. The self-regulating physical processes that work unconsciously and autonomously can then function, and the conscious psychological processes can create a beneficial environment in which that can happen.

For beneficial pain, it is helpful if we are in contact with an environment in which we feel safe, supported and understood. This should be the case in a good therapy situation in groups as well as in individual sessions.

We now know that there is immense repair potential and powers of self-healing in the whole of the human organism. There are now impressive examples of neuroplasticity[6] in the

---

[6] Neuroplasticity is the ability of nerves and brain structures to restore themselves.

nervous system and the brain (Doidge, 2015). In a hospital study, Mechthilde Kütemeyer discovered that physical lesions that were not healing properly closed after those concerned had talked about the traumatic experiences that lay hidden beneath these lesions (Kütemeyer, 2008). But there are limits here too that we must recognise:

- The crooked bone in the toe is unlikely to straighten, even if the original trauma, for instance violence experienced as an infant, has since been recognised and felt.
- The organs that have already been damaged will never recover to their original capacity prior to being affected by the trauma.
- We can never get back the kidney that has been removed in an operation.
- Teeth that have been extracted will not grow back.

Even so, it never seems to be too late to take the opportunity afforded by physical distress signals to look into their traumatic background. We should take it seriously, "when the body says 'No'", as the Canadian doctor, Gabor Maté so aptly put it (Maté, 2011). The earlier we start, the better our chances are of achieving complete healing. Particularly for infants and children, it is a blessing when the alarm signals they convey to parents and carers about their body are not dismissed as mysterious 'illnesses', but have their traumatic origins investigated and taken seriously (Nickel, 2017).

In my practice I have experienced many times that, to the astonishment of their doctors, clients with a medical diagnosis of cancer are suddenly free from tumours and cancer indications after they have arrived at the origin of their psychotrauma. So-called autoimmune illnesses suddenly disappeared when the psychological conflicts that lay behind them had dispersed. In my case too, as I have already mentioned, I have been able to heal my physical suffering successfully on many occasions.

Even at an advanced age, we can counter any further worsening of physical infirmity by treating the cause rather than the symptoms. When we bring our healthy 'I' back to full bloom and freely develop our own will, our self-healing powers can unfold. Then traditional medicine as well as alternative medical practices can contribute their support to those healing processes with regard to the organism's material and energetic aspects.

There is a possibility that we might then one day be able to die peacefully without our trauma survival parts fighting back and without having to live in the grip of dementia, or hoping for others to make the decision to turn the machines off for us.

References

Adler, R. H. et al (2017). *Psychosomatische Medizin*. Munich, Urban & Fischer.

Ammon, M. & Fabian, E. (Publisher) (2014). *Selbstfindung und Sozialisation*, Gießen, Psychosozial.

Ammon, M. (2014). *Identität – ein interpersonelles Geschehen aus dynamisch-psychiatrischer Sicht,* in: M. Ammon & E. Fabian (Publisher). *Selbstfindung und Sozialisation,* pp. 123–158. Gießen, Psychosozial.

Bauer, J. (2005). *Warum ich fühle, was du fühlst*. Hamburg, Hoffmann und Campe.

Bauer, J. (2015). *Selbststeuerung*. Munich, Karl Blessing.

Bourquin, P. & **Cortés,** C. (2016). *Der allein gebliebene Zwilling*. Innenwelt.

Broughton, V. (2013). *The Heart of Things*. Steyning, Green Balloon Publishing.

Buford, B. (2010). *Geil auf Gewalt*. Munich, Goldmann.

Chalmers, A. F. (2001). *Wege der Wissenschaft*. Heidelberg, Springer.

Dahlke, R. (2007). *Krankheit als Symbol*. Munich, Bertelsmann.

Damasio, A. R. (2006). *Descartes' Irrtum*. Munich, List.

Davison, G. C. & **Neale**, J. M. (1979). *Klinische Psychologie*. Munich, Urban & Schwarzenberg.

Dethlefsen, T. & **Dahlke**, R. (2008). *Krankheit als Weg*. Munich, Bassermann.

Dilling, H., **Mombour**, W. & **Schmidt** M. H. (1993). *Internationale Klassifikation psychischer Störungen ICD-10*. Bern, Hans Huber.

Doidge, N. (2015). *Wie das Gehirn heilt*. Frankfurt/M., Campus.

Enders, G. (2014). *Darm mit Charme*. Berlin, Ullstein.

Erikson, E. H. (1976). *Identität und Lebenszyklus*. Frankfurt/M., Suhrkamp.

Ermann, M. (2007). *Psychosomatische Medizin und Psychotherapie*. Stuttgart, Kohlhammer.

Evertz, K., **Janus**, L. & **Lindner**, R. (Publisher) (2015). *Lehrbuch der Pränatalen Psychologie*. Heidelberg, Mattes.

Evertz, K. (2015): *Psychodynamische Aspekte von Schwangerschaftskonflikten in Bildern*, in: K. Evertz, L. Janus & R. Lindner (Hg.). *Lehrbuch der Pränatalen Psychologie*, S. 270–300. Heidelberg, Mattes.

Felitti, V. J. et al (1998). *Relationship of Childhood Abuse and Household Dysfunction to Many of the Leading Causes of Death in Adults*, in American Journal of Preventive Medicine, 4, pp. 245–258.

Garbe, E. (2015). *Das kindliche Entwicklungstrauma*. Stuttgart, Klett-Cotta.

Goffman, E. (1973). *Asyle. Über die soziale Situation psychiatrischer Patienten und anderer Insassen*. Frankfurt/M., Suhrkamp.

Graeber, D. (2014). *Schulden*. Munich, Goldmann.

Gruen, A. (2000). *Der Fremde in uns*. Stuttgart, Klett-Cotta.

Gruen, A. (2014). *Der Verrat am Selbst*. Munich, dtv.

Gruen, A. (2015). *Dem Leben entfremdet*. Munich, dtv.

Heller, L. & **Lapierre**, A. (2013). *Entwicklungstrauma heilen*. Munich, Kösel.

Hoppe, G. (2014). Abtreibungen und Trauma, in Franz Ruppert, *Frühes Trauma*, pp. 105–127. Stuttgart, Klett-Cotta.

Huber, M. (2013). *Der Feind im Innern*. Paderborn, Junfermann.

Juul, J. (2013). *Mann und Vater sein*. Freiburg, Kreuz.

Kakar, K. (2015). *Frauen in Indien*. Munich, C. H. Beck.

Kohn, A. (1986). Non Contest. The Case against Competition. Boston, Houghton Mifflin Company.

Kuhn, T. S. (1976). *Die Struktur wissenschaftlicher Revolutionen*. Frankfurt/M., Suhrkamp.

Kütemeyer, M. (2008). *Die dissoziative Wunde – ein Erinnerungssyndrom seelischer Traumatisierung*, in Zeitschrift für Psychotraumatologie, Psychotherapiewissenschaft und Psychologische Medizin, 2, pp. 27–39.

Langlotz, E. R. (2015). *Symbiose in Systemaufstellungen*. Heidelberg, Springer.

Laszlo, E. (1995). *Kosmische Kreativität*. Frankfurt/M., Insel.

Levine, P. A. (2010). *Sprache ohne Worte*. Munich, Kösel.

Marx, S. (2010). *HerzIntelligenz® kompakt*. Freiburg, VAK.

Maté, G. (2008). *In the Realm of Hungry Ghosts*. Toronto, Random House.

Maté, G. (2003). *When the Body Says No*. Hoboken, New Jersey, John Wiley & Sons Inc.

Nickel, R. (2017). Chronischer Schmerz und frühe Traumatisierung, in: *Trauma*, 1, pp. 6–14

Pert, C. B. (2001): *Moleküle der Gefühle*. Reinbek, Rowohlt-Taschenbuch.

Reddemann, L. (2008). *Psychodynamisch Imaginative Traumatherapie*. Stuttgart, Klett-Cotta.

Rhodes, J. (2014). *Der Klang der Wut*. Munich. Nagel & Kimche.

Ruppert, F. (2002). *Verwirrte Seelen*. Munich, Kösel.

Ruppert, F. (2008). *Trauma, Bonding & Family Constellations*. Frome, Green Balloon Publishing.

Ruppert, F. (2011). *Splits in the Soul*. Steyning, Green Balloon Publishing.

Ruppert, F. (2012). *Symbiosis & Autonomy*. Steyning, Green Balloon Publishing.

Ruppert, F. (2015). *Trauma, Fear and Love*. Steyning, Green Balloon Publishing.

Ruppert, F. (2017). *Early Trauma*. Steyning, Green Balloon Publishing.

Saß, H., **Wittchen**, H.-U., **Zaudig**, M. & **Houben**, J. (1998). *Diagnostisches und Statistisches Manual Psychischer Störungen DSM IV*. Göttingen, Hogrefe.

Sauer, M. & **Emmerich**, S. (2017). *Chronischer Schmerz nach Trauma – ein Phänomen des leiblich Unbewussten*, in Trauma, 1, pp. 24–36.

Schneider, K. (1992). *Klinische Psychopathologie*. Stuttgart, Thieme.

Schubert, C. (2011). *Psychoneuroimmunologie und Psychotherapie*. Stuttgart, Schattauer.

Seidler, G. H., **Freyberger**, H. J. & **Maercker**, A. (2011). *Handbuch der Psychotraumatologie*. Stuttgart, Klett-Cotta.

Sheldrake, R. (1998). *Das schöpferische Universum*. Berlin, Ullstein.

Siegel, D. J. (2010). *Wie wir werden, die wir sind*. Paderborn, Junfermann.

Strauss, D. (2014). *Abnabelungs- und Wiederanbindungsprozess als letzte Phase der Geburt*, in: F. Ruppert, *Early Trauma*. Steyning, Green Balloon Publishing. Rowohlt .

Walz- Pawlita, S., **Unruh**, B. & **Janta**, B. (2015). *Identitäten*. Gießen, Psychosozial.

Weber, G. (1995). *Zweierlei Glück*. Carl-Auer-Systeme.
Wirsching, M. (1996). *Psychosomatische Medizin*. Munich, Beck.
van der Kolk, B. (2014). *The Body Keeps the Score*. New York, Penguin.
von Uexküll, T. (1976). *Grundfragen der psychosomatischen Medizin*. Reinbek,

Dr Franz Ruppert, born in 1957, is Professor of Psychology and a psychological psychotherapist. He has developed Identity-oriented Psychotraumatherapy (IoPT) on the basis of the Intention method.
www.franz-ruppert.de

HARALD BANZHAF

Trauma as the key to understanding physical suffering

Polytrauma and psychological trauma – medical and psychological realities

People associate widely differing phenomena with the word 'trauma'. As a medical doctor with emergency medical training, for a long time it made me think immediately and solely of 'poly-trauma' – a term that instinctively triggers the highest alert in the emergency services. During my time as an emergency doctor, this word alone was sufficient to send my stress hormones rocketing. Strangely enough, at these moments I appeared to the paramedics assisting me as noticeably emotionally calm in the face of the external situation, while internally I felt really alive.

Medicine has coined the term 'polytraumatised' for people who, as a result of a traffic accident or a major fall, suffered severe injuries to various organ systems. This is a case of an acute condition with primarily organic dysfunction that requires a quick and focused intervention. Those concerned are in an acute life-threatening situation that is accompanied by an excessive release of stress hormones and inflammatory mediators.

From the psychological perspective, trauma means something quite different. Here it is mainly a case of psychological consequences following an acute event that was overwhelming but has been survived, combined with mortal fear and loss of control, which the psyche has been unable to deal with, and which has left wounds leading to a profound disruption of mental and physical integrity. Psychotrauma also includes a lasting threat from external dangers, for example from a violent person, and short- and long-term physical and psychological consequences. This applies particularly to children who have been at the mercy of traumatising parents for their entire childhood.

Depending on whether the focus is medical or psychological, perceptions differ a great deal. In one case the organism with its disturbed physiological functions is central; in another the focus is primarily the psychological, emotional and mental functions. The dilemma is that in the first case a body without a psyche and in the second, a psyche without a body is treated. Although almost all scientific investigations conclude that body and psyche are inseparable, we in the tradition of western medicine still hold onto an outdated world-view, and construct our reality along these simplified lines (Maté, 2003). This makes everyday practice slightly easier, but our chances of attaining a holistic understanding of the world and of life are ruined. We are cutting ourselves off from events that we could call healthy or healing, because a real healing process can only succeed if all parts of the system receive the necessary attention and acknowledgement.

The psychiatrist Daniel Siegel, who coined the term Interpersonal Neurobiology (Siegel, 2015), talks of the triangle of wellbeing – the concordance of mind, brain and relationships. In this context 'brain' refers to the physiological component, the body as the physical organism. Integrating these three parts seems to be the key to health and healing. The manner and type of our relationships with other people play an outstanding role here. This ability to form relationships with ourselves as well as with others is shaken to its foundations by traumatic experiences. After such an experience, the brain and mind as well as the body are seriously altered. It is an attack on the centre of our being. Trauma does not generate a gradual and temporary alteration of our Self; it permanently disorganises this Self and dismantles it into parts of a jigsaw puzzle that have no coherent correlation and no connection with each other.

In this book we will come across many individual life stories and discover that every organ or organ system in its own way can become the bearer of traumatic energy, and express the related fear, panic and distress in the form of different symptoms. In order to understand that we need body, psyche and mind for a successful integration process, we have to remind ourselves that we possess a triune brain, which evolves in the course of our individual development as a human (MacLean, 1990). It forms the material blueprint for our human ability to think and feel. We are usually conscious of our cerebral neocortex ('neomammalian brain'), which combines the functions of logical, analytical thinking and deduction, and facilitates highly complex cognitive processes such as language, planning, etc. Hidden below this is, from an evolutionary perspective a much older part of the brain, the 'paleomammalian brain', which holds our emotions, feelings and everything non-verbal. And then deep within our head is the oldest part of our brain, the 'reptilian brain', which is equipped with everything we need for our physical existence: heartbeat, blood pressure, body temperature, water balance are all regulated here. This is also where we find the control centres for the functions that are essential for our survival at times of extreme need, such as fight or flight reflexes, including the so-called 'playing-dead' reflex, when neither fight nor flight seems to have any promise of success and all other strategies for coping with stress have failed.

In order to demonstrate the close connection between physical and psychological processes, and at the same time be aware that these are different categories, Walach, Wittmann and Schmidt (2017) have pointed out the concept of the complementarity principle, by which is meant descriptions that are simultaneously necessary to understand a subject. This makes it clear that in order to be human, we need both physical and mental processes. This is the reason why we are actually aware of both sides, even if our focus is sometimes directed towards the physical-physiological processes to take measurements, and at other times towards the mental-psychological phenomena in order to describe subjective experiences.

In this respect, it would be advantageous for both the medical and the psychological scientists not to close themselves off from the other position. Medicine has to recognise that there are no bodies without a psyche; and psychology should give up the idea that psychological processes are possible without a biological-physiological matrix, a body. The connection of this phenomenon is described as 'embodiment' (Storch, Cantieni, Hüther and Tschacher, 2010). With that we could leave the outdated 'machine model' of medicine behind and at the same time understand that psychological processes require a biological matrix and have a physiological equivalent.

This becomes clear in an investigation of 5- to 10-year old children in which the telomeres[7] of those children who had been subjected to abuse, mobbing or domestic violence were shortened and who were therefore aging prematurely[8]. In these cases trauma had led to a profound alteration of the body biochemistry and finally of the whole organism, combined with far-reaching negative consequences for the individual's whole life. It is now widely recognised that there is a close relationship between health, longevity and the length of the telomeres. An investigation in 2014 drew attention to the correlation between the length of the telomeres and existing stress-associated illnesses such as depression and post-traumatic stress disorder, and put forward the theory that traumatic stress not only triggers psychological illnesses, but also influences cellular aging[9]. This is a further indication of body and psyche not representing opposites but being a self-organising system. Splitting off a part of this whole will inevitably prevent healing in the broad sense.

---

[7] The technical term for the protective caps at the chromosome ends that ensure that body cells can divide.

[8] I. Shalev et al (2013): "Exposure to violence during childhood is associated with telomere erosion from 5 to 10 years of age: a longitudinal study" in: Molecular Psychiatry (2013) 18, p. 576-581; doi: 10.1038/mp.2012.32.

[9] L. Zhang et al (2014): "Telomere length – a cellular aging marker for depression and Post-traumatic Stress Disorder" in: Medical Hypotheses (2014) 83(2), p. 182-185; doi: 10.1016/j.mehy.2014.04.033.

Acute stress is life-saving; chronic stress causes illness

Nature has equipped all creatures, including us humans, with a programme enabling us to react instantly in life-threatening situations to defuse a dangerous situation and ensure our survival. Whether the threat is real or virtual is irrelevant because our brain stem does not differentiate between actual and imagined danger. If in an emergency we believe ourselves to be strong enough, we face the fight, and if we are lucky we prevail against the acute danger. If we consider our resources insufficient, we draw back and flee from the danger. Our body mobilises all the reserves of strength at its disposal. Hormones such as adrenaline and noradrenaline are secreted via the endocrine system, stimulating the cardiovascular system to a maximum. Pulse and blood pressure rise, the lungs enrich the blood with as much oxygen as possible, so that the target organs and muscles are able to work as efficiently as possible. Mental processes and the immune system are extremely active. All metabolic processes not required at that moment, such as digestion and others, are restricted. We can also describe this stress axis as a 'call to arms'. When the danger is over, all systems can return to their base level and recover. After this fight or flight situation, physiological counter-programs ensure that the stress hormones that had previously built up can be worked off and no longer flood the organism.

However, if no solution is found and the problem or danger cannot be removed, something problematic takes place in the body: a second stress axis is activated and the stress hormone cortisol is pumped into the organism via the hypothalamus, pituitary gland and adrenal gland. The immune system is weakened, the hormone system is thrown off balance and chronic inflammatory processes are set in motion. Subsequently a large number of problematic physiological changes take place. If cortisol values are raised in the long term it is damaging to nerves and toxic for the brain. In the worst case nerve cells die. A study published in 2009 showed clear differences in the density of glucocorticoid receptors in the hippocampus of people who were traumatised in childhood[10]. Sexually abused, beaten or abandoned people had significantly fewer of these receptors. These chemical docking stations for cortisol play a decisive part in a person's susceptibility to stress. The higher the number of these receptors, the better a person can deal with adverse circumstances during his life.

The autonomic nervous system, which is largely deprived of conscious control, regulates these processes. The so-called sympathetic nervous system is responsible for activation and mobilisation. Its counterpart, the parasympathetic nervous system (also termed the 'vagus nerve' after its largest nerve), is responsible for relaxation and regeneration. The younger a person is when he loses this precisely matched interrelationship between agitation and relaxation, the sooner he will develop a long-term imbalance. The sympathetic part of the nervous system then dominates, with all the signs of permanent tension, agitation, activation of the stress hormone axes and countless biochemical and molecular changes. Being constantly alert and easily irritated, experiencing muscular tension, moods of depression and sleep disorders, having an increased susceptibility for infections and chronic illnesses, are just some of the possible consequences. There is a consensus that chronic stress is the number one cause of illnesses (Lipton, 2005), because being on permanent alert means being unable to regenerate. All organ systems are then overstretched in the long term. On a biochemical level, the body's persistent insidious tendency to become inflamed ('silent chronic inflammation'[11]) is the precursor to countless chronic illnesses, and the organism's premature aging process.

---

[10] P.O.McGowan et al (2009): "Epigenetic regulation of the glucocorticoid receptor in human brain associates with childhood abuse" in: Nature Neuroscience (2009) 12(3), p. 342-348; doi: 10.1038/nn.2270

[11] B. Fougère et al (2016): "Chronic Inflammation: Accelerator of Biological Aging", in: Gerontol A Biol Sci Med Sci. (2016) pii: glw240; doi: 10.1093/gerona/glw240.

Trauma, toxic stress and the consequences for the brain

If something happens during which a person is unable to make use of his fight or flight response as all available strategies are ineffective – either because the danger is overwhelming, or his resources are too weak – then an archaic emergency programme is activated: the 'playing-dead' reflex. This is controlled via the vagus nerve, which in the form of the ventral vagal complex provides for calmness, relaxation and the activation of the 'social engagement system'. Then the evolutionarily oldest and non-myelinated part, the dorsal vagal complex, appears (Porges, 2001).

What we on a physical level call the 'playing-dead' reflex, freezing or numbing of the organ functions, is, on a psychological level, responsible for the after-effects of traumatisation. This is a state that leaves no option except complete self-abandonment, accompanied by extreme helplessness, indescribable fear followed by numbness, which means a fragmentation of normally interrelated physical and psychological functions. In other words in the face of the monstrous danger, the person leaves his conscious body, and body and psyche no longer form a complementary entity as a connected whole.

And what happens in the brain during and, above all, after such an experience of traumatic stress? The triune brain develops in the baby from the bottom upwards. The central reptilian brain with its brainstem, which is responsible for physical survival, is the first of the three parts to be fully functioning, at the very start of life. Breathing, circulation, body temperature and many other physiological and biochemical metabolic processes have to be coordinated. Then, in the course of the first years the mammalian brain with the limbic system develops. Together, the limbic system and brainstem are also called the emotional brain. Finally the neocortex, the rational brain, our cerebrum and with it the frontal lobes and the prefrontal cortex are fully developed. Throughout a person's life, trauma can endanger and affect the functioning of all three parts.

One particular part of the frontal lobes, the prefrontal cortex, which is situated directly behind the eyes, takes on a very special role. It is not only responsible for feelings of empathy, but connects the cerebrum, which is responsible for our thoughts and actions, with the limbic system, the seat of our emotions. Van der Kolk calls this part of the brain 'the watchtower' (van der Kolk, 2015). In a sense, this hugely important control centre takes on a meta position. From this higher perspective we can look at all predominant and detailed information such as thoughts, feelings, emotions and sensory impressions, including the somatic markers, the information from the so-called abdominal brain, observing, analysing, evaluating and finally deciding what is good and right for us. This part of our brain, which, from an evolutionary perspective is very young, seems to embody the characteristics we call human and which distinguish us from all other mammals.

According to Joachim Bauer (2015) the formation of self-awareness is a process that is also essentially organised from the prefrontal cortex. This becomes functional during the first three years of life and forms the prerequisite of the concepts of 'I', 'You' and 'We'. Prior to this, a dyadic relationship exists between the infant and his closest attachment figure, usually his mother. The prefrontal cortex greatly influences self-control and self-regulation by controlling the 'base' centres of lust, gratification, fear and aggression. In time, a feeling of self that encompasses different psychological parts and, at best, is able to integrate them, develops through this highly complex process of formation and cross-linking of the different parts of the prefrontal cortex. One prerequisite, however, is a successful neuro-biological relationship between 'I' and 'You'. If the prefrontal cortex is unable to develop fully due to earlier traumatisations, or if its function is impaired, then the development of a healthy 'I', an awareness of 'You' and 'We', and finally the formation of self-awareness is endangered or even rendered impossible.

On a neuro-biological level, according to Joachim Bauer, massive stress and psychotrauma can cause a physiological reduction in the networks responsible for the 'I-You' relationship. The younger a person is when they are traumatised, the greater is the danger of grave and long-term consequences. Sometimes even less dramatic circumstances have far-reaching effects. For instance, the volume of the hippocampus is reduced in children if their relationship to their primary caregiver deteriorates. Studies have shown that the brain volume of children decreased by up to 20% after they experienced violence or neglect. This also affected the prefrontal cortex.

Below the 'watchtower' is a further important 'clearing centre' in the limbic system, the thalamus. This plays a very important role in understanding trauma. All sensory impulses arising from the periphery and arriving from the thalamus via the sensory organs (hearing, sight, smell, touch) are filtered and passed on to the amygdala for evaluation.

The paired amygdala ('blue almonds') act as the central control that decides whether an impulse is dangerous or harmless for the organism. They are often called the 'smoke alarms' of the brain. If the amygdala fire and send neuronal signals to further parts of the brain such as the hippocampus ('sea horses') and the cingulum ('island'), large amounts of stress hormones are automatically released to prepare the body for fight or flight and to ensure that the greatest possible capacity is available. This balance between the emotional and the rational brain is crucial for our wellbeing and for our long-term health. Only when both parts are equally represented can a balanced state be achieved, transcending over-excitation and numbness.

Traumatic stress initiates a serious alteration in this delicate balance. When the organism believes itself to be in a real or perceived dangerous situation, or indeed in mortal danger, the brain parts revert more or less completely to lower, older functions which have stood the test of time. The rational brain is deactivated first, followed by the limbic system. This is controlled by the reptilian brain with the fight or flight reflex in the brainstem, including the playing-dead reflex as the final option. Depending on the seriousness of the threat, there is no conscious control or outside influence over these emergency plans.

It is now recognised that trauma can damage the function of the brain parts described, particularly the medial prefrontal cortex, the amygdala and the hippocampus, and can massively disrupt the individual structures. An investigation from 2014 clearly demonstrated the connection between traumatic stress, oxidative stress and post-traumatic stress disorder, as well as their effect on neuro-degeneration and cell aging[12]. According to van der Kolk (2015) the balance between 'smoke alarm' and 'watchtower' changes radically in the case of post-traumatic stress disorder (PTSD). If the prefrontal cortex loses its ability to evaluate and modulate, people are unable to control and suppress the impulses arising from the lower brain parts.

If traumatisation has caused the set points in the amygdala to change, and the majority of impulses received only signal threat and danger, then people are no longer able to feel safe, to relax or to regenerate. They are permanently in a situation where the sympathetic nerve is activated, and where a high consumption of power and energy is demanded. If the trauma continues emotionally and the prefrontal cortex is no longer able to carry out its limiting function, the ongoing release of stress hormones will continually trigger corresponding physical reactions, which are then permanently activated. This paves the way for numerous after-effects that cause illnesses due to the permanent internal overload. This permanently activated operating state ends sooner or later in exhaustion and burnout. This explains why burnout can be termed a consequence of trauma (Banzhaf and Schmidt, 2015).

Discourse: 'Burnout'

The term 'burnout' is generally defined as a triad of emotional and physical exhaustion, cynicism and indifference (depersonalisation) and the feeling of failure or ineffectiveness. The phases

---

[12] M.W Miler & N. Sadeh (2014): "Traumatic stress, oxidative stress and post-traumatic stress disorder: neurodegeneration and the accelerated aging hypothesis" in: Molecular Psychiatry (2014) 19(11), p. 1156-1162; doi: 10.1038/mp.2014.111.

leading up to being burnt out develop via increased commitment and high motivation, through withdrawal and isolation, to suicide. Most studies show a noticeable and continual increase in cases of burnout. In a medical context, burnout is a problem concerning the difficulty of coping with life, and can only be described by an additional diagnosis. There is some overlapping with the symptoms of depression and chronic fatigue syndrome (CFS). This phenomenon was first described by Freudenberger, and applied to people in caring professions who reacted to continual professional stress factors. Later it was used mainly in a professional context. Today burnout is present at all societal and professional levels. According to the German health insurance report on absenteeism in 2012, the number of working days lost due to the diagnosis of 'burnout' increased more than tenfold in the AOK insurance between 2004 and 2011.

Burnout is often seen as having a causal and direct connection with increasing stress and external demands, with professional, familial and social overload, with multi-tasking, with work intensification and having to be continually accessible. But if we allow ourselves to risk a look into the deeper connections, it is not difficult to see that the survival parts described by Franz Ruppert in his splitting model are almost identical with the patterns of people heading towards burnout. These parts, which are continually overactive and never satisfied, orientate themselves inevitably and without respite to the external world, have to continually act out and simultaneously suppress trauma feelings, are always suspicious and cannot allow themselves any rest. Burnout could therefore, according to Gabor Maté, be a clear signal that the body at some point says "No" (Maté, 2003). It could also be a very clever and perhaps final attempt by the body to slam on the emergency brakes in a driverless train that is ignoring all stop signals and racing at full speed towards a station, and whose destination is chaos, helplessness and destruction.

Burnout could therefore be on the one hand a consequence of traumatisation, and on the other the desperate attempt to stop this process of self-destruction. For this reason, my practical medical experience has shown it to be necessary to check all burnout symptoms very carefully, looking at their signal characteristics and their actual underlying causes. Often well-meant strategies and therapies that treat burnout are simply functioning to strengthen the survival parts and unconsciously fuel the process causing the person to become ill. When trauma survival parts prevent the person concerned from relaxing, and constantly demand some sort of activity, then neither a seminar on time management nor a psychosomatic course of treatment with the elements of classic stress management can offer any help. In the worst case they themselves become part of a trauma survival strategy.

The dorsolateral prefrontal cortex, which functions as a timepiece and signals when a situation has ended and is past in real life, is also highly sensitive to traumatic stress. Together with the extremely stress-sensitive hippocampus, it puts an experience into a specific context and meaning. If this function fails and a corresponding ability to evaluate becomes impossible, then those concerned are even more helpless, and less able to categorise events in a meaningful and adequate way.

In this neurobiological concert the thalamus is given the task of filtering information received from the environment via our eyes, ears, nose and skin, as well as distinguishing what is important from what is trivial, and focusing attention and concentration. Van der Kolk (2015) calls the thalamus 'the chef', who decides what is included in the soup of our autobiographical memory. The fact that, following a trauma, the person concerned is often unable to recount a coherent narrative but only an incoherent collection of different, fragmented sensory impressions, is due to an injury to the thalamus, which, because of the traumatisation, is able neither to filter nor to put everything into context. Through the dysfunctional and damaged perception filters, these people find themselves in a sort of constant sensory overload that contributes further to the overburdening, irritability and nervousness that already exist.

There is frequently no recollection of early traumatisations because they are stored in the so-called implicit memory. This is where information about our early body sensations, emotions and behavioural patterns is located. Having no memory of it does not, however, mean that what was experienced and stored is not operative. On the contrary, the explicit memory only develops from the third year onwards, after the hippocampus becomes fully functional, allowing us consciously to recall facts and experiences, to categorise them and put them into context (Levine, 2016).

We have now described a working mechanism that is able to explain the connection between experiencing trauma and the changes in our brain on a neurobiological level. This knowledge may explain the psychological, mental and emotional consequences as well as the chronic activation of the reptilian brain in the form of constant over-excitation or numbness. However, in order to understand the highly diverse symptoms of illness on a physical level, we have to take a further step, and a deeper look into the extremely complex links in the physical-mental connection. In what follows we will discover how the changes in the brain as a consequence of traumatisation are connected with the long-term effects on the whole body and its organ systems.

Cell-stress and psychological stress – two sides of the coin

Excessive stress on a physical level leads to numerous molecular, biochemical and physiological alterations. Increased values in so-called oxidative and nitrosative stress markers are measurable. This implies that the organism is unable to function optimally. At the cell level this means that the necessary supply of energy from the mitochondria (these are the power houses of the cells responsible for vital energy production) is no longer guaranteed and the cell goes into a state of emergency. We talk here of mitochondrial dysfunction. From a medical point of view it is a disrupted mitochondrial function that causes chronic illnesses.

On a physical level, chronic fatigue and continual exhaustion are caused by this disruption in energy production at the cellular level, and they are the starting point for many other symptoms and illnesses. Increased oxidative and nitrosative stress is a significant biochemical and molecular mechanism for the formation of so-called multi-system diseases. This is the term for disorders which are revealed by a superficial symptom, or relate to a particular organ, but which are actually caused at a deeper level by a general disorder of a superordinate system. For instance, illnesses of the immune system, above all auto-immune illnesses, metabolic disorders such as diabetes, illnesses of the cardiovascular system, which are amongst the most common causes of death, and last but not least, tumours.

When we talk about psychological stress, we are referring to states of rage, anger, aggression, but also depression, sadness or helplessness. If we look at a depressed person's body language, his gestures and expressions, we can see that these psychological expressions also have a physical equivalent. How closely body and psyche are linked is also shown by the fact that our brain has no separate areas for the perception and processing of physical and emotional pain.

The body's own chemical substance P (pain) is jointly responsible for pain perception in the nervous system, and in the immune system it is involved in the inflammatory reaction. These findings of psycho-neuro-immunology provide us with indications that our body with its nervous-, hormone- and immune systems as well as our psyche, form a functional entity. The measurements of the neurotransmitters, in other words the transmitter substances in the brain such as serotonin, dopamine and oxytocin, indicate that psychological phenomena have their physiological equivalent. Determining the heart rate variability shows the exact emotional state a person is in: whether he is in fight or flight mode, or whether he is relaxed and calm.

These connections indicate to us that psychological stress and physical stress are mutually dependent. Numerous research results point out these links and describe the connection of cellular stress and psychological illnesses.[13,14] Physical stress will inevitably have an effect on a psychological level, and psychological stress is expressed in physical reactions. They are two sides of the same coin.

The findings of the biochemist Martin Pall (2007) suggest that a strong trigger can lead to a biochemical vicious cycle with serious effects that can be the foundation of many chronic illnesses. Pall sees the cause of so-called multisystem diseases, such as chronic fatigue syndrome, fibromyalgia, multiple chemical sensitivity and post-traumatic stress disorder in the NO/ONOO cycle, which was named after him.[15] This clearly shows that different causes – chemical stress on the one hand, psychological traumatisations on the other – lead to one and the same biochemical process that in turn leads to increased oxidative and nitrosative stress, chronic inflammation, energy depletion in the cells, and finally to chronic disease and damage to the nervous system.

We can thereby recognise that an initial psychological injury, a trauma, can lead via the mind-body connection to massive physical illness as a result. This connection has been confirmed by the result of a 2016 investigation carried out by the University of Ulm. Increased inflammatory values were found years later in the blood of women who had been ill treated, 'abused' or neglected. The consequences were not only an increased risk of psychological illness, but also a weakening of the immune system and an increased susceptibility for age-associated physical illness. The researchers identified altered processes in the mito-chondria as one of the causes. In the first years of life, according

---

[13] G.T. Rezin et al (2016): Mitochondrial dysfunction in bipolar disorder: "Evidence, pathophysiology and translational implications", in: Neuroscience & Biobehavioural Reviews (2016) 68: p. 694–713; doi: 10.1016/j.neubiorev. 2016.06.040.

[14] T. Cikánková et al (2016): "Mitochondrial dysfunctions in bipolar disorder: effect of the disease and pharmacotherapy", in: CNS Neurol Disorder Drug Targets (2016).

[15] Sprich: "No, oh no"; http://nunm.edu/images/CE/cureabst.pdf

to the experts, the body's so-called 'stress response' develops: an interaction between the hormone-, nervous- and immune systems. This provides the basis for the ability to react adequately in acute stress situations. However, the stress response is substantially altered if, during this highly sensitive phase, children are subjected to negative experiences such as sexual traumatisation or violence.[16]

Bad genes, good genes? Epigenetics as the missing link

The genes in the chromosomes of our cells form the blueprint for the structure and function of our organism. There are different theories concerning the causes and emergence of disease and aging processes. One of these states that the genetic information in our DNA significantly influences whether, when, and which diseases we might suffer from. For a long time we assumed that mutations, or alterations, in the structure of the DNA in the cell, and thereby of the genetic material, meant that the cell was unable to carry out its original program correctly. This could lead to pathological changes and even to malignant degeneration – in other words to cancerous cells. Mutations either occur by chance or are caused by external influences (for example chemical toxins or x-rays). The DNA was considered a very stable chemical structure.

However, according to the newest scientific findings, this is only part of the story. Our genome, in other words the total of all the genes in our body, is in no way fixed and inflexible. To a great extent, our genes do remain the same all our lives; however, the information taken from them is highly changeable, malleable and adaptable. This realisation is the real revolution! This may also be the key to understanding the connection between physical illness and psychological trauma. Via the mechanism of

---

[16] C. Boek et al (2016): "Inflammation in adult women with a history of child maltreatment: The involvement of mitochondrial alterations and oxidative stress" (Abstract), in: Mitochondrion, 30, p. 197–207.

epigenetic changes[17] a transformation of psychological information (e.g. a psychotrauma) takes place on matter, in other words on our biological organism.

The second piece of good news is that, through this body-mind connection we are able to achieve change, and therefore there is hope that we can modify our legacy, our experiences and individual circumstances in the way they affect our personal lives and the lives of our descendants. There is no inevitable pre-determined destiny given to us at the beginning of our lives by our parents (and their ancestors) in the form of a defined set of chromosomes or the traumatisations we have experienced so far in our lives. Our genes are structurally determined, but the information from them, the 'gene expression' is extremely changeable. Gene expression means the regulation upwards or downwards of individual genes or their functions.

Epigenetics is the name given to this young branch of science. Epigenetics refers to everything that is in addition to genetics. From a biological point of view 'epi' means everything that encases and envelops the genes. These are protein structures and other chemical substances that can protect the DNA on the one hand, and on the other hand can transform and modify the information contained within them. The epigenetic structure overall is referred to as the epigenome.

It is remarkable that all signals that reach our brain and our mind, and are sent out by them, can directly influence the gene expression. In other words, they can regulate our genes and the information they carry for our body upwards or downwards, or switch them completely on or off. Everything we think, feel or do has a physical effect!

This so-called soft heredity through the constantly variable gene expression explains for the first time at a biological-physiological level the long-suspected mechanism of intergenerational heredity, whereby information, characteristics or patterns of

---

[17] Biochemical changes based on external influences, not contingent on the genetic code.

behaviour are transferred from one generation to another without the genetic material having to change.

Just as the DNA in our genes has served as a (collective) storage medium for millions of years of evolution, so the epigenome is the store for all short-term changes in our individual biology and our unique lives. Our personal experiences are directly coded here without having to take a detour via our predetermined genetic code.

A study by the psychiatrist and neuroscientist Rachel Yehuda, analysing holocaust survivors, has spectacularly demonstrated and explained the transfer mechanism of trauma experience to offspring via the biochemical path of so-called DNA-methylation.[18]

DNA-methylations are markers that allow our cells selectively to use areas within the DNA for various processes. We can think of DNA markers as similar to the text formatting in a book: if a key word in a dictionary is highlighted in some way, it has a different meaning for the reader than the same word in running text. The different patterns and degrees of methylation play an important role in whether and how the information contained in a gene is read.[19]

This process of gene expression therefore determines the form and the effectiveness of genetic information. Via the path of epigenetic change, the personal experiences of a living being can be transferred to their offspring. And due to the epigenome, our genes also react to experiences that other people have made. Thus neither bad nor good genes exist. However, the form and activity of genetic information are extremely variable, and not only through the experiences of our ancestors, but also and above all through our own personal experiences.

In a study with traumatised soldiers who had seen duty in Afghanistan, a direct correlation became apparent between

---

[18] R. Yehuda et al (2016): "Holocaust Exposure Induced Intergenerational Effects on FKBP5 Methyation", in: Biological Psychiatry (2016) 80(5), p. 372–380; doi: 10.1016/j.biopsych.2015.08.005.

[19] https://de.wikipedia.org/wiki/DNA-Methylierung

trauma and the aging process. The personal and individual experiences from the war zone had led not only to some massive psychological symptoms, but had also manifested themselves on a cellular level, identifiable by the conspicuous biological markers for the physical aging process.[20]

Firstly, we are embodied beings with a highly complex physiological organism. Secondly, we also possess a psyche that lets us think, feel and remember. Both condition and form each other. And at this point we can also state that, due to epigenetic changeability, it seems that not only our psyche, but also our cells can store memories.

With the epigenetic alteration in the cell function through a different gene expression, we seem to have found the missing link between psyche and soma, between emotion and body. Now we can understand why psychological injury, traumatic experiences and difficult emotional states manifest themselves on a physical level and are able to influence and trigger organic diseases.

Because psychological injuries, via the mechanism of methylation or demethylation, alter the gene expression of numerous genes engaged in the metabolic process, those molecules are upregulated that disrupt the finely adjusted balance between oxidative and antioxidative substances in the body, and lead to increased biochemical stress. This can be measured and made visible in the blood via biomarkers. Thus a meta-analysis published in 2015 demonstrated a significant correlation between childhood trauma and an increase in inflammatory transmitters as a sign of dysregulation of the immune system in adulthood.[21] Chronic stress, caused, for example, by caring for chronically ill children, provokes alterations in the mothers' cells

---

[20] M.P. Boks et al (2015): "Longitudinal changes of telomere length and epigenetic age related to traumatic stress and post-traumatic stress disorder", in: Psychoneuroendocrinology (2015) 51, p. 506–512; doi: 10.1016/j.psyneuen.2014.07.011.

[21] D. Baumeister et al (2015): "Childhood trauma and adulthood inflammation: a meta-analysis of peripheral C-reactive protein, interleukin-6 and tumour necrosis factor-a", in: Molecular Psychiatry (2016) 21(5), p. 642–649; doi: 10.1038/mp.2015.67.

through an alteration in the telomeres of the immune cells, which in turn accelerates the aging process (Chopra and Tanzi, 2015).

If chronic psychological stress is able to cause such changes, we can easily imagine what happens when traumatic experiences have an impact on people, particularly if, as with infants or children, the nervous system, immune system and endocrine system are not fully developed.

A study from 2004 showed that baby rats whose mothers cared for them assiduously, had more glucocorticoid receptors in the hippocampus later on in life, and therefore behaved less anxiously and less aggressively. The variations in care received by the young resulted in an altered gene expression, which affected stress regulation via the hypothalamic-pituitary-adrenal axis, which affected the whole of their later life.[22]

According to van der Kolk, after a trauma experience "the body bears the full force of the trauma".[23] If we have to assume that the number of unrecorded cases of people suffering from trauma is much higher than official figures would have us believe, then we get an idea of the possible resulting illnesses that are triggered and remain hidden. According to a study carried out in 2014 by the European Union Agency for Fundamental Rights (FRA), more than 30% of all women in Europe over 15 years old have become victims of physical and/or sexual violence.[24]

On the one hand a trauma experience is overlaid with extreme shame, on the other the fear of renewed traumatisation plays a key role, which is why victims often say nothing. If children, infants or unborn children become victims, they often have no conscious access to this experience in later life. Although the experience is stored in their implicit memory, it cannot be

---

[22] E.W. Fish et al (2004): "Epigenetic programming of stress responses through variations in maternal care" in: Annals of the New York Academy of Sciences (2004) 1036, pp. 167–180.

[23] B. van der Kolk (1994): "The Body Keeps the Score: memory and the evolving psychobiology of posttraumatic stress", in: Harvard Review of Psychiatry (1994) 1(5), pp. 167–180.

[24] FRA – European Union Agency for Fundamental Rights (2014): "Violence against women: an EU wide survey. Main results report".

deliberately recollected. Those concerned are therefore unable to talk about it. Even so, these experiences cause the epigenetic changes described above, with serious consequences for further mental, emotional and physical development. Activation of the hypothalamic-pituitary-adrenal axis, initiation of the biochemical vicious cycle through the creation of aggressive free radicals and the accompanying altered gene expression, leads finally to epigenetic change and with that, the creation of not only physical but also psychological imbalance culminating in manifest and serious illness.

If psychological injuries find no tangible resonance in our consciousness, then they seem to express themselves in physical symptoms until the person concerned perceives them as an illness. With that they become tangible, and can be diagnosed and treated according to conventional medicine's current understanding. However, if the illness only reflects the symptom, and the cause remains hidden, no interventions, however persistent they may be, can provide lasting recovery or in-depth healing.

Different neuronal areas and nerve fibres are involved depending on the maturity and development of the brain at the time of the traumatisation. The active fibres are particularly susceptible to a disruption of their normal growth. This fact is particularly relevant for the different symptoms that arise. The so-called regulative neuronal networks are particularly likely to prevent integration in the developing brain if they are affected by an overwhelming trauma experience. These include the prefrontal cortex, the hippocampus and the corpus callosum (the band connecting the two cerebral hemispheres). The prefrontal cortex is substantially involved in the formation of meaning and emotion and connects the higher parts of the brain with the limbic functions and the brainstem. It possesses a central integrative function. We only have access to our emotional brain and thereby to our self-awareness by activating the medial prefrontal cortex.

The hippocampus is responsible for, amongst other things, memory, control of the 'I'-function and emotional assessment. And by connecting the two cerebral hemispheres, the corpus callosum enables the exchange of information between the left side, which is more linear and logical, and the right, which is more holistic and non-verbal. Investigations have shown that recalled traumatic experiences tend to activate the right hemisphere and deactivate the left (van der Kolk, 2015). In the right hemisphere, which develops in the womb before the left, touch, sounds and smells are stored with the emotions connected with them. This can explain why traumatised people can have perceptions based on traumatic experiences, which then trigger a flashback experience, while the corresponding mental memory is completely missing. It is not difficult for us to imagine the long-term negative consequences if, while the brain is still maturing, disturbances occur in this highly sensitive area.

Joachim – chronically ill or traumatised?

Joachim came to my practice with the confirmed diagnosis of Lyme disease, also known as Lyme borreliosis. Lyme disease is an infectious disease caused by bacteria of the Borrelia type (*Borrelia burgdorferi*) spread by ticks or other biting insects. Joachim had become infected several years previously and he was suffering a great deal as the infection had become chronic and had led to a number of physical symptoms. At the same time further tests had identified other stresses on his body, above all a significant heavy metal contamination, presumably caused by earlier amalgam fillings in his teeth. However, Joachim had also had a very problematic childhood. His father, a professed Nazi, severely abused him, both physically and psychologically. His mother was unable to protect him during his childhood, and instead made him the scapegoat for her own unfortunate biography.

In our context, what was remarkable was the fact that the Lyme disease only improved permanently after he drastically reduced his heavy meal contamination by means of a detoxification therapy. Channelling these toxins out of his body only succeeded after he had worked intensively, using the constellation method to reveal his psychological traumas, worked through them and gradually healed them. Joachim's chronic pain has gone now, his nightmares, his anxiety and anger have largely disappeared and he has rediscovered his creativity, and his pleasure in composing and writing, and he has found his inner peace and, according to him, he has lost his fear of dying.

There is no question that there are illnesses that, at least superficially, need no previous psychological traumatisation. Being involved in a traffic accident, being poisoned or subjected to a toxin, for instance mercury, for years, or suffering an infection following an insect bite or sting and the transfer of a disease-causing pathogen, these are all possible regardless of any psychological predisposition. However, we ought to bid farewell to the 'either/or' position, which is not helpful. Often we are unable to say definitely what was there first. When body and psyche form a system where one is dependent on the other, it is logical for the individual parts to be able either to support or impede one another. If we enable the body to go through an optimum metabolic process, we prepare the ground for successful and healing inner work. The neurotransmitters in our brains that are necessary for our wellbeing, such as serotonin, our happiness hormone, require an adequate supply of other chemical substances (B vitamins, vitamin C, magnesium, to name a few). Finally, a healthy gut with its microbiome, an unimaginably large number of bacteria, is the basis for the production of serotonin and other important neurotransmitters. Over 90% of the body's serotonin is produced in the gut (Enders, 2014).

When we carry out inner trauma and healing work, we relieve and free the body at the same time of obstructive emotional blockages that can interfere considerably with its regular functioning. In this context we should bear in mind the chronic activity of the biological stress axis resulting in increased cortisol values in the organism due to a constant indeterminate fear based on an earlier traumatisation.

Joachim's case history goes to the heart of the dilemma we can find ourselves in if we only look at one side of the coin. For a doctor and an expert in environmental medicine, finding a chronic bacterial infection, contaminants and a lack of micronutrients, and treating these, would suffice. A psychotherapist would probably be content with having discovered a severe psychological traumatisation and would treat its consequences. By doing that, however, we would have succumbed to a split that we should be removing. From this perspective Joachim was not only traumatised but was also ill. He was traumatised due to the stress of his experiences in childhood. He was ill as a result of Lyme disease that had become chronic, contamination with heavy metal and the countless biochemical consequences. It is entirely possible that Joachim's early experiences had caused a change in his whole biology and had created a predisposition towards his susceptibility to other related illnesses, ostensibly having purely physiologically causes.

The possible connection could be that via the mechanism of altered gene expression as a result of epigenetic adaptation, the traumatisation could have caused countless molecular changes that influenced the immune response following the infection, the mechanism of endogenous contaminant detoxification, and the regulation of endocrine metabolic processes including the balance of micronutrients.

Many of these fundamental questions are unanswered in the context of current medical science and require a closer look and further research. But the saying: "We only see what we know" is also valid. If we are ourselves split and can only see with one eye, or only want to see with one eye, then we miss a part of reality. We are physical beings with a consciousness. This fact is increasingly taken into account by the new scientific discipline of body-mind medicine.

Energy results from awareness

The consequences of a trauma experience often last a lifetime and affect all areas of the person's life. The adjusting screws regulating the nervous system are misaligned, the endocrine and hormone system become imbalanced, the immune system is weakened, and as a result of the altered gene expression, dysfunctional proteins are formed which, in the worst cases, activate so-called tumour genes. Neuronal processes are negatively influenced on a functional level as well as a structural level.

Both emotional and mental processes are obstructed. The interaction of the different neuronal networks is thrown out of sync. Memories concerning the trauma are stored in fragments in the brain, in different places that can be far apart from each other. As a result, the conscious memory of the trauma experiences is limited or non-existent.

As well as psychotherapy work on traumas, and supporting the organism, as illustrated above, we have a further highly efficient tool to help prepare for recovery and healing. By focusing our awareness on a single, and initially neutral object, the activity of our autonomic nervous system is calmed down. The parasympathetic part with nerve fibres responsible for relaxation and regeneration is activated, and at the same time the sympathetic continuous excitation is reduced. This is shown by a reduction in the release of acute stress hormones (for example noradrenaline), an improvement in the heart rate variability, and also in a decreasing amount of cortisol in the blood.

Through 'focusing' our awareness we can calm our highly active survival parts and regulate the autonomic nervous system into a less stimulated mode. To this end, the method of mindfulness-based stress reduction (MBSR), which was developed over 30 years ago by the molecular biologist Jon Kabat-Zinn (2013), is, for several reasons, helpful and supportive. This method can be used without any spiritual orientation. The concept of mindfulness has been well studied scientifically and is deemed effective. It is being used more and more in the treatment of trauma. Simply concentrating on one's own breathing, as the overarching physiological rhythm-setter for a number of organ systems, supports the activation of the parasympathetic nervous system. A study in 2014 showed that one eight-hour meditation reduced inflammation and relieved pain via an alteration in the gene expression, and also rapidly normalised the level of cortisol.[25]

---

[25] P. Kaliman et al (2014): "Rapid changes in histone deacetylases and inflammatory gene expression in expert meditators", in" Psycho-neuroendocrinology (2014) 40, pp. 96–107; doi: 10.1016/j.psyneuen.2013.11.004.

Thus we have an extremely effective tool that intervenes in the biochemical cycle, harmonising what has to a great extent been disrupted by traumatic life experience. From other studies we know that mindfulness training supports the stability of the hippocampus and calms the amygdala.[26, 27] MRI scans have shown that just eight weeks of training in MBSR result in an increase in density of the hippocampus and a reduction of density in the amygdala. This means that mindfulness meditation enables, from a functional as well as a structural point of view, the integration of previously non-integrated consciousnesses in the brain. As the alarm signals in our limbic system are able to be less active and the hippocampi, which are also responsible for memory function, are supported, we can bring previously unrecalled memories into our consciousness. These can then be worked on step by step and in the long term their emotional charge can be deactivated.

Through the practice of mindfulness we can learn gradually to extend our window of tolerance for mental and emotional experiences, which can also be of a traumatic nature. Focusing on the moment can help us avoid falling into old patterns, not being once more dragged into the surging waves of traumatic experiences and their memories, and not allowing their momentum to drag us down and cause us to dissociate. Van der Kolk (2015) identifies mindfulness as an important element in any trauma therapy, because the medial prefrontal cortex, the 'watchtower' is strengthened.

Joachim Bauer (2015) describes the prefrontal cortex as the seat of self. Strengthening it, therefore, has an immediate effect on our self-awareness. This awareness and knowledge of self, which is able to unite all the elements of our personality and to encourage the various actors within us to concentrate all our

---

[26] B.K. Hölzel et al (2011) "Mindfulness practice leads to increases in regional brain gray matter density", in: Psychiatry Research (2011) 30:191(1), pp. 36–43; doi: 10.1016/j.psychresns.2010.08.006.

[27] B.K. Hölzel et al (2010) "Stress reduction correlates with structural changes in the amygdala", in: Social Cognitive and Affective Neuroscience (2010) 5(1), pp. 11–17.

strength and resources on wholeness and unity, is a vital part of the healing path and process. It has been shown that mindfulness training is able to stabilise and strengthen the prefrontal cortex that is such an important integrative central part in this process.

Mindfulness promotes the so-called vertical integration of sensing, feeling and thinking. The input from the brainstem, the most primitive part of our brain, and the one responsible for controlling the survival reflexes of fight/flight or freeze, can be modified by the younger limbic elements that can create feelings such as security and protection. These can eventually be integrated through the most recent part of our brain, the neocortex, which is able to carry out a new evaluation and a re-evaluation of events. It allows us to become aware that what we have experienced is in the past. At the same time, horizontal integration is possible, in which both hemispheres of the brain with their different preferences are synchronised, allowing mental and emotional content that has been stored to be connected again to a transparent and understandable entity.

In this context we need to refer once more to the preeminent function of the hippocampus, which plays a definitive part in the integration of memory. If this integration is disrupted, implicit memories will not be pieced together with the actual experiences. With traumatised people this has the effect of emotions, physical sensations or perceptions being experienced as new and happening in the present, and thus able to lead to a re-traumatisation, although the 'story' is in the past and no longer current.

A trauma can only be healed if people in their whole being experience that "it is past" and that they are in safety. It is not enough for a person to be able to tell their own story mentally. The visceral emotions, which means those belonging to the limbic system, have to give the signal that there is no longer any mortal danger, that there is no need any more for anxiety, fear, desperation and terror. To do this it is necessary for the self-system, consisting of brainstem and limbic system, to be assigned the importance it deserves. Therapy that is purely cognitive-oriented overlooks this fundamental connection.

Modern neuroscience confirms that our self-awareness and

our self-perception are rooted in our body (Damasio, 2000). This means that we should not regard the body as an annoying appendage that is damaged and produces chronic illnesses as a result of a psychotraumatisation, but should rather place it at the centre of the therapeutic process. It is at the end of the frequently long history of suffering following a trauma experience, and is simultaneously the starting point for recovery and healing.

Body-based exercises and yoga elements support the medial prefrontal cortex in observing and regulating physical sensations without losing themselves in them or being carried away because the amygdala are firing too strongly. This check, known as 'bottom-up regulation', is designed to calm the frequently predominant over-excitation, as it activates above all that part of the nervous system responsible for tension release and composure, the vagus nerve.

But now for the ventral part, the myelinated part: the importance of this part of the autonomic nervous system is shown by the direction of its fibres. About 80% of the nerve fibres are afferent, which means they run from the body and gut towards the brain, and give the brain feedback from the periphery of the body (Porges, 2001). The anatomic structure of our nervous system shows the immense importance of the body and its signals. We should not just see it as a victim and a diseased organ, but should include it in the healing process.

If we learn to focus our awareness, we strengthen mechanisms that help us process and overcome traumatic experiences from a psychological-emotional point of view, and give positive support to our physiology and biochemistry.

The development of body-awareness is the connection between the external world that still seems threatening, and the internal world, that is closed, separated and fragmented. Traumatised people have to learn to allow their own body sensations again, and to trust them. Only then are they able to confront their own past without being in danger of becoming the victim of re-traumatisation, of collapsing or freezing.

Richard Schwartz (1997) believes that, despite every traumatisation, deep down there is a mindful self, an undamaged essence that can help to reorganise and heal the inner system. All current studies about including mindfulness in the therapeutic process confirm Schwartz's assumption on a neurobiological basis as well.

The power of mindfulness cannot be overestimated, also in view of the resulting compassion. Only when we are capable of showing the smallest measure of understanding, affection and goodwill towards parts within us, can we set foot on the difficult path of our own injuries and scars. Compassion towards ourselves is the healing elixir for our own wounds (Banzhaf, 2010). Luise Reddemann (2016) also points emphatically to the importance of compassion. Mindful awareness also allows a form of composure and patience in view of the slow progress and small steps that are frequently all that is possible in the healing process.

Finally, the quality of acceptance, that is formed through regular mindfulness training, is helpful. The moment we accept what has happened the fight-flight mode collapses, if we simultaneously recognise that the trauma belongs in the past and we are in a safe place and equipped with resources that were unavailable to us back then. This must not be confused with the playing-dead reflex or freezing, for which there was no alternative at the moment of traumatisation. Acceptance is a form of extreme self-compassion and an expression of deep wisdom, because what has happened cannot be undone. Any resistance to this fact mobilises anew all emotional, mental, biochemical and molecular defence mechanisms that result in the triggering of a psychological re-traumatisation or physical chronification.

Trauma therapy from an integrative viewpoint

We have seen that through traumatic experiences, emotional wounds as well as alterations on a molecular and biochemical level and hence dysfunctional metabolic processes arise, which manifest themselves physically and can encourage or cause disease. Looked at in this way, numerous physical symptoms can be seen to be the consequences of psychological trauma. Based on the knowledge we have today, the dualism of 'either/or' that is still valid in scientific practice, is outdated and should be replaced by '... as well as ...'. As already stated, of course there are illnesses without a prior psychological traumatisation. Even so, much points to psychotrauma also being able to explain physical symptoms that were previously seen as purely organic. The classic paradigm is that of a monocausal cause-and-effect relationship on a purely pathophysiological basis. At best, the discipline of psychosomatics, as an extension of internal medicine, recognises certain connections for a limited number of illnesses and their diagnoses as (also) having a psychological cause. The term psychotrauma is still not recognised here either.

As psychological processes need a material basis, we cannot disregard the material organism. Findings from molecular biology, neurobiology and epigenetics point to the complementarity principle described above. Our brain as the central hub for physiological, emotional and mental processes is dependent on being supplied with chemical substances. Neurotransmitters as well as neural pathways require macro- and micro-nutrients. Nerve cells can only work at an optimum level if they are provided with the appropriate nutrients. To create new synapses – those junctions that allow a connection between different axons (nerve fibres) – there have to be material building blocks.

It has been known for some time that not only do our neurons change, but also that new neurons can form. This process, known as neurogenesis, establishes the prerequisites that on a material basis are necessary to heal a trauma.[28] New interconnections form and new neuronal patterns emerge, initiated by altered mental and emotional experiences during the therapy and healing process. New experiences in therapy as well as in everyday life cause neuronal structures to change, which permit altered mental and emotional modes of behaviour and experience. Thus it would be foolish for us not to supply the organism with all the materials and substances it needs to

---

[28] H. Song et al (2002): "Astroglia induce neurogenesis from adult neural stem cells", in: Nature 417, pp. 39–44.

operate at an optimum level. If our brain lacks anything material it will not be fully able to achieve the extremely demanding task of trauma integration.

If our brain requires a good supply of macro- and micronutrients even under 'normal' circumstances, how much more will it need in times of emergency and extreme stress?

Not infrequently difficult life situations mean that unborn children, infants and post-birth children do not receive sufficient micronutrients to enable their brains to function at an optimum level. In this connection, the psychiatrist Günter Seidler in an interview points to the fact that children in war zones such as Syria have suffered pre-natal brain damage through lack of nutrients.[29]

Numerous pollutants and poisons forming additional stress factors are the price we pay for our highly industrialised society. These can seriously disrupt or damage the maturing process of the brain as well as the function of the neurons (Wilks, 2015). Traumatised people of any age need to be well supplied with care and nutrients, and the more serious the traumatisation, and the younger the person was when it was experienced, the more urgent this is. In view of eating habits with fast food and junk food, there is a shortage in the supply of important vital substances such as zinc, selenium, B vitamins and many more. For example haemopyrrollactamuria (HPU) is characterised by a significant lack of zinc and vitamin B6. Subsequently, amongst other things, the memory of trauma is impaired. Our clinical experience has shown that, with the substitution of zinc and vitamin B6, the conditions for a successful psychotherapeutic intervention can be improved.

Other metabolic disorders, for example a genetic variant in the COMT gene (catechol-O-methyltransferase), influence the physiological reduction of acute stress hormones. As a result, the autonomic nervous system remains in a state of increased alert for a long time after a stress situation. This metabolic reaction

---

[29] www.spektrum.de/news/ich-bezweifle-dass-es-dort-je-wieder-eine-funktion-ierende-zivilgesellscaft-geben-kann/367283

causes an extremely high consumption of vital substances and predisposes to an increase in exhaustion or burnout. Connections have been described between COMT polymorphism[30] on the one hand and traumatisation at a young age on the other, as well as the development of post-traumatic stress disorder or depression.[31]

An interesting question would be whether the HPU or COMT polymorphism given as examples can be traced back to a traumatic cause. That would mean that physical metabolic alterations that have life-long physiological effects, are triggered by early traumatic experiences. Numerous studies have shown that the more coherently the cells in a biological system function, the healthier the system is.[32] In a medical context we talk of coherence when blood pressure, heart rate and breathing are synchronised and aligned. In our context, coherence could mean that body and psyche, material and non-material, form an entity and thereby the basis for a person's health and wellbeing. When individual systems in a larger whole, such as a human organism, are split from one another, we cannot expect them to function optimally.

The way in which traumatic experiences, genetic influences through polymorphisms and their effects on brain structure are connected, is shown by a study of the level of the brain-derived neurotrophic factor (BDNF) in the blood.[33] In carriers of a

---

[30] Polymorphism is the appearance of different gene variants and with that the production of different gene products (e.g. proteins or enzymes).

[31] S.J. van Rooij (2016): "Childhood Trauma and COMT Genotype Interact to Increase Hippocampal Activation in Resilient Individuals", in: Frontiers in Psychiatry (2016) 7, p. 156; doi: 10.3389/fpsyt.2016.00156.

[32] M. Trousselard et al (2016): "Cardiac Coherence Training to Reduce Anxiety in Remitted Schizophrenia, a Pilot Study", in: Applied Psychophysiologie and Biofeedback (2016) 41(1), pp. 61–69; doi: 10.1007/s10484-015-9312-y.

[33] L. Gerritsen et al (2012): "BDNF Val66Met genotype modulates the effect of childhood adversity on subgenual anterior cingulated cortex volume in healthy subjects", in: Molecular Psychiatry (2012) 17(6), pp. 597–603; doi: 10.1038/mp.2011.51.

certain gene variant of this factor that is responsible for the protection and growth of neurons, damaging and stressful experiences in childhood led to a reduced volume in the area of the prefrontal cortex.

Heavy metals such as mercury (one of the most toxic substances and a major component of amalgam fillings) block enzymes, bring metabolic processes to a standstill, cause cell stress and damage the energy generation in the mitochondria, the little powerhouses in every cell. For example, there is a study[34] that suggests a connection between toxic heavy metals and the locus ceruleus, a core area in the hindbrain. It is responsible for the release of the neurotransmitter noradrenaline that prepares the body for fight or flight, playing an important role in the stress reaction cycle. A disturbance in this area inevitably affects the body's reaction to stress and its adequate coping mechanisms.

The hippocampus, which has been mentioned several times already, is extremely sensitive to stress, and to numerous environmental toxins, while at the same time playing an exceptional role in processing traumatic experiences. If harmful environmental substances have previously damaged this area, traumatic experiences can lead to a further reduction in function, thereby negatively affecting the real purpose of this part of the brain. The effect of psychotherapeutic interventions will then be unsatisfactory, if the neuronal structures that are necessary for the healing process are themselves impaired or damaged functionally or structurally.

Hans-Ulrich Hill (2014) emphasises that the practice of separating psychological and organic illnesses is outdated, and that all diseases of dementia possibly have common causal factors that must be sought not only in genetics but also primarily in the environment. These include chronic psychological and traumatic

---

[34] R. Pamphlett (2014): "Uptake of environmental toxicants by the locus ceruleus: a potential trigger for neurodegenerative, demyelinating and psychiatric disorders", in: Medical Hypotheses (2014) 82(1), pp. 97–104; doi: 10.1016/j.mehy.2013.11.016.

stress and also harmful environmental substances, allergic and autoimmune reactions as well as chronic viral and bacterial infections. These factors foster inflammation in the brain that can end in a progressively degenerative process. It is probably the interaction between these different factors that have already been mentioned that explains the increase in neurodegenerative diseases, particularly Alzheimer's disease. In our practical work with identity-oriented psychotrauma therapy we recognise, not infrequently, that a psychological split is so profound that the person concerned prefers to banish it completely from their memory rather than face their extremely painful traumatic past. At the same time the stress experienced with numerous damaging substances in the environment permanently increases. This unholy alliance of psychological and physical stress factors leads via the mechanisms previously described to disorders that we call disease, and that manifest themselves chiefly in the very stress-prone nervous system and in the brain.

Recognising and implementing this requires first and foremost an awareness process that can be supported by careful perception and understanding. However, this means for each of us recognising our own splitting and, related to that, our restricted and limited view of the world, and being prepared to remove this step by step. The sooner and more completely the conditions for inner work are fulfilled, the more comprehensively this process can show its effects externally. The internal and external are not independent of one another. They belong together intrinsically and require mutual appreciation and regard in order to act together coherently. In doing so, they create the basis for what we call integration, i.e. health and healing of body and psyche.

Recognising diseases as the consequences of psychotrauma is a paradigm shift in medicine. From a medical point of view it is essential to consider psychotrauma and the most diverse facets of its appearance when searching for the root cause of symptoms. Not infrequently, traumatic experiences for newborn babies and their mothers begin during birth. This phenomenon, which is seldom the subject of discussion in public, and which can be triggered by a supposedly routine procedure in modern obstetrics such as a caesarean section, an episiotomy, or induction, can be the start of a lifelong trauma (Ruppert, 2014, Mundlos, 2015).

Experiencing a trauma means experiencing traumatic, i.e. toxic, stress. Traumatic stress is able to generate cellular stress. Cellular stress for its part activates via an altered gene expression a series of epigenetic modifications and forms the basis for numerous dysfunctional metabolic processes that, over time and depending on the seriousness and intensity of the traumatisation, lead to chronic disease. First of all, the weakest link in the chain becomes visible. It is therefore not expedient to cling to individual diagnoses, or to focus on symptoms, because cardiovascular diseases, rheumatic disorders, autoimmune diseases or cancer can, on a physical level, be the final phase of a long illness development and dysfunctional change that originates in a hidden place of psychological traumatisation. It is therefore sometimes essential to return to the start of the chain if we are aiming for lasting health and healing. Everything else is simply suppressing or displacing the symptoms. It is of course necessary to take into account and treat all accompanying factors, reinforcers or contributing causes. This process has then earned the name of 'integrative' therapy.

For therapists this means having to deal with both body and psyche. Students of medicine, in their six years of training, learn virtually nothing about psychotrauma, and psychotherapists often know little about the material organism. Both groups leave the other field to the other contingent.

When people complain of psychological symptoms and are given a purely organic-medical diagnosis, they will quickly grasp that it makes sense for them to refer initially to physical symptoms, so that they are at least listened to. On the other hand, my many years of clinical experience as a practising doctor have shown that it is not infrequent for physical symptoms that are at first glance inexplicable and do not fit any textbook pattern, to be hastily classified as psychosomatic, and for the patients concerned to be offered a therapy that is exclusively psychologically oriented. Yet in these cases there is still little consideration given to trauma-specific backgrounds. Although behaviour-therapeutic interventions sometimes facilitate a lessening of the symptoms, profound healing cannot take place because the causes remain hidden.

The above shows that our body itself can become seriously damaged by psychological trauma experiences and that numerous diseases arise as a result. On the other hand, this body is the link to the healing of the trauma. This happens primarily through the visceral sensations in the gut, heart or the neck. This is where the narratives with all their unspeakable experiences are stored physically; and that is where we have the possibility of restoring the connection between the events that have been split off and the fatal consequences for our whole being. We can only experience peace when these physical sensations give us the signal that we are safe and no longer in danger. It is precisely because we are physical beings that it is essential for us holistically to include the body as a feeling and knowing organ in every form of therapy or intervention.

In our individual human existence, the earliest experiences we make are on a physical and sensory level (Janov, 2011). Physical touch is seen as taboo in many psychotherapies, particularly when the therapy follows traumatic sexual experiences. However, turning to the body in a way that is respectful, individually tailored and provides safety, a connection that has been cut off for a long time or permanently suppressed can be made or re-established. Through touch, we become aware that not only do we have a body, but also we are actually embodied, and our organism has its own vital physical needs. From my own clinical experience as a manual therapist I can confirm that many patients have an immense longing for contact and physical touch. This finding is all the more important because in our modern, highly technical field of medicine it happens less and less frequently that a doctor actually will touch the patient. As one of my professors once said jokingly to us as junior doctors when talking about forming a diagnosis: "... as a last resort, take the extreme measure of examining the patient..."

Body therapies based on mindfulness can help to become

aware of emotional energies that have been trapped and frozen by experiences of trauma, to become familiar with them, in order finally to let them go and in the best case to resolve them. According to Peter Levine (2010), the trapped energies that are not completely discharged also lead to the after-effects of trauma with their diverse symptoms. He talks of the trauma being trapped in the nervous system.

The telomeres play a key role in influencing our health and longevity. We have seen that traumatic experiences can cause lasting damage to them. Numerous scientific findings [35, 36, 37, 38,] have established that the relevant protective factors can be positively influenced by physical activity, by a certain diet and by mindfulness meditation (Chopra and Tanzi, 2015).

On a practical level this means that we look at a complete set of data concerning a patient's vital substances and replace specific micronutrients according to the laboratory results. At the same time we screen for possible toxins in the body, which can then be channelled out where appropriate. Parallel to this we encourage patients to be physically active and tell them about a form of nutrition that supports regeneration and healing processes on both physiological and psychological levels.

One significant aspect we offer patients, if their medical history is appropriate, is to make their symptoms visible and to work on them and their deeper causes with constellations using the Intention Method. On the basis of the insights mentioned

---

[35] A. Ludlow et al (2008): "Relationship between Physical Activity Level, Telomere Length, and Telomerase Activity", in: Medicine & Science in sports & Exercise (2008) 40(10), pp. 1764–1771.

[36] C. Werner et al (2009): "Beneficial Effects of Long-term Endurance Exercise on Leukocyte Telomere Biology", in: Circulation (2009) 120, p. 492.

[37] D. Ornish et al (2013): "Effect of comprehensive lifestyle changes on telomerase activity and telomere length in men with biopsy-proven low-risk prostate cancer: 5-year follow-up of a descriptive pilot study", in: The Lancet Oncology (2013), Vol. 14, No. 11, pp. 1112–1120.

[38] L. Carlson (2015): "Mindfulness-based cancer recovery and supportive-expressive therapy maintain telomere length relative to controls in distressed breast cancer survivors", in: Cancer (2015), Vol. 121, Issue 3, pp. 476–484.

above, we encourage our patients to treat themselves and their situation with sympathy, empathy, and mindfulness, and they receive directions on mindfulness exercises. Our experience has shown that this strengthens the person's motivation and ability to face up to their own traumatisations. We have developed a programme for this that we call the *A4-Concept* (Banzhaf and Schmidt, 2015). The four 'As' stand for *Auffüllen, Ausleiten, Aufstellen and Achtsamkeit* (replenishing, channelling out, constellations and mindfulness).

In summary we can say that a psychological trauma damages the body-mind coupling that is necessary for physical and psychological wellbeing and healthy growth. As a result of the experience, brain and body are flooded with stress hormones, and with that the initial psychological event has become materialised. This in turn has huge consequences for the biochemistry and the neurobiology of the whole organism, for body, brain and psyche. By initiating a biochemical vicious cycle, this toxic stress alters numerous metabolic processes via the gene expression at the epigenetic level, resulting in serious functional and structural changes. The path is then clear for countless physical and psychological symptoms. Virtually all areas of the body, all organs or organ systems can be affected. They are actually only representatives for something that is underlying, split off or suppressed – for the trauma.

The method of identity-oriented psychotrauma therapy is able to merge the fragmented parts of the trauma-damaged 'I', thereby re-connecting body and psyche. The organism then no longer has to produce signals that we call 'illness' to point to its distress. The gene expression that has been altered following a traumatisation can be modulated, disrupted biochemical and neurobiological circuitry can be brought into balance, and the body's chronic readiness to become inflamed can be regulated. The unbalanced relationship between arousal and relaxation can be brought into equilibrium.

Even in the brain, molecular and structural alterations are possible. An experiment by Nader shows clearly the extent to which our brain can be shaped, thereby altering our whole self.[39] He established that every time memories are recalled, they are actualised afresh, and thereby altered. Jonah Lehrer writes: "Every time we think about the past we are delicately transforming its cellular representation in the brain, changing its underlying neural circuitry."[40] This means nothing less than that we can re-form and re-shape our reality by the way we look upon things and recognise them, our emotional perception and cognitive assessment, and the inclusion of our physical sensations.

Recognising psychotrauma in medicine for what it is, namely a huge disruption in the integrity of psyche and body, would amount to a paradigm shift. We would then have to recognise that, although treating the symptoms can sometimes save a life, treating the underlying cause in therapy would be much longer-lasting, healthier and less expensive. This would have far-reaching consequences in medicine as well as in psychotherapy for diagnostics as well as for therapeutic interventions. But above all it would be a major and significant step towards integration and healing.

References

Banzhaf, H. (2010). *Achtsamkeit und Mitgefühl in der Therapie*, in Deutsche Heilpraktiker Zeitschrift, 1, pp. 64–67.
Banzhaf, H. & **Schmidt**, S. (2015). *Meditieren heilt*. Freiburg, Kreuz.
Bauer, J. (2015). *Selbststeuerung*. Munich, Blessing.
Chopra, D. & **Tanzi**, R. E. (2015). *Super-Gene*. Munich, Nymphenburger.
Damasio, A. R. (2000). *Ich fühle, also bin ich*. Berlin, List.
Enders, G. (2014). *Darm mit Charme*. Berlin, Ullstein.
Hill, H.-U. (2014). *Umweltschadstoffe und Neurodegenerative Erkrankungen des Gehirns*. Aachen, Shaker.
Janov, A. (2011). *Vorgeburtliches Bewusstsein*. Munich, Scorpio.
Kabat-Zinn, J. (2013). *Gesund durch Meditation*. Munich, Knaur.

---

[39] K. Nader & E. Ö. Einarsson (2010): "Memory reconsolidation: an update", in: Format Annals of the New York Academy of Sciences (2010) 1191, pp. 27-41; doi: 0.1111/j.1749-6632.2010.05443.x.
[40] www.wired.com/2012/02/ff_forgettingpill

Levine, P. A. (2010). *In an Unspoken Voice.* New York, North Atlantic Books.

Levine, P. A. (2015). *Trauma and Memory: Brain and Body in a Search for the Living Past: A Practical Guide for Understanding and Working with Traumatic Memory.* US, North Atlantic Books.

Lipton, B. H. (2005). *The Biology of Belief.* San Rafael/CA, Mountain of Love Productions, Inc. and Elite Books.

Maté, G. (2003). *When the Body Says NO.* Hoboken, New Jersey, John Wiley & Sons Inc.

McLean, P. (1990): *The Triune Brain in Evolution.* Heidelberg, Springer Science & Business Media.

Mundlos, C. (2015). *Gewalt unter der Geburt.* Marburg, Tectum.

Pall, M. L. (2007). *Explaining Unexplained Illnesses.* Binghamton, NY, Harrington Park Press.

Porges, S. W. (2001). *The Polyvagal Theory: Phylogenetic substrates of a social nervous system,* in International Journal of Psychophysiology, 42, pp. 123–146.

Reddemann, L. (2016). *Mitgefühl, Trauma und Achtsamkeit in psycho-dynamischen Therapien.* Göttingen, Vandenhoeck & Ruprecht.

Ruppert, F. (2017). *Early Trauma.* Steyning, Green Balloon Publishing.

Schwartz, R. C. (1997). *Systemische Therapie mit der inneren Familie.* Stuttgart, Klett-Cotta.

Siegel, D. (2012). *Pocket Guide to Interpersonal Neurobiology.* USA, Norton.

Storch, M., Cantieni, B., Hüther, G. & Tschacher, W. (2010). *Embodiment.* Bern, Hans Huber.

van der Kolk, B. (2014). *The Body Keeps the Score.* New York, Penguin.

Walach, H., Wittmann, M. & Schmidt, S. (2017). *Neurobiologische Grundlagen der Osteopathie,* in J. Mayer & C. Standen (Publisher), Lehrbuch Osteopathische Medizin. Munich, Elsevier.

Wilks, J. (2015). *Choices in Pregnancy and Childbirth.* London, Singing Dragon.

Dr. med. Harald Banzhaf is the Medical Head of the Healing Centre Zollernalb in Bisingen/Hohenzollern with his own practice for integrative medicine, and lecturer at Tübingen University. He works with the Identity-oriented Psychotrauma Therapy developed by Prof. Dr. Ruppert and is a trainer in mindfulness and an accredited MBSR teacher.

DAGMAR STRAUSS

My heart, my love, my trauma

Our heart – a central organ

There is no organ in the human body that has inspired as many idioms over hundreds of years as the heart. In everyday speech we use phrases such as: "From the bottom of my heart", "It broke my heart", "Dear to my heart", "My heart leapt", "Wear one's heart on one's sleeve", etc. In almost all cultures the heart is seen as the seat of love and the centre of our life energy. Our heart reacts immediately to every emotional feeling. We feel love in our heart, not in our brain. What goes "right to the heart", what we "take to heart" and what "touches our heart" affects us in the centre of our being.

The heart is the central organ of our human expressiveness, of our relationship and attachment wishes. It expresses our need for human closeness and love. "The heart is the central organ for a person's emotional confrontation with himself and his environment." (Peters 2014, p. 37) When we are close to a loved one, our heart begins to beat "faster". In contact with a loving person, we can relax. We become calmer because we feel accepted, safe and secure. We open ourselves, "our heart leaps" and a warm feeling flows through our whole body. But it is not only feelings of love that affect the function of our heart. Disgust, anger and fear also alter our heartbeat. A client with 'cardiac arrhythmia' summarised the way he feels about his heart with this sentence: "My heart is the centre of my I-awareness".

From the beginning to the end of our life, our heart is the driving force. It is the organ that begins to beat from the third week of our development as an embryo in the womb. When, from the fifth week, our hands and arms grow from the sides of the heart, they push themselves further around the heart until the fingers touch.

Anatomy and function of the heart

Our heart is a hollow organ the size of a fist. It weighs between 300 and 500 grams and lies at a slightly slanted angle on the left side of the chest. At rest, an adult heart beats 60 to 80 times a minute, which is about 4,000 times an hour and three billion times in a life of 70 years. Depending on height and weight, a human being has five to six litres of blood. Every day, the heart sends this amount of blood about 1,200 times through the whole body.

The heart has two atria and two ventricles, separated by the septum. It is connected with every cell in the body by a dense vascular network and ensures that all the cells are supplied with oxygen, nutrients, hormones and information. Even the brain is dependent on the heart because it would not be able to perform its work if it did not receive a reliable blood supply at all times. The heart not only supplies the whole organism with blood, but also supplies itself, via the coronary vessels, which branch off immediately behind where the aorta issues from the left ventricle.

The cardiac muscle movements are not controlled by the brain; the sinoatrial node, a small cluster of nerve cells, is responsible for generating electrical impulses in the heart and is known as the heart's pacemaker. This node is situated in the right atrium, and its cells build up electrical impulses, which discharge over the whole organ making the heart beat. Because it is the centre of the whole organism, it works in conjunction with the influences it receives from the brain and, via the blood, from the body's periphery and its interior.

Heart rate variability

In recent years groundbreaking discoveries have been made in heart research concerning the function and capacity of the heart. Researchers at the Californian 'HeartMath Institute' have discovered that feelings have a direct effect on our cardiac rhythm.[41] A healthy heart never beats in regular time like a soldier, but oscillates actively about an individual mean. If we feel our own pulse at the wrist, we have the impression that it is completely regular. However, if it is measured with more sensitive measuring techniques, we find that the intervals between the beats are of different lengths. In the recovery phase, the pause between two heart beats, the organism oscillates particularly strongly. A heart that beats in regular time is 'frozen' and can no longer adapt to internal and external conditions. This is a sign of a serious illness. The more flexible the heart movements are, the healthier the person is.

In order to determine a person's individual cardiac rhythm, the intervals between the beats are measured. That is called the heart rate variability. It denotes a person's ability continually to alter the frequency of his cardiac rhythm. Variability in the interval between two heart beats is desirable and shows a good ability to adapt to environmental influences. A rhythmically oscillating heart frequency variability indicates a positive emotional state. The heart frequency variability becomes disorderly when we are dominated by emotions such as anger, resentment, anxiety and frustration. The heart frequency becomes harmonious when we experience feelings of affection, sympathy, gratefulness and joy.

Breathing also has a significant influence on the heart. The tip of the heart rests on the diaphragm. When the lungs raise and lower the ribcage, the heart oscillates with the rhythm. Breathing in speeds up the pulse rate; breathing out slows it down. A client of mine once had an internal picture in which she saw that "her heart was moved up and down like a boat carried by the breath's gentle waves".

---

[41] www.heartMathinstitute.com

Heart-brain and heart-field

In recent years neuroscientists have discovered that our heart has its own nervous system with over 40,000 neurons. As these neurons not only receive information from the body's interior, but also act like a brain and transfer information to the head's brain and the body, we speak of a 'heart-brain' (Peters 2014, p.24). The heart-brain's information is sent specifically to those areas of the head-brain that deal with emotions. Our heart-brain is able to feel, to remember, to learn and to make decisions. It influences our perceptions, our feelings, our thoughts and ultimately our actions.

Researchers at the HeartMath Institute have detected that our heart produces a pulsating electromagnetic field whose waves transport information over long distances. A direct exchange of information can therefore take place between two people at the level of the heart. Scientists have concluded that, just like an 'antenna', our nervous system is able to receive information that is sent unconsciously by another person. The heart's electrical field is 60 times greater than that of the brain, and the magnetic element of this field is even 5,000 times higher than that of the brain; it can be detected at a distance of several metres from the body. According to the researchers, sympathy is the emotion that affects our environment most strongly. The electromagnetic waves of information produced by one person's heart can be detected in the brain waves of a second person (Peters 2014). In other words, our heart's activity continually passes information to our environment, and we receive similar information from other people – in most cases unconsciously.

Peters (2014) describes an experiment in 1989 in which white blood corpuscles were taken from the mucous membrane of a Pearl Harbor veteran's cheek, preserved in a nutrient solution, and taken to a place far away. Then the veteran was shown a film depicting the attack on Pearl Harbor. While he watched the film, his electromagnetic activity and that of the extracted cells was measured. The test subject had a strong physical reaction to the traumatic air attack. The extracted cells, far away, showed the same reaction as the body from which they had been taken. It all happened with no measurable time lag. In a further experiment the cells were shielded by a Faraday cage – and the same thing happened. The cells reacted just as if they were still in the body. Another experiment confirmed this result. The DNA of extracted cells also reacted simultaneously to the test person's artificially generated stress symptoms at a distance of more than 500 kilometres. Atomic clocks were used in the experiment to ensure that the timing was exact (Peters 2014. p.81 ff).

The heart and the autonomic nervous system

In addition to the sinoatrial node, our heart is also influenced by the autonomic nervous system. Although the sinoatrial node also pulsates without the autonomic nervous system, it needs its influence and impulses to adapt the cardiac activity to the changing needs of the organism. The autonomic nervous system is responsible for all involuntary functions in our organism. It is regulated by two large nerve complexes, the sympathetic and parasympathetic. Tension and stress activate the sympathetic nervous system, and calm and relaxation activate the parasympathetic nervous system. Their interaction ensures a dynamic balance in our organism. Information from both parts of the autonomic nervous system passes through the spinal cord and lead fibres from the organs to the brain and vice versa. The sympathetic nervous system increases the heart rate, while the parasympathetic calms the heart. The parasympathetic nervous system is associated with recovery, calm and regeneration, a slow heart rate and interpersonal relationships and love. If a person is under stress, the activity of the ventral vagus nerve is reduced and he is no longer capable of establishing attachment or relationship contact.

The polyvagal theory of Stephen Porges

In order to gain a deeper understanding of the heart function and the development of 'heart diseases', we have to look more closely at the parasympathetic side of the neural heart supply.

Stephen Porges (2010) discovered 20 years ago that mammals possess a divided parasympathetic nervous system. He has concluded that human beings and all other mammals, but not reptiles, possess three separate autonomic neural circuits that are embedded into the overall nervous system. They have evolved successively and are built upon one another. The PNS is chiefly represented by the vagus nerve that divides into a front and a back branch. The front part of the vagus nerve ('ventral vagus') influences in particular the heart and the activity of the lungs. According to Porges the ventral part of the vagus nerve is responsible for the social interaction between humans. He therefore calls this the 'social engagement system' (SES). It is closely connected to our emotionality and our relationships. For this reason, as well as supplying the heart, the ventral vagus is also responsible for the neural supply of the facial muscles, in particular the ciliary muscles of the eyes, the auditory ossicles, the larynx, the pharynx, the throat, the lungs and the gut. It supports our ability to interact socially with other people via eye contact, facial expression, tone of voice, and listening. It slows the heartbeat when we are in comfortable contact. We then relax mentally, emotionally and physically.

Our feelings are reflected chiefly in the upper half of the face. By supplying the facial muscles, the ventral vagus provides the connection between heart and face, particularly the muscles around the eye. The nerves that regulate the face and voice are connected with the heart. That is why feelings of the heart can be seen in the eyes and heard in the voice. When we come into contact with a person we first look at the eyes before we look at the rest of the face. It is in the eyes that we can see whether this person is well disposed towards us, and whether we can feel safe with them.

Babies look at their mothers' eyes and watch the muscles around their eyes to find out her emotional state. If the eyes show joy, warmth, love and attentiveness, the child feels safe and can relax with his mother. Someone whose mouth is smiling, but whose eye area remains frozen and whose gaze is unfriendly, is unconsciously seen as threatening. We will therefore avoid any contact with him. Only when the smile is connected with the heart, in other words when the eyes 'smile' too, do we unconsciously recognise that we can feel safe. Smiling can be learnt; it does not have to be connected with our heart.

We read aggressive behaviour in the lower half of people's faces. We are social beings who feel good with physical closeness, because through it we can calm ourselves if we feel agitated. However, this is not possible if this need has been damaged early on in life by the caregiver (for instance by physical and sexual violence). Traumatised people are not able to calm themselves with the help of physical contact, and instead, as a survival strategy, withdraw and isolate themselves. Traumatised people often have frozen facial features. They show little facial expression in situations of social contact.

The older part, in terms of evolution, of the parasympathetic nervous system Porges has termed the back ('dorsal') vagus. It steps in when, faced with a dangerous situation, we can react with neither fight nor flight and it seems inevitable that we will die. The dorsal vagus ensures that the energy mobilised by the sympathetic nervous system is quickly reduced. It is instrumental in psychologically and physically freezing the whole organism, as a last resort. This state of immobilisation is accompanied by breaking off contact to any bodily sensation. It stops all perception and numbs awareness. It prevents the person from feeling his own experience of the current situation. It is almost as if we go into physical and mental 'hibernation'. Below the outward calm the intense fight or flight energies mobilised by the sympathetic nervous system are still raging. They are completely suppressed by the dorsal vagus and are held captive and frozen with no loss of intensity.

According to Porges, the ventral vagus complex forms the physiological basis of our ability to interact socially. It allows us to calm ourselves and to remain relaxed. If the ventral vagus is well developed and possesses a high vagal tone, it supports us in our 'I'-strength, ensures robust health and helps us establish loving interactions with attachment figures. If we are open to our own feelings we can also express our emotions outwardly.

In a resting state, the heart is influenced by the ventral vagus. It acts as an intermediary between our body and our psyche. Research groups have found that vagus activity is important for a person's emotional and social development (Sroka 2011). A childhood full of sensitive and loving interactions with the mother leads to a vital emotionality and to openness towards the person's own feelings. A well-developed ventral vagus also ensures a high degree of stress tolerance. A high baseline vagal tone in childhood is associated with better cognitive ability and with good physical health.

Early traumatisations in particular cause us to lose the ability to activate the ventral vagus. We are constantly on the defensive, have problems with social interactions and are unable to calm ourselves down. Hyper-vigilance, unrest and over-sensitivity are the result – as are so-called 'heart diseases'.

Case Study: Lina

Lina has been coming regularly to group constellations with me for many months. She has severe attachment trauma and suffers from having been sexually traumatised. Today she wants to look at her illusion of love with a man with whom she has fallen in love, but with whom she cannot form a healthy relationship. Her intention is: *"Wie fühle ich mich mit Hannes?"* "How do I feel with Hannes?" [Word for word translation: How feel I myself with Hannes?]

In contact with her 'I' the first thing that comes up is her aversion to sexual contact. Then Lina brings in a representative for 'myself'. The representative immediately feels a pleasantly animated beating of the heart but also feels slightly shaky. 'Myself' feels very affectionate towards Lina and both look expectantly at one another. After a while 'myself' feels a bright ray of love travelling from her heart to Lina's heart. Lina looks irritated and her chest feels constricted. The pain in her heart is overwhelming. The pain is so severe that Lina is unable to suppress it and begins to cry loudly. She breathes heavily and it is clear that her old trauma feelings have been activated. I support her with a calm voice and encourage her not to suppress these feelings now, but to try to stay in contact with them. While she opens herself to these old painful feelings, I ask her to maintain eye contact and physical contact with 'myself' so that she does not lose the present position and is able to link the previous pain with the adult Lina. While she gives this pain space in her chest, the 'I' comes and puts her hands in a loving and supporting way on Lina's shoulder blades. Held in this way by 'myself' and the 'I', and supported by me, she can give herself up to the massive love-pain of the little, abandoned and lonely child within her. I encourage her to stay in eye contact with 'myself' (in order to continue to activate the ventral vagus), while simultaneously feeling the pain.

As a child, Lina was alone with her pain and, in order to survive had to split it off and lock it away in her heart. Now, however, an adult counterpart is there, Lina's 'myself', who is supporting her efforts to be able to stay in contact with her childhood pain. In doing so she has brought an early-traumatised part of herself into the present. The pain no longer forces her to retreat internally.

After Lina has been able to calm herself through the feeling of 'being well supported', for the first time she feels the desire to lay her head on the shoulder of 'myself' and relax. She is very surprised at this impulse, as she has never before been aware of this feeling of trust in herself.

After the constellation Lina says that the pain from the heart was so intense, because it was so terrible that this great love could not reach its target. She was never allowed to express this love because her mother could not bear it. "Where can I go with the love that is so powerful within me that there are no words for it?" She had therefore given up and locked her heart and her love away from herself and the world.

'Heart diseases'

In 2014 in Germany, 338,056 people died of cardiovascular diseases. This diagnosis is given as the most frequent cause of death.[42] Biologically oriented medicine considers that the best way to prevent 'heart disease' is the right diet, a healthy lifestyle and sufficient exercise.

Medicine divides the general term 'heart diseases', and differentiates between 'functional heart diseases', such as 'cardiac arrhythmia' and 'angina', and those accompanied by organ change, for example 'narrowing of the coronary arteries' and 'heart attack'. Functional heart diseases usually show symptoms such as palpitations, irregular heartbeat, tachycardia, sharp pains in the region of the heart, burning and hot flushes of the heart apex, twinges, pain and aches in the left side of the chest. These symptoms are often accompanied by panic attacks and mortal fear. At the organic level there are usually no detectable defects. According to statistics, 10 to 25% of the population suffer from these 'indefinable heart symptoms'. (Morschitzky and Sator 2013, p.42)

Organic heart disorders occur when there are problems with the blood and oxygen supply to the cardiac muscle. When the coronary arteries are narrowed by the build up of plaques there is an insufficient blood supply to parts of the cardiac muscle, either temporarily or permanently. Temporary coronary circulatory disorders also manifest themselves in different forms of 'tightening of the chest'. Those concerned feel sudden oppressive pains behind the breastbone that extend to the left side of the chest and the left arm. A severe attack can lead to sudden collapse, combined with nausea, difficulty in breathing, sweating and a feeling of mortal fear. Usually these attacks only last a few minutes. 'Heart attack' is the most frequent cause of death, although the heart attack rate has decreased in recent years, due to improved acute treatments and preventative medicine (Sroka 1987, 2006). A heart attack is no longer a 'manager's disease', as

---

[42] German Federal Statistical Office, www.destatis.de

it was termed some decades ago. It now affects lower social classes much more.

From the viewpoint of conventional medicine, coronary circulatory disorders arise from calcification of the vessels that are supposed to supply the cardiac muscle with blood and oxygen. According to conventional medicine, these vessels become less and less elastic, and their volume and thus the blood supply to the heart is reduced, with the result that the tissue is no longer supplied with sufficient blood and oxygen, leading to a deficiency, particularly when there is increased stress. A heart attack might also be caused by a blood clot suddenly closing a coronary vessel. The tissue behind it would then abruptly lose its supply of blood and oxygen and would die within a few seconds. If only a small part were affected, the attack might often go unnoticed. Inferior scar tissue would be created to replace the tissue at the spot where the heart attack happened. If a large blood vessel were affected, the consequence could be fatal. As the signs usually go unnoticed by the person concerned, the heart attack would be experienced as sudden and unexpected.

In his books about 'heart diseases', and particularly 'heart attacks', Sroka (2011) puts forward a different theory: that the blood circulation in the coronary arteries is often not in the least reduced by any narrowing. If the coronary vessels slowly became narrower through calcification, so-called collaterals would be formed. In other words, a 'detour circulation system' would be created in order to guarantee the supply to the heart. There would usually be a drastic drop in the ventral vagal tone immediately preceding a heart attack. This suspension of vagal heart activity is what causes the sudden lack of blood circulation, or even ischemia of the heart muscle.

'Heart-attack personality' as a trauma survival strategy

Psychosomatic medicine often describes a person suffering from a heart condition as a personality characterised by ambition, restlessness, hard work, competitiveness, an urge to dominate, single-mindedness and impatience. This person constantly puts himself under pressure and is always short of time. He tends to be a perfectionist, suffers from high levels of self-control and extreme obsessiveness. He tries to gain control of his environment. He suppresses feelings, particularly fear, and tends towards rationalisation. He struggles to be able to relax as his inner tension constantly drives him on. He suffers from hyperactivity.

Patients suffering from a 'heart condition' find it difficult to endure feelings of dependency and passivity. They do not experience any fulfilment outside their professional life, and try to avoid rest periods. They do not outwardly show anything of the feelings that drive them and influence their behaviour.

Psychosomatic therapy usually consists of a diverse range of relaxation techniques such as autogenic training, yoga or breathing therapy. However, this is not sufficient to heal the underlying trauma, because the different behaviours are typical for what in Franz Ruppert's theory is termed a 'trauma survival strategy' for the 'trauma of love' (Ruppert 2010).

Case history: Moritz

Moritz wants to look at his irregular heartbeat today. His intention is: *"Ich will die Ursache meiner Herz-Rhythmus-Störungen kennen."* [Word for word translation: "I want the cause of-my heart-rhythm-disturbances to know."] "I want to know the cause of my cardiac arrhythmia."

Moritz's 'I' is neutral to begin with and is curious to see what the process brings. The representative for 'heart', which was set up separately from the 'rhythm-disturbances', feels as if it doesn't belong to Moritz and has not been invited by him. It would like to be closer to Moritz but cannot reach him. The representative for 'heart' knocks repeatedly on the wall trying to draw attention to himself. He has the feeling Moritz isn't hearing him. The 'heart' begins to cry, is profoundly sad and feels under pressure. It has the feeling Moritz has decided to go through life without his 'heart'. It feels abandoned and lonely. It wants to try and reach Moritz.

The representative for 'of-my' has a strong feeling of melancholy and a deep longing for the mother, with a need for warm connection. He has a heart-felt longing for warmth, tenderness and sensibility. He asks Moritz how he has come to distance himself so far from his heart.

During the constellation, the 'heart' feels increasingly weak, and keeps losing energy. He looks at Moritz and tells him that he likes him a great deal, even loves him! 'Heart' says he would have liked to have had a mother who expressed her feelings and said: "I love you!" But that never happened. Today 'heart' wants to be loved by Moritz and to be seen by him. Moritz cannot yet give his heart this love. As an observer of this scene it is touching to see how difficult it is for Moritz to open himself up to his own heart and how *'heart'* looks pleadingly at him.

Moritz now comes to the group regularly and wants to learn to fall in love with his own heart.

The 'trauma of love'

From the perspective of Identity-oriented Psychotrauma Therapy (IoPT), which was developed by Franz Ruppert, the basis for the overarching need for recognition, and the willingness to give everything to achieve it, is born in childhood in the child's relationship with his parents. A baby who is not seen by his mother with his needs, and does not receive sensitive responses to his signals, experiences this as an emotional catastrophe. Later as an adult, he is likely to spend his whole life trying to gain his mother's love by, for example, striving for professional success. In the case of Moritz there was no possibility of reaching his mother and being seen and accepted by her. The consequences of this were emotional withdrawal, avoidance of attachment relationships and rejection of his own gentle feelings. Thus the longing for love and security is split off.

The basis for the personality profile of the 'heart attack patient' is therefore a lack of maternal love and sensitivity. Instead, the child has to follow the stipulation of being "quiet and good". Later the 'heart patient' submits to the hostile values of a competitive society. This results in an excess of suppressed anger and aggression with which the 'heart condition' patient holds back his wishes for security, tenderness and love in his life, which then has a destructive effect on his heart.

Olga Bazhenova and Stephen Porges carried out an experiment with five-month old infants (Sroka 2011, p.44). A positive feeling triggered by positive attention was shown in a corresponding joyful facial expression in the child, and was connected with being calm and relaxed and with high vagal tone. As the ventral vagus reacts to gentle touch, loving physical contact is essential for a baby. The higher the relaxed vagal tone, the greater was the ability of children aged eight to eleven months to remain attentive in social interactions, and the greater their resilience to stress. Withdrawal, depression, aggressive behaviour and sleeping problems at the age of three years old were statistically significant in connection with a lowered ventral vagal tone.

In this study it was shown that it is very important for the development of the ventral vagus that the parents possess the ability to regulate the child's emotions and intense feelings. So that the child can successfully co-regulate, the parents have to have good contact with their feelings and possess a stable 'I'-structure to avoid being overwhelmed by the child's feelings. A secure attachment relationship with the parents teaches the child to regulate his feelings himself in adulthood and to enter into good social relationships. Looking after and maintaining interpersonal relationships has a significant influence on our wellbeing and our psychological and physical health. Sroka (2011, p.48) concludes that disturbances in the development of feelings and relationships in childhood predispose the person in later life, through a weakness in the vagus, to heart attacks.

As Franz Ruppert has found out, a 'trauma of love' occurs when a mother cannot give her child love and security because of her own traumatisation (Ruppert 2010, 2014). This lovelessness can extend to rejection of the child, which then leads to an irresolvable dilemma in the child's psyche. The child would like to oscillate with the mother in a 'cycle of love' from heart to heart. An emotionally-healthy mother can joyfully accept her child's love, connect it with her own feelings of love and allow her love to flow in return to her child through her loving gaze, her soft touch, her gentle voice and her vitality. She focuses her attention in a healthy way on her child, looks after him with sensitivity and holds him comfortably and securely in her arms. The child can thus feel safe and secure. A strong and binding love develops between the two, that neither space nor time can separate.

When a baby has the deep sense of having his needs recognised and understood by his mother, the basis of his own self-perception is formed and he learns in the course of his development to regulate his fears and stressful feelings himself. He then experiences the world as a place where he is welcome and which gives him everything he needs for a good life. He develops into a clearly defined personality who is able to have good social contacts and enter into loving relationships.

However, if the mother rejects the love that every fibre of her child's being transmits to her, the child feels helpless, desperate and powerless. It is then impossible for the child to form a good attachment to his mother. Through her own 'trauma of love', the mother is incapable of giving her child warmth and security. She therefore causes a trauma for her child, and the coldness of her heart inflicts profound emotional wounds on him.

We should therefore not only focus our attention on physical violence, but also on silent emotional violence, which is frequently not externally visible. A child experiences a lack of respect in the form of rejection, attributions, expectations, punishments through lack of contact, etc. in the same way as with physical violence. As van der Kolk (2015) emphasises, a child feels the same pain if he experiences emotional rejection as he does if he is physically beaten. The sympathetic nervous system is greatly activated and his fear increases to panic.

Maria's constellation illustrates the consequences of neglect and emotional violence.

My Body, My Trauma, My I

Case history: Maria

Maria has had massive heart pains for several weeks. Medical tests have clarified that there are no organic causes for her symptoms. For her intention she formulates: *"Ich will spüren, was hinter meinen Herzschmerzen steckt."* [Word for word translation "I want to-feel, what behind my heart-pains hides."] "I want to feel the reason for the pains in my heart."

The representative for the 'I' immediately experiences strong palpitations, feels panic, arousal and feelings of trauma, and struggles not to fall over. She feels nauseous, and as if she is going to faint. She experiences powerful pressure on her neck and a constricted feeling in her chest. She feels very afraid, which makes her whole body shake. The 'I' seems to slip away internally, and feels as if life is leaving her. Maria says that she had a great many suicide fantasies during puberty and was only able to balance them out by sleeping a lot. She had thus "got rid of" herself in another way than actually taking her life.

The representative for 'heart' joins them. Her whole body shudders and she feels as cold as ice. When Maria looks at her, all emotion drains from her; she feels as if she has a heavy burden. I encourage her to make eye contact with her 'I' in order to stabilise herself, which she does. Contact is established between the two of them, which brings Maria back into the present and makes her feel clearer. The 'I' says she feels calmer when the 'heart' is there.

The 'heart' now starts moving from one foot to the other like clockwork, saying "tick tock, tick tock". While doing that the representative has to breathe deeply. She says she feels cold but still functioning, but it's reduced to a minimum. 'Heart' feels that she is a little baby without social contact. She is alone and abandoned. Maria says that she grew up on a farm and her mother didn't look after her at all. There were just unfamiliar maids who 'provided' for her. Her mother was never really there for her.

The 'I' now feels very connected with the 'heart' and keeps looking across at it. They are both concentrating intensely on each other. The 'heart' now wants to breathe for the 'I', and now the representative for 'pain' joins them and says she feels threatened from outside. The 'I' then says that it is a matter of life and death.

150

When the representative for 'behind' arrives, its heart starts racing and it wants to run away. It reveals itself as the survival part that wants to have nothing to do with anything and would prefer to be outdoors. This statement upsets Maria so profoundly that she begins to cry, because being outdoors in nature was the one place she felt safe as a child. When Maria shows such strong emotions the 'heart' turns to her for the first time and looks at her. They make eye contact for the first time and recognise each other. Now the 'I' can open its eyes again and look around. Finally all three look at each other: Now it all seems fine for Maria.

A baby on his own can neither fight nor flee. In order not to die of over-stimulation, he has to split off his overwhelming fear and unendurable pain. Trauma fear is mortal fear! This is why the dorsal vagal complex is activated. It down-regulates the whole nervous system and guides the infant into a state of numbness. The dorsal vagus takes the lead and the Social Engagement System (SES) is disabled.

A mother who closes her heart to her child, and shows no feelings of love and keeps her trauma survival strategies behind impenetrable walls, becomes a threat to her child. Her eyes look at the child impassively, or she looks through the child with an empty, faraway gaze; she projects her fears, rejection and anger as well as her own unfulfilled wishes onto the child. There is no gentle look from her eyes to accompany her smile, and the child will never see himself reflected in the shine of his mother's loving eyes. He never feels welcome, seen and accepted.

Thus the child then loses contact with himself by breaking off access to his own needs, his heart and his own 'I'; there is no healthy and stable 'I'-awareness with an early attachment trauma. The infant loses contact with his own 'I', closes himself away from his own feelings, and all his senses are then hyper-attentively directed outwards. He keeps looking towards his mother and tries with his limited opportunities to establish eye contact with her. If the mother is not with the child in her feelings, the child then has to be with the mother as she is. If the mother is not sensitive to the baby's inner world, the child has to try to fit in with the mother's inner world and align himself with her needs rather than his own. The baby learns that contact with people is only possible through the abandonment of himself and his needs; he increasingly loses himself, becoming increasingly tense internally and externally, continually trying to deal with the dilemma of his need for contact and his fear of closeness. A truly relaxed, sincere and warm connection can never be achieved.

A person who has suffered an attachment trauma throughout his childhood because of his mother's unloving behaviour has to lose his own physical and emotional self-awareness in order to survive. This is the only way the child can have any contact with the mother who emotionally rejects him. The price for this survival is the relinquishing of his 'I'. The seed of his 'I' that was planted is unable to germinate and develop into a strong and empathetic person.

Many conflicts that have arisen from traumatisations have often persisted over many generations in the psyches of family members. The essential biology of the bonding drive forces the child to identify with the trauma feelings of his mother and her ancestors. We normally bond with those people with whom we feel safe, but when we are forced to bond with a person who is a threat to us, we have to identify with their suppressed trauma feelings. In order to continue to exist in this hostile environment, the child develops more and more survival strategies over the years, ones we can identify as the assumed character structures of a 'heart-attack' patient.

Case history: Sonja

Sonja comes to see me on a one-to-one basis because she is suffering from intense angina pains, cardiac arrhythmia, and burning sensations in her chest, all of which worry her greatly. Her intention is: *"Ich möchte die Ursache wissen, woher die Herzbeschwerden kommen!"* [Word for word translation: "I would-like the cause to-know, whence the heart-complaints come!"] "I would like to know the underlying cause of my heart complaints!"

I act as the representative for her 'I' and immediately have the feeling that Sonja is an empty shell with nothing inside her chest. I can't connect with her and she looks at me with empty eyes. Then I become dizzy and I get intense images of a baby lying alone and abandoned in her bed. A great fear arises in me and my heart beats very fast. I see an elastic band that reaches from my heart to the mother's heart, which is pulled tight and suddenly and violently snaps, lashes back into my heart, constricts my chest and creates in my image a large, open wound. This wound produces a deep, agonizing and unbearable pain. All this is accompanied by a profound fear that the mother is abandoning me and never coming back. From now on as this representation I know there will not be one moment of relaxation. I am distraught and begin to cry, and I tell the client of my sadness, my loneliness and the fears that I will have to die alone.

Sonja listens to me, unmoved, and when I look into her eyes it is as if all my feelings are suddenly blown away and I am unemotional again. I feel nothing any longer. All other feelings have disappeared along with the trauma feelings: there seems no vitality, hope or desire any more. I feel as if I am empty inside. My experience is as if that from now on I will be a quiet, withdrawn and good child, making no demands and not expressing any needs. My mother is pleased at such an easy child.

Sonja says that that resonates somewhere deep within her but she doesn't feel anything, nor has she any sympathy with me in my representation. She does confirm, however, that she never experienced her mother showing any sort of feeling; in her childhood there was no joy, no sadness, no desire and no vitality.

Since then Sonja has been coming regularly to the group and she is gradually realising what a 'child-hostile' environment she grew up in. She wants to come into her own feelings in order to find a way out of her apathy and lack of willpower. Her heart complaints have disappeared in the course of working therapeutically on her early childhood bonding trauma.

Identity-oriented Psychotrauma Therapy (IoPT)

In order to accompany clients into a regulated and stable 'I'-state, it is essential that the therapy should activate the ventral vagus nerve. Restoring a healthy relationship to the person's own original 'I'-state provides the healing in the therapy. The development of a loving bonding contact within herself helps the frozen and traumatised 'I'-state to thaw and to feel again.

Through a client's work in coming into contact with his 'I' through the representative process, with respectful and empathetic support, new relationship experiences can come. Slowly, step-by-step, the client can open himself to his heart and his gentle feelings. The ventral vagus complex then switches on, the chest area opens and the tension is increasingly eased. This relaxation is shown in the release of body and facial muscles, a more gentle voice, open look and deep exhalation.

In working with the representative process, the ventral vagus is the neurobiological centre of the therapy, and intense 'social interactions' can take place. The goal is the integration of parts of the person's identity that have been split off, suppressed and frozen during the process of trauma survival. This happens through re-connection to the child parts of the psyche that were kept out of the person's awareness and stranded in the past. These emotional parts have remained in the old trauma situation from early childhood and need to be integrated into the adult in the present. The child elements that remain caught in the past need a healthy adult counterpart within the client who can enter into deep empathy for the traumatising plight of the child at that time.

In order to do this, the fact of the person's trauma has to be taken seriously and recognised. Trauma therapy is always a gentle and controlled encounter with the fears of the past. The trauma experience has to be integrated into the person's own life, calmed down emotionally, and then, through the person's empathy with himself, integrated into the personality. In this way a complex picture of the person's own life and his experiences is created little by little. Thus an identity can emerge that provides strength, empathy, self-confidence and assurance.

The client has to be able to hold onto his healthy adult present-time awareness so that he does not fall into a regression, from which there can be no re-connection of the traumatised child parts to the here-and-now awareness. It is about creating a space that can differentiate between the present and the past. The client in close contact with his healthy 'I' has this ability. The client has to be able to hold his 'I'-structure in order to integrate his traumatised child parts. If he confronts his trauma too soon, without an 'I'-connection, the client might fall completely into the trauma feelings of the situation in the past. This would be a re-traumatisation.

It is therefore important for integration that the client develops a dual self-awareness. That means that he can remain in contact with himself even if the pain from the past rises from hidden depths within himself and forces its way into his felt awareness. It is helpful for this process if a strong, healthy, supportive and curious 'I' accompanies the process alongside the client. Today he is no longer alone in confronting the situation that was unendurable for him as a little child. In trauma integration it is not the pain that is the problem, but the little child from back then who was unable to deal with the pain in his loneliness. He therefore needs an adult healthy counterpart who can physically take the pain and hold it, just as, back then, the baby would have needed a stable, adult body to provide a calming influence. The stable 'I' provides the support in the here and now for the traumatised child from the past, and helps to understand that the child's fear was justifiable then, but is no longer necessary today. From this secure environment the client can address his traumatised child part with emotional sympathy, and open himself to his frozen trauma feelings from the past. During the whole of the integration process, the client can remain supported by the physical contact with his 'I' and thus work through the old traumas within him to heal them. Thus a bridge can be built within the client from the traumatised child parts of himself to the adult healthy structures.

We have heard that empathy activates the ventral vagus and stirs the blood of anyone seeing the distress of a little child whose physical symptoms 'cry out' for attention. This is the challenge that trauma integration has to overcome: the client has to feel something that, because of their attachment trauma, they never experienced before, and so were unable to develop in themselves – empathy. IoPT work is thus emotional development work.

When working with representatives in the resonance-driven interaction with the person's own 'I', the client's Social Engagement System (SES) is doubly activated. Through face-to-face contact in our relationship with our own 'I' and simultaneously with another representative, who, as the unfamiliar person or the 'you', is automatically present, we encounter our 'I' in 'you'. The client recognizes his 'I' in the representative, who emotionally mirrors the client's feelings through words, facial expressions, gestures and movements. Good bonding contact to the 'I' or the 'close to I' parts, such as 'to me', 'me', 'my', and 'of my', is the best resource for trauma confrontation and trauma integration, as it builds up healthy structures through supportive and empathetic contact.

A stronger healthy 'I' can develop in a person through this bonding contact to himself. From this secure internal position the client can begin to explore his own life history step by step. His own identity develops naturally through encountering and integrating split off and suppressed parts. When I am emotionally ready, I can encounter these parts in a representative and invite them into me in the present through loving and empathetic interaction through eye contact and feelings. These subtle, interpersonal internal contacts encourage activation of the social nervous system. If integration work is to succeed, it is necessary for the client to be able to recognise his healthy 'I' in the representative, and thus to look himself in the eye and establish contact. He can now give himself everything that he needed so badly as a child from his mother in order to be seen, accepted, loved and feel secure. The ventral vagus tone then gradually increases and his ability to enter into relationships with others can begin to develop.

In many encounters between the client and his 'I', I have witnessed how the client's anxious, numbed, narrow and mistrusting gaze is transformed under the loving attention and understanding of his 'I', and how the client was able to release himself slowly from his numbness. When looking at his 'I', the client's gaze gradually becomes more gentle and trusting. Thus structure-forming self-recognition is achieved, coupled with deep relaxation.

Case history: Erich

Erich has had a right bundle branch block[43] for several years that as yet displays no symptoms and was only discovered by chance during a general medical examination. Nevertheless, he would like to make this his topic of exploration. His intention is: *"Ich will die Ursache meines Herzfehlers verstehen."* [Word for word translation: "I want the cause of-my heart-defect to-understand."] "I want to understand the cause of my heart defect."

The 'I' representative is ready to look at Erich's 'heart matters' with him. The 'I' is very familiar with Erich and feels close to him. In contact with his 'I', Erich feels something that is very far away and scares him. When the 'I' hears that, his heart begins to race and he confirms what Erich is saying. The 'I' now feels weak, because it is frightened. Erich downplays this fear and thinks he can 'conquer' it. He says that he often causes himself problems in life by this attitude.

The 'I' now becomes desperate and sees no escape for himself. Something unbearable is there, and now the 'I' has to lie down because he is getting weaker and weaker. He closes his eyes because he can't watch any more. Now the 'I' feels like a little baby, and it is increasingly difficult for the 'I' to stay present. The 'I' feels fear, resistance and desperation. He feels the distress of an infant that had no chance. The 'I' lies curled up on his side like a little baby and says that his heart hurts him so terribly, but he has to endure it. He is so little that he is unable to turn over onto the other side. Erich wants to come into contact with him but doesn't know how to go about it, and lays his head on the shoulder of the

---

[43] In a medical sense, a right bundle branch block is not termed a heart defect.

'I'. This is too much for 'I'; he cannot support the adult Erich, and Erich is not yet able to have eye contact with his baby-'I'. The 'I' feels lonely and abandoned and has the feeling that he is somehow wrong, a 'mistake'. However, he doesn't want to see himself as a mistake. Both begin to cry.

Erich now lies down next to his 'I' and cautiously touches his hand. The 'I' wants to be held by his right thumb just like a baby. Erich becomes increasingly gentle and tender towards the 'I', which gradually feels that he has a heart connection with Erich. Erich himself increasingly relaxes with the contact; his 'I' appreciates the gentle touch, and is now able to relax. Both lie there for a while in gentle contact with one another. This then was enough for Erich, a big step of getting in this touching contact with his 'I'.

Regardless of the symptoms and complaints with which our heart tries to warn us, it is never too late to open ourselves to our own suppressed and split off feelings. Even if we have had to separate ourselves off from our 'I' at an early age, our heart will show us the healing way back to our healthy identity. Then we can lead a loving, 'I'-centred existence, in which all emotional experiences of our life history have their place. Our heart beats in good contact with ourselves – in pulsating vitality for us and in relationship with other people.

References

Morschitzky, H. & **Sator**, S. (2013). *Wenn die Seele durch den Körper spricht*. Ostfildern, Patmos.

Peters, M. (2014). *Gesundmacher Herz*. Kirchzarten, VAK.

Porges, S. W. (2001). *The Polyvagal Theory: Phylogenetic substrates of a social nervous system*, in International Journal of Psychophysiology, 42, pp. 123–146.

Ruppert, F. (2012). *Symbiosis & Autonomy*. Steyning, Green Balloon Publishing.

Ruppert, F. (2015). *Trauma, Fear and Love*. Steyning, Green Balloon Publishing.

Sroka, K. (2006). *Herzinfarkt – Neue Wege*. Norderstedt, Books on Demand.

Sroka, K. (2011). *Herzinfarkt vermeiden*. Tübingen, Psychosozial.
Sroka, K. (1987). *Herzkrank*. Hamburg, Rasch und Röhring.
van der Kolk, B. (2014). *The Body Keeps the Score*. New York, Penguin.

Dagmar Strauss, was born 1962, is married and has three grown-up sons. She is an alternative practitioner, with an independent practice since 1991. 2009-2012 she trained in Somatic Experiencing according to the work of Peter Levine. 2010, 2012 and 2013 she trained with Franz Ruppert in Identity-oriented Psychotrauma Therapy (IoPT) and with the Intention Method. Since 2012 she regularly leads constellation groups. 2015-2017 she trained in Neuro-Affective Relational Model (NARM) according to the work of Laurence Heller. 2016 She trained in attachment psychotherapy according to Karl-Heinz Brisch. www.lebenssinn-wandlung.de

EVELYN HÄHNEL

Food, the digestive system and trauma

Eating, nourishment and food

Finding, producing and processing food is one of the principal activities of humans. A person with nothing to eat or drink will suffer from malnutrition, and eventually will die of hunger or thirst – and this does happen worldwide thousands of times a day. 795 million people today do not have enough food to eat. More people die each year from hunger than from Aids, malaria and tuberculosis combined.[44] Industrial food production only solves part of the problem, and in itself creates other challenges. In the developed countries the populations are becoming increasingly overweight and are developing food allergies; children eat too much and are becoming overweight when still very young. Drinks containing too much sugar and alcohol are frequently consumed to quench thirst, with the corresponding toxic effects for the whole organism.

Gene manipulation, radiation, chemical additives, flavour enhancers etc. have increased in almost all foods. Nutrition has become a science in itself (Pudel and Westenhöfer 1998), has gained much detailed knowledge and is able to give state authorities and individuals many useful tips on how to eat appropriately. For example, not to eat at night when the organism is wired for digestion. There is no lack of advisors who want to help with suggestions, diets, and nutritional ideologies. However, this should not absolve each of us from our own responsibility of finding the best daily nutrition for our children and ourselves.

---

[44] http://de.wfp.org/hunger/hunger-statistik, taken from website 10.2.2017.

160

Eating together promotes social interaction. This ranges from a meal at the family table to a wedding celebration, from the company Christmas dinner to a state banquet. Cultural and individual eating customs can also create deep divisions if the form of nutrition is declared a characteristic of the individual's religious or political identity, and those who do not adhere to it are branded 'unbelievers' or traitors of community values. The best meal does not taste good and becomes indigestible if familial conflicts make the atmosphere at the dining table unbearable.

Our digestive system

Mouth, oesophagus, stomach, small intestine and large intestine are the organs of the digestive system; the liver, gall bladder, spleen and pancreas are also part of this. More than 30 tons of food and 50,000 litres of liquid make their way in a sensitive interaction through the digestive system in a life spanning 75 years. The first stage of digestion begins in the mouth when we chew our food. It is a long way to the anus where the undigested remains are eliminated from the body. The small intestine alone, with all its villi[45] and protrusions, is four to six metres long. Its task is to sort the food into material that the body can absorb and material that has to be passed on to the large intestine as waste to be excreted.

The intestinal brain

Millions of chemical substances have to be analysed in the digestive system, thousands of toxins identified and rendered harmless. Scientists are now talking of an intestinal brain with over 200 million neurons that copes with all these demands (Gershon 2001). In evolutionary terms the intestinal brain is

---

[45] **Villi** are specialised for absorption in the small intestine as they have a thin wall, one cell thick, which enables a shorter diffusion path. They have a large surface area so there will be more efficient absorption of fatty acids and glycerol into the blood stream.

much older than the brain in our skull; there is no area in the latter that has any responsibility for digestion. The gut works independently. We therefore have little conscious influence on our digestion; it is mainly controlled by unconscious processes. The vagus nerve keeps our brain informed of what is happening in the gut. When digestive problems occur over an extended period of time it is important that the person concerned influence the activity in their digestive system by addressing the issues that lie behind these problems, and for that to happen they need a healthy 'I' and a will of their own.

Gut instinct and stress

"A person in love has butterflies in their tummy." "The way to a man's heart is through his stomach." We often make decisions based on our "gut instinct". Someone who is afraid can "be scared shitless". Our digestive system reacts immediately to emotional states and can easily be disturbed by them. In stressful situations when feelings emerge, such as pressure to perform, feelings of fear, anger or grief, the gut is also affected. It begins with bacterial miscolonisation – the population of more than 500 known types of bacteria become confused and negatively affect the digestive process (Enders 2014).

Under stress the sympathetic nervous system releases adrenalin, a hormone secreted by the adrenal medulla, which increases heart rate and blood pressure in order to give the body energy so that it can react quickly. At the same time this process suppresses the peristaltic movements of the digestive tract. Situations of constant stress and longer periods of slower peristalsis can lead to major digestive problems.

Digestion and the immune system

80% of our immune system is located in the gut, and the gut bacteria contribute to the development of a healthy immune system. Part of the immunisation begins in the womb, delivered to the baby via the placenta (Enders 2014). Children born by caesarean section have a lower immune defence and a higher allergy risk. These children have missed out on the mother's vaginal bacteria that contribute to the development of their immune system. After birth the infant receives antibodies via the mother's milk. If the child is not breastfed, these first antibodies will be lacking. The infant is then stimulated to produce his own antibodies through contact with bacteria and pathogens in the environment. The quality and freshness of the nutrition therefore are crucial for a healthy immune system. However, there are many mothers who no longer cook fresh meals, with the result that their children do not learn how to deal with fresh food and their eating behaviour suffers.

Vomiting, diarrhoea and constipation

Whatever arrives in the stomach has to be digested. The only choice the stomach has is to send the food back up, which means vomiting or spitting it out, or to digest it. In digestion the food is mixed with gastric juices, containing, amongst other things, hydrochloric acid for disinfection, and is then transported into the small intestine for sorting and digestion. If the small intestine is overloaded with substances that it cannot identify, it is unable to cope and does not carry out the sorting process well. We can imagine what happens then: some of the good material is mistakenly sent on to excretion, and some waste products are retained in the body.

We can see the gut as symbolising our life flow: it takes everything we, or others, give it to digest, processes it as well as it can and excretes anything that is undigested. If poor-quality, or even poisonous, food is eaten it can upset the way the gut functions in the same way as if we are constantly subjected to psychological threats, as for example a lack of emotional security in our relationship with parents, partners or our own children, that we are unable to 'digest'. It is then impossible to filter enough nutritious content from this input for our own healthy life. Only two possibilities remain: either we dispose of this poor quality food straightaway (diarrhoea) or we keep it inside us too long (constipation). This is often the cause of skin problems, which can be a further attempt by the body to free itself of waste products or other problems. The body tries to get rid of substances that cannot be digested through the skin, which has a major excretory function and is the body's interface with the environment.

Inflammation, ulcers, 'cancer' and medication

In the case of gastritis or a stomach ulcer, we have to question why the stomach feels so threatened that it produces too much acid. According to conventional medicine, the bacteria helicobacter pylori are responsible for this, although 50% of all people have helicobacter in their stomach. In other words, it is a bacterium that is carried by many people who do not have a stomach ulcer, or any other stomach complaint.

In many cases a violent experience lies behind a stomach ulcer. A study by the German Ministry for Family Affairs has revealed that stomach ulcers are one of the most frequent consequences of domestic violence, after cardiovascular problems and headaches.[46] Often such people live in an abusive relationship. Women in particular often live in a constant state of alert and keep their own behaviour under the extreme control in order to avoid angering parents or partner.

Cortisone is often prescribed for acute and chronic inflammation. However, the frequent use of cortisone itself results in many side effects that upset the digestion, for example

- a reduction in the production of the stomach lining, which can lead to stomach ache and inflammation of the stomach lining;
- increased blood sugar levels, which can lead to diabetes;
- increased blood pressure;
- increase in weight;
- water retention in the tissues.

---

[46] www.re-empowerment.de/haeusliche-gewalt/folgen-haeuslicher-gewalt

People who regularly take painkillers and anti-inflammatory medication are particularly at risk of getting a stomach ulcer, the likelihood of which quadruples on such medication. 'Crohn's disease', a chronic inflammation of the gastrointestinal system, can appear from the oesophagus right through to the anus. Conventionally this condition is nearly always treated with cortisone when it flares up. It mostly occurs in people between the ages of 15 and 35 and leads simultaneously to constipation and diarrhoea.

All medication affects what happens in our intestines. We are also often assimilating medications (such as antibiotics, painkillers, beta blockers, hormones, etc.) in foods such as milk, meat, fish and eggs, through the mass production of these foods. If we then try to treat a cold, say, by suppressing our immune system with antibiotics, we are cultivating unhealthy bacteria in our intestines on a massive scale. Anti-depressants and sleeping pills also upset our digestion. All this leads to a vicious cycle of increasing dependence on medication, and with every additional pill, new symptoms and side-effects are tackled but also created.

I also suspect a connection between types of 'cancer' in the digestive system and perpetrator-victim dynamics in which those concerned are trapped. The perpetrator sits deep 'in the gut' and cannot be released. This is the case with sexual traumatisation when one part of a daughter is still emotionally attached to her father, even though he raped her as a child. As one client said, her father "sits in her stomach like lead" and no matter how much she vomits, she cannot get rid of him.

Digestion and mother-attachment

The intestine is one of the first organs to develop in an embryo. In the third month of pregnancy the unborn child already possesses a complete digestive system. This reacts to the child's emotional attachment with his mother and even at this stage of development is particularly susceptible if the emotional relationship with her is disturbed (Brisch 2014, Ruppert 2014). After birth, breast milk is the child's natural first food. However, if the contact between mother and child is disrupted by an early trauma (for instance through medication, drugs, alcohol, violence, rejection, an attempted abortion or just the thought of it), the baby might not tolerate his mother's milk or might unconsciously reject it. Feeding 'baby food' that has been augmented with chemical processing agents and preservatives can induce increased sensitivity and intolerance to certain food-stuffs throughout the individual's life. Food intolerances such as gluten-, fructose- and lactose-intolerance, and celiac disease can actually be intolerance of the mother; the child's own mother is indigestible to the child, yet the child's attachment to her is crucial for his survival.

My mother-trauma

A trauma of mine began six weeks after I was born. In the 1960s that was the usual breastfeeding period and statutory pregnancy leave. When the six weeks were up, my mother put me into a crèche without further ado in order to return to work. My caregiver and my diet changed instantly. A massive adjustment for me that I was almost unable to cope with. I was later told that the nurses in this crèche took my mother aside one day and told her that they could not guarantee my survival. They said that I was not eating and was not able to retain my food, that I was becoming increasingly frozen, that there was "increasingly less of me" and that I appeared lifeless. They advised her to take me home and to look after me herself so that I gained strength again, which my mother did, luckily. This traumatic episode was trotted out throughout my childhood in order to blame me, saying that, even as a baby I had made my will felt and had blackmailed my parents. I was thus made into a perpetrator, even though I was actually the victim!

I was unable to resolve this early threat to my life caused by being separated from my mother and having my attachment to her disrupted. As a child I was always afraid of being abandoned by my mother. Which was something that kept happening, because her traumatisation meant that several times she went to hospital or a sanatorium for some time. Even today, as an adult, I need a great deal of trust and security in order to enter into attachments and develop intimacy. I am always mistrustful of new contacts.

Children's distress

Children are quick to have a 'tummy ache'; they react immediately to any internal imbalance, feeling a lack of, or a surfeit of emotion. They sense if they are alone, if they have love-pains or are afraid, if they cannot reach their mother, or have no space of their own because their mother overwhelms them.

In my opinion, the foundations are laid in childhood for problems we may develop within our digestive system. These are all the times when we were not seen, we did not receive enough attention or were not sufficiently comforted and loved. Being hastily fed, or sometimes having to wait too long for our sustenance, are reasons in later life to link food with stress and trauma.

Parents tell their children that they were wanted, but at the same time often do not manage to satisfy their children's basic emotional needs. Reality shows that food is often used as a consolation, to keep a child quiet. Food is used to compensate for a child's emotional need for physical contact. Later on food is used as a replacement for attention.

'Diabetes'

In a constellation in my practice a client diagnosed with 'type 2 diabetes' encountered his *'illness'* when represented as a powerful survival part. He was under the illusion that with the illness he could control himself. In his childhood he had been completely isolated from any sort of attachment and no one had been there for him. He spent his life in a storeroom with no one offering him healthy relational contact. He was never allowed to develop his own 'I'. When the constellation brought to light that a traumatised part was the motivator for this 'diabetes' dynamic, he immediately wanted to establish contact with this part.

However, the part withdrew in fear. The client was offended by this and remarked that this part did not want him, and he again lost interest in it.

In the conversation that followed he recognised the scenario as a recurring pattern in his life. For him sugar acts as a replacement for the lack of emotional contact and calms him so that he does not have to feel the pain and fear from being abandoned as a child. These feelings are pushed down deep and suppressed, and sweets cover his need for loving contact.

According to the WHO 2014 (World Health Organisation report), the number of diabetes cases has quadrupled in the past 35 years. There are now 422 million people worldwide with this diagnosis.[47]

Children's traumas

If children are rejected, either consciously or unconsciously, if they do not fulfil their parents' expectations, if they are moulded to their parents' wishes, if they have to support their traumatised parents, if they experience violence and sexual attacks, then their eating and drinking behaviour is likely to be maladjusted, and they will have problems with their digestive system. Verbal violence, silence, lies, pretence that everything is fine, breaking contact – behaviours such as these confuse children, who cannot distinguish what is real and what is not. The apparent contact with their parents is actually non-existent and they are emotionally starved. If in such a family they have to behave at table as if everything is fine, it is not surprising that a child will either have no appetite or that he eats more than he should out of misery.

Adaptation to the extent of self-abandonment

Traumatic experiences caused by emotional attacks from the survival strategies of mother or father, result in the child being unable to develop his own 'I'. The child is only tolerated in order

---

[47] www.who.int/diabetes/global-report/en, taken from website 10.2.2017.

to support his parents, or to be used by them so that they can endure their own life. Children in such a situation do everything for their parents to the extent of total self-abandonment, in the hope that in the end they will receive their parents' love. Unconsciously they may believe they have no right of their own to live. They learn that the way they are is wrong, because, if not, would their mother have given them away, beaten them or not protected them from the father's violence?

Many children have been brought up in this way, in the service of their parents and unable to know their own needs and to meet them. Being good means eating everything on their plate. If the child does make his own demands, he is punished. The children are supposed to be grateful, to step back, and to betray their own wants and needs so that the connection with their parents that they need can continue to exist. As a result their willingness to adapt is reinforced, they are quick to accept blame, they try to please everybody, they put themselves last, their emotional attachments are dysfunctional and they easily develop physical symptoms in their digestive system as well.

Disorders in the digestive system can be the result if emotional abuse is constantly repeated. Children suffer for example from vomiting and diarrhoea because unconsciously they experience these contacts with their parents as being poisonous. As long as contact with the parents as an adult continues, it has the effect of constantly repeating the traumatisation. Unfortunately many people find it very difficult to stop contact with traumatising parents. Conscientiousness, a guilt conscience, hostility and well-meant manipulation by relations and friends make it difficult for them, and unhealthy contact seems better than no contact at all.

Not to feel one's own vitality can become a deeply ingrained experience. It can become the main issue of a person's life, which is often hidden behind diagnoses such as 'anorexia', 'bulimia' or 'obesity'. In order for these extreme forms of eating disorders to develop, sexual traumatisation is often a factor in addition to a 'trauma of identity' and a 'trauma of love' (Ruppert 2014).

Finally becoming 'I'

If an individual is unaware of these unconscious relationship patterns, it is very likely that they repeat them in new relationships. The new relationships then will also have the effect of retriggering and retraumatisation and these continually frustrating experiences will often end in isolation. It is essential that people with such traumatised child parts develop their own healthy 'I' in therapy and make a decision to begin their own life and stop being in the service of others' survival strategies; to attach importance to their own 'I' and to treat themselves with care, even at the risk of distancing themselves from their current caregiver. That is a transformational and often painful process. We have to take responsibility for ourselves, which is often not easy. However, we can develop our healthy 'I' step by step to become autonomous and make positive changes to such self-harming behaviour. How often do we remain silent when we ought to say something, for harmony's sake? How often are we afraid of slipping into feelings we do not want to feel, because they are painful? How often do we flee internally because we cannot endure the pain? How often would we like to belong, and so submit to rules made by others that we do not necessarily agree with? And what else in our lives can we still not digest?

In identity-oriented psychotrauma therapy these correlations are examined, understood and felt. This triad touches all levels and cells of our being – with a lasting effect. The individual with his own trauma biography comes increasingly to himself, to his original 'I' and step by step can begin to walk a self-determined and healthy path.

Let's begin to be honest with ourselves. Let's begin to respect and love ourselves. Let's start to pay attention to our split-off traumatised parts with their frozen feelings and integrate them back into ourselves. It is never too late to explore ourselves and trust ourselves more. Let's decide to develop inner autonomy that does not create any mutual dependence in our relationships, but encourages a healthy give and take, then we can pass on this self-responsibility to support children and adults in developing freely within secure boundaries. So that they can feel their healthy 'I' and use their own will to develop it.

Finally I would like to illustrate the fundamental themes in this article with a case history.

Escape from the struggle with food and digestion

Monika is 51 and lives on her own. She has a brother who is two years younger with whom she has little contact. Her father died 13 years previously. Her mother is still alive and her mother's helplessness constantly provokes Monika to look after her. For as long as Monika can remember she has lived in 'survival mode', that is, her financial situation is also just enough to survive. She is very afraid of becoming incurably ill and dying. Her mother had had ectopic pregnancies before she was born and after her brother. Monika often suffers from constipation combined with painful wind. Conventional medicine has diagnosed 'diverticulitis' – small bulges or pockets in the lining of the intestine in which faeces become trapped.

Monika's first intention is: *"Ich möchte gerne, dass mir meine Verdauung friedlich + entspannt dient."* [Word for word translation: "I would-like gladly, that to-me my digestion peacefully + relaxed serves."] "I would really like my digestion to serve me in a peaceful and relaxed way." She starts with the word 'digestion' and immediately the representative says that she does not want to serve, but would like cooperation. Monika resists and does not want to have to bother with this problem as well. Thereupon the 'digestion' withdraws, hurt. Monika feels that she is the victim and is overwhelmed with the situation in which she finds herself as perpetrator.

Suddenly a strong, angry perpetrator part arises in Monika: she wants to kick someone and wants someone to atone and suffer for what was done to her, not having had a childhood, always being alone and having to be there to be of use to her mother. The representative for 'digestion' becomes afraid of her and Monika scares herself with the extent of her destructive part.

Monika now talks about being continually overwhelmed by

171

her mother's demands and those of her other relatives. She is unable to sort out this unfamiliar mixture of feelings and detests the pattern of always having to serve, and always having to be ready to satisfy the needs of others. Contact between 'digestion' and Monika now becomes more trusting and more understanding.

The next word 'serves' turns out to be her maternal grandmother, who was a strong woman with a magnetic personality, a ruler who Monika still secretly admires and who has her full attention, even though she has been dead for 15 years. During the further course of the conversation Monika recognises that she has to decide between her grandmother and 'digestion' to create the conditions necessary to be able to look after herself.

Three weeks later Monika comes to the practice again. She said she was paying more attention to her eating and not shovelling so many sweets into herself. Her digestion alternates between 'alright' and 'mediocre'. Her new intention is: *"Ich möchte mich mit meinem Magen unterhalten, was ihn drückt."* [Word for word translation: "I would-like me with my stomach to-talk, what him presses."] "I would like to talk to my stomach to find out what the matter is." She begins with the word 'stomach' but is unable to identify it as her stomach. The 'stomach' then feels rejected. For a brief moment both think that the situation from the first constellation with the perpetrator-victim split is going to be repeated. But nothing dramatic happens.

The next word 'my' is a large part of her family system including her relations, which completely possesses her and in which she is not seen as a person. There is nothing of her own; she disappears in the needs of the others. What might be hers belongs to the others. The question then arises in Monika: What is mine and what is not? When something arrives in her stomach she realises it cannot be identified and sorted out; it has to be digested because it's already inside her. She recognises the necessity of pre-sorting, psychologically and physically. Previously she had only noticed something after it was inside her and already causing problems.

She sets up 'presses'. This word stands before her like a monument and demands that she differentiate precisely what she eats before she eats it, otherwise there is a danger that not only foreign substances but also her own, what is good for her, might be rejected, and then nothing would nourish her.

Two weeks later Monika comes to the practice again. She says that her digestion has become more peaceful and lighter. She no longer shovels her food into herself, does not swallow her anger as much, and eats far fewer sweets. Overall she is much more attentive and empathetic towards herself. Her new intention is: *"Ich will nix Fremdes mehr schlucken."* [Word for word translation: "I want nothing foreign more swallow."] "I don't want to swallow anything foreign any more." She begins with 'nothing'. That is a part that doesn't actually exist and that she doesn't know. Monika again feels that she doesn't want to deal with it. 'Foreign' is more familiar to her than what is her own. 'I' and 'want' have no contact with each other; in fact all parts have relatively little contact with one another. 'Want' knows, however, that it has a choice, which makes Monika relax visibly. She wants to leave it there, developing a feeling of being able to choose for herself.

Several weeks pass before Monika comes back to the practice again. She says that she is digesting better, that is, "more is coming out". When she feels bad, her eating behaviour also becomes bad. Overall she is sorting substances out better. Sometimes she feels as if her intestines are at war. Her new intention is: *"Was drückt mich im Enddarm?"* [Word for word translation: "What presses me in the rectum?"] "What is the pressure in my rectum?"

The 'me' is relatively indifferent, but wants to assimilate the 'rectum' that has also been set up. The 'rectum' hides under a cover and does not want to have any contact. It says something has happened to it. The 'presses' is a small, traumatised part that has no contact with anyone else, and in its helplessness joins 'rectum' under the cover. On the other side 'in-the' is standing. It also has no contact and feels great anger inside, together with having images of sexual abuse and anal sex. 'What' is alternately scared and empathetic towards the different parts of Monika. Finally the 'question mark' is there and is completely overwhelmed with the information that Monika's mother had an ectopic pregnancy before her, and another one after Monika's younger brother. It recognises the split in Monika and stays in between.

The parts have little or no contact with each other. That means that no stable 'I' exists that can coordinate psyche and body. This is also shown in Monika's sentence of intention, which does not contain an 'I'. The hidden subject of sexual trauma can only manifest itself when the parts connected to it have the confidence to show themselves. This can only happen when a healthy 'I' is present. Until then, anger will rule as a survival strategy, and splits off the trauma feelings that are stored in the rectum. In order to be seen and recognised as truth, these have to make themselves felt as pressing symptoms.

Monika already has access to her 'trauma of identity' and her 'trauma of love'. Her 'trauma of sexuality' is still waiting for her to recognise it and feel it.

References

Brisch, K. H. (2014): *Säuglings- und Kleinkindalter*. Stuttgart: Klett-Cotta

Enders, G. (2014): *Darm mit Charme*. Berlin: Ullstein

Gershon, M. (2001): *Der kluge Bauch*. Munich: Goldmann

Pudel, V. & **Westenhöfer**, J. (1998): *Ernährungspsychologie*. Göttingen: Hogrefe

Ruppert, F. (2015). *Trauma, Fear and Love*. Steyning, Green Balloon Publishing.

Ruppert, F. (ed.) (2016). *Early Trauma*. Steyning, Green Balloon Publishing.

Evelyn Hähnel, who died in 2017, was an alternative practitioner with her own practice from 1994. She studied and practised psychotrauma and identity therapy, body therapy according to Traditional Chinese Medicine, yoga teaching and nutrition counselling. From 2000 to 2017 she trained in Identity-oriented Psychotrauma Therapy and Theory according to Professor Dr. Franz Ruppert. From 2007 to 2017 she led self-encounter and therapy groups, and from 2015 to 2017 she led training seminars with Franz Ruppert in Bilbao, Spain.

BEATE HERRMANN

Severe constipation

Standstill since childhood

Since my childhood I have suffered from severe constipation; it is often so bad that I cannot open my bowels for up to four to six days at a time. When the bowel movement occurs, it happens suddenly, regardless of where I am. And when it happens there is no stopping it. That is very difficult to manage, because I am not always at home when the spasms start. I then suffer the whole day and am physically and psychologically exhausted.

Up until three years ago I successfully suppressed my constipation problem and told myself it was one of those women's problems, and that as my mother also suffered from it, it was inherited. I never asked why I was constipated. In our family being constipated was considered 'normal'. Several visits to doctors confirmed my inherited women's problem; so as far as I was concerned, the cause was clear. As the years passed, my periods of constipation became longer and more unpredictable. Sometimes I had normal bowel movements for three to four months, then again for five to eight days I would have severe constipation. It didn't occur to me to tune into myself regarding my physical symptoms.

Thanks to taking part as a representative in some advanced training in 2014 with Franz Ruppert (I represented the word 'Stillstand' or 'standstill' in someone else's work), I became aware that the contents of my intestines were at a standstill because something was holding them up. In my representative role I could not move from the spot, however hard I tried; I simply could not move. Something in the constellation stopped me. In the work, when I was confronted by another representative looking at me, I clearly saw my mother, just like my own mother, standing before me and demanding that I look after her.

"I would like to hear what my constipation wants to tell me"

Good; I now knew that my gut problems had something to do with my mother, but there was no change in my suffering. The agony of my digestion remained and so I was happy when I was able to go into resonance with my intention in a seminar one day in spring 2015: *"Ich möchte hören, was mir meine Verstopfung sagen will."* [Word for word translation: "I would-like to-hear, what to-me my constipation to-say wants."] "I would like to hear what my constipation wants to tell me." My aim was to get a little bit closer to myself and find out what my constipation was saying to me. Almost all words in the self-encounter were very active. They all talked at the same time and ran about, shouting. An absolute madhouse! The 'constipation' and I (Beate) stood quite still, not moving, as if cemented to the spot. The representative for my 'I' had gone, and was hiding in the corner of the room and was very quiet. To begin with I didn't notice my 'I' and didn't even miss it. My attention was 100% focused on the other words. I was so occupied with coordinating them, organising them, controlling and listening, trying to understand all of them and everything that I did not sense either myself or the 'constipation' and I still had no contact with my 'I'. "Just hang on until they've all calmed down", that was my motto, hold on, just hold on. I recognised myself in my early childhood, and then I also saw my 'I' crouched in the corner, shy and helpless. In this family madness, I started to get a raging headache and stomachache. I felt inside me how my small intestine contracted; as usual I ignored it and continued trying to orient myself in the never-ending madness.

The 'constipation' then said to me: "It's not about me! You want me to say something to you! You don't look at me, you ignore me; your family distracts your attention from yourself." I couldn't get any further in this self-encounter. I had no chance of reaching my 'I'. The distance was huge. But I did see the full reality of my family; that was really the way it was! Everything that showed in the work was true. All I could do in my family

177

was "keep still, endure, hold on, don't move too much, withdraw". But I did take on board the sentence "your family distracts your attention from you", and was happy to have realised this.

Regular bowel movements until . . .

My constipation disappeared shortly after this self-encounter, and I had some regular bowel movements. For the first time in my life I felt freer and more mobile. Four months later however my guilty conscience was plaguing me because I hadn't looked after my mother for a while. After the representative role in 2014 I had broken off all contact with her and my siblings. That did me good but at the same time it hurt. My feeling of 'not belonging' was still there, and on some days I could bear it better than on others. I finally went to see my mother when 'belonging' won the upper hand in me.

Due to her psychiatric diagnosis and the phases of schizophrenia, she lived in an old people's home and needed full-time care, which her partner and we children could no longer provide. I had only been with her for two hours when I had exactly the same symptoms as I had during my self-encounter. My whole small intestine contracted and my head ached. I was sad, but as I could now deal more consciously with myself, I tried again to come into contact with my 'I'. I noticed that, once more, it was not about me. Again, I drew myself back completely – and as a result, I was massively constipated following the visit to my mother, for nine whole days!

During the pain and cramps that accompanied defecation I remembered my first self-encounter work and I realised that, when in contact with my mother, I exhausted myself trying to do everything right for her, to do everything that she wanted, and as far as I was able to be there for her, emotionally, financially and materially. But when I do that I don't have any connection with my 'I' and I become submerged in her traumatic experiences. This fact really hurts me, both physically as well as emotionally. It became increasingly clear to me that there was no chance for me of having my own 'I' when with my mother, and that instead I was subjecting myself, and my body, to an impossible task. I wanted always to do everything for mama, to be the mother to my mama. I had always held myself back, just like the content of my intestines. I clearly felt two parts in me: the little Beate who longed for mama and contact, and the older one who lives in the here and now. They could not have been more different.

Grief and the pain of loss for the family

I had taken a step closer to myself and my 'I', just as I had wanted to, but I had the feeling that I had lost my family. One year and several constellations later, I noticed that I had never had a family at all in reality. I had been unable to develop an attachment to my mother in her womb; emotionally she wasn't there. She was offensive, aggressive and disparaging towards me, shifting the anger she felt towards her own mother, onto me. I had let that happen for all those years and had withdrawn more and more so as to protect myself. I hadn't noticed what my mother, my father and my siblings were doing to me. I longed endlessly for contact, in whatever form.

It was only with Franz Ruppert's method, which I had got to know about in 2009, that I could approach my reality. Further self-encounters followed; I didn't give up, and kept working on the process around my digestion. I began to feel more, and to understand my situation better. I felt how bad it was for me, not having had a mother. I still want contact with my mother, but I have to turn away because it is unbearably painful for me. I had to split and split and split in order to survive, until there was almost nothing left of me.

My mother was psychologically ill, traumatised by war, and had spent half her life in a psychiatric ward. In any contact with my family everything is insane and confused, but my family only had to beckon and I was there doing whatever I could. Afterwards I was always utterly distraught because the connection wasn't good for me. Play the game and you have a family – find your 'I' and you're out. All this was causing my constipation!

And the more I found myself, the more I became, according to my family, the bad one, the cold one, the hard one, who didn't look after everyone else, but, egoistically, only after herself. There were no end of demands, accusations and reproaches. No one wanted to hear me or understand why I wasn't able to sustain the contact any longer. It was very difficult for me not to split my 'I' off again and give in to the demands of my family. Again and again I told myself that I had to withdraw from my family. It's not me who's the perpetrator; it's them!

Deciding to choose me

I made the decision to choose myself, and then I let in the grief and pain at the loss of my family. "Stay with me; don't be distracted; make contact with my 'I'; take myself seriously" – I repeated these words to myself until I could feel them, and it felt very good. My bowel movements gradually became more regular. I was alone, with no contact to my family and yet my defecation was suddenly a daily occurrence. Insane? No, normal!

I was happy, but then things changed. On 10th November 2015 my mother had a heart attack and was taken into intensive care, and my digestion stopped once more. For ten days I feared for my mother's life. I stayed with her day and night, just as I had done as a child. I was focused on her and again I was away from my 'I' and my body, which again reacted by massively holding back.

My mother died with all the family members around her – all except me. I wasn't there. That hurt so much. Why wasn't I? I grieved not just for my mother; I also grieved for myself, for little Beate who had tried for half her life to be with mama, to make contact with her, to be seen and loved by mama. So many injuries have surfaced, from very early trauma up to today. It was all there again.

Today, almost a year later, I perceive my little Beate. I love little Beate as she is, and my constipation too. It is not completely gone, because my intestine shows me straightaway if my environment isn't good for me. The best thing is that I now listen to what it tells me. Franz Ruppert's method 'self-encounter with the help of the sentence of the intention' has activated much in me, and brought me closer to my own 'I'. I continue on my path to autonomy. A strong word; the goal I am aiming for.

Beate Herrmann, born 1965, has diploma in Talk- and Family Therapy with Systemic Competence (DGfS) (*Deutsche Gesellschaft für Systemaufstellungen* German Society for Systemic Constellations). She has completed further training in Identity-oriented Psychotrauma Therapy (IoPT) with Prof. Dr. Franz Ruppert, and has had her own practice since 2006 with individual clients, children and adolescents as well as couples using the intention method. www.anliegenaufstellen.ch

INGRID PERG

When traumas affect the kidneys

"On the psychological level we are all healthy!"

In order to recognise links between trauma and kidney diseases, psyche and body have to be understood as an entity. This approach cannot be taken for granted; it is scarcely rooted in our consciousness. During my research on a dialysis ward, I wanted to know if patients were interested in discovering the psychological background to their kidney disease. Most patients were amazed at this question and couldn't imagine such a connection. One middle-aged woman told me during her dialysis: "My kidney disease is purely hereditary. My mother had it, and my daughter is showing signs of it. I don't want to look into the causes on a psychological level. In that respect we're all healthy!" This statement is illustrative of the taboo in dealing with possible psychological causes of physical illnesses.

Gabor Maté writes that it is well understood in Chinese medicine and in the Indian and shamanic cultures that psyche and body correlate with each other. He relates that, based on medical studies and his own experience, he is in no doubt that suppressed feelings and psychological stress can trigger physical illnesses (Maté, 2003). Babette Rothschild also emphasises that in the healing of trauma, the body and the psyche have to be given equal attention (Rothschild, 2002). I can confirm this assumption based on my long years of working in this field: I have been working for many years with a holistic philosophy and I make use of physical signals as a means of surfacing hidden psychological processes into consciousness. If we use our implicit body memory, where all our experiences are stored from the beginning of our lives, we can come closer to a healthy identity.

Kidney function and kidney disease

Anatomically kidneys are a pair; their main function is to recognise which substances are beneficial for the body, and which breakdown products have to be eliminated from the body as poisons via the urinary duct. They regulate the acid-alkaline balance and are substantially involved in the body's metabolism, hormonal processes, and the circulatory system (Cheers, 2000).

Kidney functions may fail due to anatomical defects, inflammation, infection, narrowing of the efferent urinary tract or through illnesses such as diabetes, obesity and high blood pressure, or if the individual is dependent on kidney dialysis or has to have a kidney transplant. There are currently 80,000 people in Germany who are permanently dependent on a kidney machine, and the number is rising by 5% every year. In 2015 there were 2,195 kidney transplants in Germany alone.[48]

According to conventional medicine, a kidney transplant from a donor within the person's own extended family is most likely to be successful, since the blood and tissue characteristics are the best possible match. In a discussion with Prof. Dr. Otto Mehls, former head of paediatric nephrology in the University Children's hospital in Heidelberg I was told that there could be a considerable risk for an adolescent, if they were in the middle of the process of separating from their parents, and at the same time were to receive a transplanted kidney from one of the parents. In such a situation there seems a possibility of the organ being rejected. If on the other hand a sibling were to donate a kidney, they would often be acting from a sense of duty so as to ensure the survival of their brother or sister. Then the person receiving the kidney might experience a conflict of identity, as he will feel indebted to the donor (Appelsmeyer, 2001).

---

[48] *www.dso.de/organspende-und-transplantation/transplantation/nierentransplantation.html?tx_zvmgallery_pi1%5Baction%5D=download&cHash=791b8b891f54106773a80ae570f64eeb*, www. German Organ Transplantation Foundation / organ donation and transplantation / transplantation / kidney transplantation . . . , taken from website on 15.12.2016.

If infants are born with kidney disease the necessary medical steps must be taken, and psychological causes are not usually considered, although it would be sensible to examine the physical information from a psychological perspective. Epigenetics research shows that traumatic events leave traces in the DNA and can thus reshape the gene activity, which can have an effect not only on the person directly concerned, but can also be transferred to subsequent generations. These modifications can be commonly found in genes that are connected with the metabolic processes of stress hormones, such as cortisol, which is produced by the adrenal gland.[49] Brian Dias and Kerry Ressler successfully demonstrated the inter-generational transfer of trauma with the help of an experiment. They subjected mice to the scent of cherry blossom, which is a smell they usually like, and at the same time gave them little electric shocks. The mice learnt to fear the scent, and repeated contact with it made them fall into a frozen state. Up to the fourth generation of descendants of these conditioned mice reacted with fear to the scent of cherry blossom and also fell into a frozen state, just as if they had been conditioned themselves (Dias and Ressler, 2014).

It has to be presumed that humans inherit these traumas similarly. The traumas of parents and grandparents shape our psyche and can find expression in their children in the form of pathological conditions of the body such as kidney disease. The effects of trauma on the next generation are currently the subject of intense discussion (Baer and Frick-Baer, 2010; Ruppert, 2014). Peter Levine describes how absurd the idea of multi-generational transmission of trauma seemed in the 1990s, however in the last few years research has succeeded not only in demonstrating the existence of such a transfer, but also in documenting the epigenetic, molecular and biochemical mechanisms responsible for it (Levine, 2016).

---

[49] *www.welt.de/gesundheit/psychologie/article122488828/Psychische-Belastung-wirkt-sich-auf-die-Enkel-aus.html.* www. world.de / health / psychology / article122488828 / psychological stress also has an effect on the grandchildren.

The following two case histories illustrate the connections I have found between the traumas of previous generations and the kidney disease of children and grandchildren.

Symbiotically entangled with father and grandmother

Anita came to my practice to discover what the underlying reasons were for her kidney issues as a small child, which had remained undetected for years. They had always been dismissed as stomach aches. This incorrect diagnosis was disastrous for her. The situation became acute when she was four and she lost her right kidney, while an operation on her left kidney restored its function. When Anita looks at pictures of herself as a child at that age, she is unable to identify with them. She told me that she frequently has the feeling of not being able to experience or feel herself, and of not knowing who she really is. She works in a rehabilitation clinic for children who have had a kidney transplant. She is happy with her work. She has a daughter and has been through a bad marriage and now lives alone. In her marriage she had to endure mortal fear, and did not feel that she was seen by her husband. She never had a deep attachment to her mother, who she was now looking after; it was her father who had always been most important to her.

As her intention for therapy work Anita chose the sentence: *"Der Hintergrund meiner Nieren-Geschichte."* [Word for word translation: "The background of-my kidneys-history."] "The background to the history of my kidneys". She didn't write this sentence word after word in a row, but wrote each word vertically one below the other on a piece of paper. She chose a man to resonate with the word 'the', who immediately felt agitated and in turmoil. He said to Anita: "I have to let go of your hands." Anita had seen this man as authoritative and depressing and said that she became very nervous of him. When Anita set up her next word 'background', she chose a woman who stood in a dominant position facing the 'the' and laughed at him. 'The' believed that this representative was his mother and out of fear he had to hold eye contact with her, because otherwise he was frightened of her. He also had backache. Anita confirmed that her father didn't have a good relationship with his mother.

She then chose someone for the 'of-my' in her intention. The person she chose told her that she felt small, and experienced pain and fear that no one could see her, that she was cold and could not see anything in the room. Anita was moved because she recognised herself in this part: "That's what it was like for me back then and what it's still like for me today; I remember." 'Of-my' felt seen and began to cry. 'The' (it seemed to be Anita's father) now remarked that the 'of-my' (Anita as a child) was relieving him of his burden and that his pain was subsiding. He wanted to help her. He felt psychologically better now but was not physically able to help her because he couldn't feel his hands any more.

'Background' (presumably Anita's grandmother) then said that something was pulling her backwards and she was afraid that she would fall into nothingness if she gave in to this pull. Anita then remembered that her grandmother had experienced a lot of violence during her difficult childhood. Her marriage hadn't been a good one either. There was a great deal of violence in her marriage and both she and her husband had been unfaithful to each other.

The client set up the next word 'kidneys-history' as two separate words, as she had written them separately in her intention. The representative for 'kidneys' felt small and abandoned, her heart was racing and she didn't know where she belonged. She sat down in the room next to 'of-my' (Anita as a child) and the two crouched together. Anita said to 'kidneys': "I can't feel you, although I can feel the 'of-my'."

When someone else went into resonance for 'history' they felt like a scared little girl who could not feel herself and had the sense of being stamped into the ground. The resonator insisted that she belonged to 'background', in other words, to Anita's grandmother. She began to whine that no one was there for her and she was completely alone. 'History' (the grandmother as a child) said to 'background' (adult grandmother) that when she speaks she got strong kidney pains, she felt alone and no one would help her. 'The' (the father) then became active again and wanted to take care of and look after the 'history' (his mother as a child). He suddenly felt his hands again and was busy rocking and holding the little one. He said if he could protect 'history' he wouldn't be afraid of the 'background' (his mother) any more.

The 'background' (grandmother) still felt that she had to resist the pull from behind her and stayed beside 'the' (father) and 'history' (grandmother as a child). The grandmother felt as if someone behind her was hitting her on the back. She held onto her son in panic and transferred her child part to him, wanting him to protect her.

Anita's split off parts ('of-my' and 'kidneys') lay weak and alone on the other side of the room. Anita now made contact with both these parts and talked to them. All the other parts watched without interacting with them.

Through Anita's case history we can see that she, through the symbiotic entanglement with her father, who was in turn entangled with *his* mother, was drawn into their unresolved traumas. As a child, Anita's father was afraid of his mother and clung to her childish trauma structures, thus entangling himself symbiotically with her. Then, as a child, Anita in her distress sought emotional contact with her father, as her mother was not emotionally accessible to her. She thus entangled herself in her father's trauma energies. This symbiosis had relieved the father, but he was unable to help her in return because his hands were tied. This constellation also brought to light that Anita was not yet able to feel the part of herself represented by 'kidneys' as it was still too strongly split off from her awareness.

In subsequent sessions, Anita tried to make contact with her own split-off parts, but in order to do that she first had to look at her trauma of identity. Only then could she take the further step and address her 'trauma of love' in which she was entangled with her father.

The most important thing is that my son is OK!

Betty, the mother of a young man, wanted to know why he had had to have a kidney transplant as a child. In her constellation the client chose a woman as a representative for her son. It became obvious that this woman actually represented her, not her son. Only then did it occur to the client that she had also spent months in hospital as a child because of a kidney disease. However, although Betty had been reminded of her own childhood trauma through the work, she was not prepared to go into this realisation any further. She told me in a follow-up discussion that she didn't want to work on that any more. She wanted to leave things as they were for the moment because her son had come through his transplant well.

I can understand this mother very well because, as parents, how do we react when we discover that our children and grand-children are actually expressing our own unresolved traumas with their physical ailments? How do we behave when we realise that our kidney disease is the expression of our ancestors' unre-solved traumas?

To realise that this multi-generational transfer exists is the first step to being able to free oneself from it. However, it also requires a definite decision on our part to confront our own trauma biography. Only then can we come into contact with the 'I' that we have abandoned due to our attachment to our trau-matised parents. Only then can we re-discover ourselves and come to know ourselves as we really are.

References

Appelsmeyer, H. (2001). *Transplantation und Identität*, in Psychomed (2001) 1, pp. 42–45.

Baer, U. & **Frick-Baer**, G. (2010). *Wie Traumata in die nächste Generation wirken*. Neukirchen-Vluyn, Semnos.

Cheers, G. (2000). *Anatomica – Körper und Gesundheit*. Willoughby, Global Book Publishing.

Dias, B. G. & **Ressler**, K. L. J. (2014). *Parental olfactory experience*

influences behaviour and neural structure in subsequent generations, in
Nature Neuroscience (2014) 17, pp. 89–96.

Levine, P. A. (2015). *Trauma and Memory: Brain and Body in a Search
for the Living Past: A Practical Guide for Understanding and
Working with Traumatic Memory*. US, North Atlantic Books.

Maté, G. (2003). *When the Body Says No*. Hoboken, New Jersey, John
Wiley & Sons Inc.

Rothschild, B. (2000). *The Body Remembers*. USA, W. W. Norton &
Co.

Ruppert, F. (2012). *Symbiosis & Autonomy*. Steyning, Green Balloon
Publishing.

Ruppert, F. (ed.) (2016). *Early Trauma*. Steyning, Green Balloon
Publishing.

Ingrid Perg, was born in 1965, and is married with three children
aged 26 (twins) and 10. She has a diploma as a life coach and
social counsellor, is a certified healing masseuse, and has a
diploma as a hypnosis practitioner. She works in her own
practice in Lienz, Austria with individuals and in groups with
trauma-oriented body therapy and with the intention method of
Franz Ruppert. www.ingridperg.at

PATRIZIA MANUKIAN

My breathing, my lungs, my trauma

Breath and breathing

We gasp for air, we wait with bated breath, something takes our breath away, we breathe a sigh of relief, or we breathe fire. We all know the many expressions that are used in everyday language in connection with feelings of fear, joy, insecurity, pain, loss, disappointment and grief. When we are excited we are short of breath. Our breathing is closely linked with our speech, because our voice is formed through our breath. Speaking is voiced exhalation, and vocalisations such as moaning, sobbing, gasping or sighing are expressive variations of breathing.

Many old languages use the same word for breath as for the psyche, the soul or the spirit. In Latin, for instance, *spirare* means 'to breathe' and *spiritus* means 'spirit'. We use the term 'inspiration' (inhalation) when we have a brilliant idea. In Greek the word *psyche* means 'breath' and 'soul'. In Indian teachings the word *atman* (that which breathes) stands for the foundation of the body's vitality (*prana*).

Breathing takes place rhythmically, and consists of two phases: inhalation and exhalation. This constant change gives life its rhythm. Breathing quickly speeds up the heartbeat and more oxygen is carried to the organs; slow breathing slows the heartbeat down. Breathing happens involuntarily. If we hold our breath for a while we soon start to feel mortal fear. Breathing is life; without breathing life stops.

Evolution of the lungs

There are three germinal layers in the embryonic period, from which a human being develops. The innermost layer (*endoderm*) forms the gastro-intestinal tract with the digestive organs, the thymus gland, the thyroid and parathyroid glands, the urethra and the respiratory tract. The middle layer (*mesoderm*) forms muscle and thus involuntary movement. The outer layer (*ectoderm*) forms the central nervous system and the skin. The organism can thus separate itself from its environment and can make contact with the outside world.

The development of the child's lungs in the womb begins from the 30th day from the ventral part of the frontal intestine. This is responsible for the epithelium (epithelial and gland tissue), which lines the respiratory structures. The nascent lung divides into a right and left branch, later becoming the lobes of the lungs. From the 5th week to approximately the 17th week the major elements of the lungs are created, including the bronchi, followed later by the alveoli. From the 13th week of pregnancy the ciliated epithelial cells become visible and the lungs begin their important prenatal function: the production of up to 15ml amniotic fluid daily. By the 26th week the lungs are sufficiently mature for the lung parenchyma[50] to be ready to function at birth.

In the nine months of pregnancy the baby receives all the important nourishment as well as oxygen via the placenta and the umbilical cord. For a short time after the birth, the baby is still supplied with oxygen via the umbilical cord. If the newborn baby and his mother are given enough time to bond externally, the transition from placenta breathing to lung breathing happens naturally and gently (Strauss 2014). The newborn baby gradually calms down from the stress of the birth and the lungs begin a gentle up and down movement and for the first time the alveoli gradually fill with oxygen until they are functioning completely. When this is accomplished, the umbilical cord stops

---

[50] The *parenchyma* is the term in biology for the functional parts of an organ.

the supply of oxygen, no longer pulsates and collapses. The placenta can now be expelled and the umbilical cord cut. From that moment on the newborn baby breathes independently. The lungs start their life-securing function.

The Swiss midwife and nurse, Brigitte Renate Meissner (2001) describes complications arising from caesarean sections that also affect the lungs. During a natural birth the child is squeezed while passing through the birth canal, which presses the amniotic fluid out of the lungs. However, with a caesarean section the baby may have an increased risk of breathing problems caused by 'wet lungs'. Also the emotional shock of the sudden opening of the amniotic sac, being ripped out of the womb and the immediate cutting of the umbilical cord can cause the newborn's breath to come to a halt through the sudden drop in pressure, and lead to feelings of suffocating or drowning as the lungs can still be full of amniotic fluid.

The anatomy of the lungs

The left and right lobes of the lungs are sponge-like tissue. They are spread out due to the negative pressure in the thoracic cavity, which is created in the pleural cavity between the inner layer around the lungs and the outer layer lining the inside of the thorax. The lungs extend upwards a few centimetres above the collarbone and downwards to rest on the diaphragm; they are protected all round by the ribs. Mouth and nose are the two entrances into the lungs, both of which lead into the trachea. Thanks to the larynx and the epiglottis, the trachea is protected from substances entering it that are not gaseous. The trachea guides the inhaled air into the bronchia and then further down into the two lobes of the lungs and then into the increasingly fine branches, the alveoli. The inner surface area of the lungs is up to $70\text{-}80m^2$. In comparison, the surface area of our skin is only about $1\frac{1}{2}\text{-}2m^2$. Our lungs are therefore our body's largest contact organs.

The lungs are covered with two important layers of membrane: the inner pleura lines the surface of the lungs and the outer pleura lines the inner wall of the rib cage. There is a cavity between them that is covered with an extremely thin layer of pleural fluid, which allows both layers to move freely against each other and yet sticks them together, securing the lungs to the costal pleura and ensuring the lungs remain spread out. When the lungs expand and contract in normal inhalation and exhalation, the pressure in the lungs falls and rises and both pleura slide past each other with no friction. If air enters this space it causes the lung to collapse.

Lungs and breathing

The lung is the organ responsible for the exchange of oxygen and carbon dioxide and also for regulating the amounts of each in the blood. Both gases are basically poisonous: oxygen because it can have a caustic effect, and carbon dioxide because it steers the acidic content of the blood into the alkaline range. With each breath we take into our lungs a specific mixture of approximately 21% oxygen, 0.03% carbon dioxide, 78% nitrogen and 1% inert gas.

A breath begins with the inhalation: the thorax lifts and the diaphragm moves downward. In the case of a deeper breath the intercostal muscles contract, thus further increasing the volume of the thorax. Exhalation happens passively through relaxation of the contracted muscles, pushing the air rich in carbon dioxide out of the lungs. The most important control centre of our breathing process lies in the medulla oblongata and consists of an inhalation and exhalation centre. In this area specific neurons control the breathing, thanks to various signals. One is the extent to which the alveoli, which are equipped with receptors, are stretched. The other factors are the chemoreceptors, which measure the composition of the fluid in the medulla oblongata and register the pressure of oxygen and carbon dioxide in the breathing area. This regulates the diaphragm's contraction.

The vegetative nervous system and its two branches regulate the breathing process: the parasympathetic nervous system creates more physical calm and relaxation through the narrowing of the trachea and the contraction of the bronchial muscles. The sympathetic nervous system allows the trachea to widen and the bronchial muscles to slacken, which increases the elasticity of the bronchial tubes and makes the inhalation deeper.

'Diseases of the lungs'

Within the European Union 'diseases of the lungs' are responsible for an eighth (12.5%) of all deaths and at least six million admissions to hospital.[51] In the EU 600,000 deaths are caused every year by a 'lung disease'. More than half of these deaths are put down to 'lung cancer' or 'COPD2016' (chronic obstructive pulmonary disease) – usually in connection with nicotine consumption.

Modern medicine does recognise that there are also risk factors for lung disease in early childhood, for instance not breastfeeding, the mother taking paracetamol during pregnancy and complications during the birth. But medicine does not research any further into the reasons for this and what effect these traumas have on the psyche and the body of the newborn baby or the toddler. Tobacco smoking is also a trauma survival strategy that can have been caused by an early trauma.

Breathing rhythm and breathing therapies

Observing the rhythm of our breathing and our lung symptoms can help to identify important information concerning our psyche and our emotions (Morschitzky and Sator, 2013). When we cry, our diaphragm moves fitfully, thereby allowing the inner organs to relax. The outward breath that follows helps us to let go of the grief. The same thing happens when we laugh. If a person can no longer laugh or cry, he is unable to express his feelings. He is not allowed to let go, to say no or to accept something he would like to. He has difficulty breathing, and

---

[51] www.europeanlung.org/assets/files/small_whitebooks/lung_health_in _europe_facts_and_figures_master_german_aw.pdf, taken from the website on 27.12.

respiratory diseases develop accompanied by intestine issues such as constipation and a weak bladder. He neither dares to let go nor to let himself go.

Attempts to alter the breathing have led to many forms of therapy and different techniques. From India come, for instance, kundalini yoga and hatha yoga, where 'connected breathing' plays a key role. Wilhelm Reich based his body therapy on breathing, followed later by bioenergetic and biodynamic therapeutic approaches (Lowen, 1979). Breathing is used in different forms to retrieve early emotional experiences. Two examples of this are 'holotropic breathing' and 'psycho-energetic breathing'. Both methods come from rebirthing, when hyperventilation is used to enable adults to immerse themselves in their birth experience (Dahlke and Neumann, 2000). Eva Middendorf's breathing therapy has also made a significant contribution to the deeper understanding of breathing (Marlock and Weiss, 2006). However, we do have to bear in mind that the form of our breathing can constitute a reaction to trauma. In such a case it makes little sense to work only on the symptoms without looking at the underlying trauma. Breathing therapy without reference to the trauma only addresses the symptoms and not the cause.

'Asthma' and contact

The deeper origin of so-called 'asthma' lies in a person's lack of touch, contact and relationships, or in their fear of relationships. 'Asthma' is a spasm in the exhalation of breath. Exhalation can be seen as relaxation and release, and as a desire to open up to someone. However, if we are afraid of someone, we cannot breathe out in a relaxed way in their presence, and we feel the need to protect ourselves from them and to close up.

Some of my constellations that have related to the asthma-dynamic have shown that it can be a case of constraint and suffocating closeness. When breathing in there is also the danger of sucking in the trauma energies of another person. With small children it is usually the trauma energies of their own mother, the impact of which can take their breath away.

The following is an example from work with a client:

Giovanni's intention is to discover why he has continually had chronic asthma attacks since his childhood and why he suffers from severe hay fever every spring. During the constellation the events of his birth and his relationship dynamic with his mother come to light: he was born at seven months, together with his stillborn twin sister, who died at five months. The birth was very traumatic and the client spent the first three months in an incubator. His mother was also traumatised and in a state of shock as she had not been aware until then that the other child would be stillborn. She developed a high fever and it was only after four days that a treatment for intra-amniotic infection was considered. During this time Giovanni had no contact at all with his mother.

His mother's traumatic experience is shown in the constellation as a part that lies with its whole weight and the pain of its loss on the newborn child and almost suffocates him. Only when a healthy part of the client pulls the small newborn child out from under the mother can the client finally breathe out and free himself from the state of shock.

Pneumonia and loss of attachments

Pneumonia, or inflammation of the lungs, is often the expression of deep despair that can lead to the loss of the will to live, because the individual feels abandoned by a loved person (Rainville, 2010).

Roberto, 48, comes to my practice wanting to know why he got severe pneumonia twice in quick succession when he was 36. Since then he has frequently had respiratory infections. The client first chooses a representative for '*pneumonia*'. The representative feels his breathing is restricted, but has no direct connection with the client. Asked what he had experienced before his illness, the client replies that his boss had told him a short while before that he would be transferred to a new department the next day. Thus, after working for 15 years with the same colleagues, a completely new environment with new colleagues awaited him. The next day he got the first symptoms of pneumonia: severe bouts of coughing. He then spent two months in hospital, where he was able to recover from this shock and the feeling of powerlessness concerning his transfer.

As further representatives, he set up his 'I' and the 'why'. His 'I' immediately had unpleasant feelings towards the 'why'. The latter seemed to him to embody a sinister person. Roberto said it could be his father, but that he didn't have any real connection with him. The 'why' feels he is an authoritarian man who denies any blame. He feels like a headmaster. Roberto now starts to recall his father's life history: At the end of the war, when Roberto's father was five months old, his own father was killed by a bomb attack outside his front door and before his mother's eyes. When he was 10 years old, his father was sent to boarding school.

For the 'I' this information is liberating and he finally connects with Roberto. It becomes clear that the pneumonia expresses a symbiotic entanglement with the shock his father experienced. The violent death of the grandfather caused Roberto's father endless pain, the more so as the whole family fell into a state of shock from one moment to the next. Going to boarding school had robbed the young boy, who frequently had respiratory problems, of his last hope for familial contact. His transfer to another department had triggered in the client his unconscious entanglement with the feelings of his father. With his pneumonia he unconsciously re-enacted the situation of powerlessness and desolation.

"Why do I choke ...?"

A little while ago I did a constellation myself with the intention: *"Warum verschlucke ich mich selbst am eigenen Speichel?"* [Word for word translation: Why choke I me myself on own saliva?] "Why do I choke on my own saliva?" My 'I' was immediately in my pre-birth trauma. It lay on the floor, hunched up and breathing heavily, coughing and gasping for air. It held its hands on its navel and stammered: "I'm suffocating. My body is being poisoned. I'm dying ...". The closer the due date of my birth came for my mother, the more her fear and stress levels increased. I was her fifth pregnancy and the first one to make it alive to the birth date. After two miscarriages and two stillbirths, my mother's fear of giving birth to another stillborn child was indescribable. Fear initiates the release of adrenaline that constricts the vessels and causes all the muscles to tense. The supply of nourishment and oxygen was thus increasingly strangulated. My mother was also given sedatives that increased my suffering immeasurably. As a result of my pre-birth distress, the doctors carried out a premature emergency caesarean section, which was an additional shock for my mother and for me.

The violent episodes, where I choked and almost turned blue, have since become more infrequent. If, today, saliva occasionally gets into my windpipe, I can cope with it much better and more quickly.

References

Dahlke, R. & **Neumann**, A. (2000). *Die wunderbare Heilkraft des Atmens*. Munich, Integral.

Lowen, A. (1979). *Bioenergetics: The Revolutionary Therapy That Uses the Language of the Body to Heal the Problems of the Mind*. USA, Penguin.

Marlock, G. & **Weiss**, H. (2006). *Handbuch der Körperpsychotherapie*. Stuttgart, Schattauer.

Meissner, B. R. (2001). *Geburt – Ein schwerer Anfang leichter gemacht*. Winterthur, Brigitte Meissner.

Morschitzky, H. & **Sator**, S. (2013). *Wenn die Seele durch den Körper spricht*. Ostfildern, Patmos.

Rainville C. (2010). *Il grande dizionario della metamedicina*. Mailand, Sperling & Kupfer Editori S.p.A.

Strauss, D. (2014). *Abnabelungs- und Wiederanbindungsprozess als letzte Phase der Geburt*, in F. Ruppert (Publisher) *Early Trauma*, (2016). Steyning, Green Balloon Publishing.

Patrizia Manukian was born in Zurich in 1967 and graduated as an alternative practitioner, kinesiologist, craniosacral therapist and counsellor. She has lived and worked in Italy since 1991. She has attended advanced training with Prof. Franz Ruppert, and since 2010 has worked with constellations for groups and individual work in Italy. www.ritrovaresestessi.com

AURORA WOLF

My eyes, my trauma, my I

What our eyes say about us

We come into the world with our eyes and our vision. We see
shapes, movement, colours, we have spatial perception, we
explore our environment, analyse and make contact. We can see
objectively or with 'heart'. Contact through sight lets us connect
with others. Often a single moment is all that's needed, for
instance 'love at first sight'. We can turn our gaze inwards, look
inside and speak with our eyes. We look through rose-tinted
glasses, are blinded by love, don't deign to look at the other
person, we scowl, make ourselves invisible, have our own
viewpoint. We say the eyes are the reflection of the soul. We say
we can see the character of another person in their eyes. What
shines through in our eyes are feelings from the present or the
past. Here we see the eyes of a child, shining with joy, or
someone who looks desperately unhappy; there a piercing
glance, demanding or angry; then eyes gentle and wide.

A trauma is also clearly visible in a person's eyes: his gaze is
empty and frozen, as if one could see through him. He is in shock
and full of horror. Longing and fear are written in his eyes. These
are eyes that look dead; they are recognisable when a person
laughs but his gaze says something completely different.

How our vision functions

Our visual organ possesses a tremendous ability to transform
visual impressions into images we can use. Light enters the eye,
goes through the pupil and falls onto the retina. There, light-
sensitive sensory cells turn optical stimuli into neuronal signals.
The information is transmitted through the optic nerve to the
visual cortex in the brain, where the images are processed. The

optic pathways from the right and left eyes cross at the hypophysis in the diencephalon. We are able to see with just one eye, but it is only with two eyes that we can see spatially. To enable this, the two images from both eyes have to merge; otherwise it leads to squinting or double images. Physically, the blink reflex protects the eye from foreign bodies; psychologically, the eyes are closed when the visual impressions are overwhelming.

The quality of our vision is connected with our mental state and is dependent on our habits. Vision is closely linked with our sense of balance, our posture and movement. A tilted head, tense neck muscles, pelvic misalignment or abnormal foot position result in an imbalance in the tone of the eye muscles and influence the vision. Orthodontic treatment can affect vision. Pressure and stress in the body increase the intraocular pressure. The proximity to the brain, the connection with the cerebral membranes, the cranial nerves, the proximity of the optic pathways to the hypothalamus and the hypophysis reveal that the eye function is involved in many processes of the body.

The eye is formed on both sides of the head at the end of the neural groove when the unborn child is just two millimetres long (Blechschmidt, 2012, p.112). If stress affects this stage of development, it is significant for the further development of the eyes and the quality of vision. In the mother's womb the child can perceive light and dark as well as soft red tones through his still-closed eyes. From the seventh month the child opens his eyes, is able to identify shapes and blinks as a reaction to a light source. After birth the child has to continue to practise his vision. The infant learns to focus, to differentiate between faces and to see spatially. When the child is two to three years old the learning process is almost completed. From the first moment, the child seeks eye contact with his mother. Her eyes are an important fixed point for his future life. His mother is the most important person, the one he bonds with and who provides direction. She is the model for his emotions and behaviour. His mother's eyes are his mirror. He forms his 'I', his identity, on her. The child reads his mother's eyes and senses her feelings. The child even perceives things the mother is unconscious of, things she has suppressed. If his mother's eyes show joy, sorrow, anger, fear, emptiness, absence, or rejection, the child will orient himself according to these feelings to be close to his mother.

Eye disorders and natural vision

Eye disorders range from refraction anomalies such as near-sightedness, far-sightedness, astigmatism, night-blindness, squinting, glaucoma, cataracts, and inflammation of the optic nerve papilla through to physical phenomena that also affect the eyes, such as diabetic retinopathy, eye disease with tinnitus and cold extremities, diseases of the central nervous system in connection with apoplexy, tumours, metabolic disorders, and sexually transmitted diseases. Surgical procedures, accidents, tension in the system of cerebral membranes, can all result in eye problems.

Nowadays in industrialised nations, poor eyesight is the norm. Natural vision is 80% distance and 20% near. In industrialised nations it is the opposite. According to the Allensbach study of 2014, 63.5% of the population wear glasses, 5.2% wear contact lenses.[52] In 2010, a survey of Bavarian company health insurers identified that, of 850 kindergarten children, every third child had problems with their eyesight. Eye tests carried out on nomads in Tibet and Morocco revealed that these indigenous peoples frequently have very good far and near eyesight into old age (Büchler and Becker, 2011, p.139). Frank Schaeffel points out in FOCUS Online that only 5% of the Amazon Indians are shortsighted. That the eye can be very flexible is shown by the example of the Moken people, who are able to narrow their pupils to such an extent that they can also focus under water.[53]

---

[52] www.zva.de/brillenstudie, www.zva.de / glasses study, taken from website on 14.12.2016.

[53] *www.focus.de/gesundheit/ratgeber/sehen/fehlsichtigkeit/kurzsichtig/kurzsichtigkeit _aid_20649.html*, www.focus.de / health / vision / defective vision / shortsighted / shortsightedness, taken from website on 27.11.2016.

Methods of healing eye problems and defective vision

Ophthalmology: Ophthalmic medical practitioners prescribe glasses for short- and farsightedness. Astigmatism is corrected with cylindrical lenses. Eyes are lasered and operated on and a lot of money is earned. Medication is also frequently prescribed. Conventional medicine still disregards the fact that muscles move the eye, and muscles can be under tension or over-flexible, and that the whole body is involved in visual function, which is dependent on the condition of the individual.

Holistic methods: Common to all holistic methods is the fact that nutrition, physical and movement behaviour, and the immune system all play a role in good vision and the health of the eyes. Suggested treatments are cleansing and intestinal detox. In Chinese medicine the functional cycle of the liver is closely connected with the eyes. Boel's eye acupuncture is supposed to stimulate self-healing. Nutritional supplements are provided for eye therapy. There are also options combined with psychology such as kinesiology, Feldenkrais forms of movement therapy and training with body, voice and eye coordination. From an osteopathic viewpoint as well, treatment of the eyes is only meaningful with a holistic approach.

The foundation of all eye training is the method of Dr W Bates. Vision trainer Leo Angart, who also refers to Bates, points out: "It is important to work on difficult issues from the past, otherwise it can happen that one experiences short-term phases of clear vision, although these are never permanent." (Angart, 2004, p.73)

My experiences with the intention method

Why am I shortsighted? Why is my field of vision restricted? Why are my eyes inflamed? Why is my internal eye pressure too high? How long have I had the problem? How has my quality of life been changed by it? Working with the intention method according to Prof. Ruppert, I have learnt a technique that I regard for both myself and my clients as the fundamental element in health work with people, and which can give me answers to such questions.

In identity constellations, relating to one another happens via eye contact. There are comments such as: I can see you clearly. I can't see you, there's just emptiness. I can see through you. One eye looks right; the other looks left. I can't look at you. Eyes are shut, look down to the ground or upwards. The lack of reference becomes perceivable. Working with the sentence of the intention is a huge chance to become clear about oneself; to live with all the qualities of one's own identity. The relationship to oneself is reflected externally.

In my professional and personal life I have always looked for ways to uncover the reasons for physical symptoms in order to be free of them. My experiences with eye issues and vision problems have shown that the causes lie:

- in the pre-, peri- and postnatal areas,[54]
- in the lack of, or weak 'I'-structure,
- in the confusion of identity,
- in the trauma of love,
- in the lack of contact and reference,
- in the perpetrator-victim dynamic.

It is also clear that eye problems can be caused by the use of medication, drug- and alcohol addiction, or for instance by the mother suffering from measles during pregnancy.

The steps to health are:

- perceiving and accepting one's own truth,
- deciding for oneself,
- finding reference to oneself,

---

[54] Frühgeborene: Früher Schmerz hinterlässt langfristige Spuren' (2010), *www.innovations-report.de/html/berichte/medizin-gesundheit/fruehgeborene-frueher-schmerz-hinterlaesst-163385.html* 'Premature babies: Early pain leaves lasting scars' (2010), www.innovations-report.de / html / reports / medicine-health/premature-early-pain-leaves-163385.html.

- connecting with oneself,
- becoming aware of oneself anew, and in general
- working on one's own trauma biography.

A symptom often has several levels and needs several attributions. We have to continue to work on it until the symptom is no longer required.

Below are the case histories of two people I have worked with over an extended period.

Case history: Anna

Anna has had a squint since early childhood. She has 60% vision with glasses. The usual treatments had not been successful. Anna saw everything double. When she was 18 she had an operation to shorten six eye muscles, which went well, but the cause of the squint was not resolved. Anna was also always ill. There was no flow to her life. She had physical therapy and psychotherapy, but it was not until she experienced the intention method that the cause of her eye disorder was revealed and her difficult life explained: At the very beginning of her life she had experienced not being wanted, and her mother taking medication during the pregnancy. The birth process itself had also had a direct bearing on her squint.

In certain situations, Anna noticed the way one eye slipped inwards and her vision became significantly more blurred. On one occasion when she was driving on the motorway, she suddenly saw almost nothing with her left eye. In her constellation on this subject it became clear that Anna had been helplessly sandwiched between her parents and their perpetual arguments. The small child within her was loyal to her father and looked to him for skin contact. But her father had sexually traumatised Anna when she was a baby. She had been orally raped and her left eye was pushed forcefully inwards. Anna lost consciousness and, close to death, she withdrew.

Anna now sees 100% with glasses. She is becoming increasingly stable in herself, which has resulted in sharper, clearer vision. Both eyes are now definitely in focus.

Case history: Zoe

Zoe suddenly became shortsighted when she was 40. Professionally she was a successful woman in a male-dominated profession. She says of herself that she is lacking a life of her own. She has had a lot of experience of therapy and has been becoming familiar with the intention method for a month or two. She writes on the whiteboard: *"Ich möchte Kontakt zu meinem Augenleiden"*. [Word for word translation: "I would-like contact to my eyes-disorder"] "I would like contact with my eye disorder". The following process then develops:

'I' takes Zoe's hands and says: "I am not looking at you. It's strange: my eyes are looking mainly upwards. I would like to have everything under control. It's like that . . ."

Zoe: ". . . because there was nothing below."

'I': "Yes. What am I doing here?! It hurts my eyes if I look downwards. I prefer being Johnny Head-in-Air."

Zoe takes a soft toy for 'eyes' and a yellow ball for 'disorder, and puts them down a metre away. 'Eyes' are very close to 'disorder'.

'I': " I feel better when the 'eyes' are there. I can look at them. They're neutral. 'Disorder' makes me angry."

A representative replaces the yellow ball as a resonance for 'disorder': "I can hardly lift the ball. It's unbelievably heavy. That's my belly."

Zoe laughs.

'Disorder': "That's not funny. I'm touching the ball as if it's a raw egg. I feel a bit proud. It feels like being pregnant."

'I': "It has something to do with me. It draws me to it."

'Disorder': "I'm not proud any more. What's happening to me?"

Zoe's head hurts.

'Disorder': "It's already very big and a burden. If I were pregnant it'd be quadruplets. Breathing is difficult."

'I': "Progesterone."

'Disorder': "I can only stand or lie."

Zoe says: "I had a miscarriage when I was 35 and afterwards the doctors convinced me to have IVF. They told me it'd be great. The hormones were too much for me. I went from a size 10 to a size 18. I felt pumped up."

'Disorder': "Hugely pregnant. It paralyses my arms and legs. I'm getting pressure in my head, behind my ears."

Zoe: "Tons of injections. I couldn't take it. Hormones changed my body and my psyche."

'I': "That's too much for the eyes! They've been affected by it!"

'Eyes' looks up for a moment, and sticks closely to 'disorder'.

Zoe: "I was a guinea pig. It was the early days of IVF treatment. The hormones were more important than the woman receiving them. The doctors ended up only talking to my husband. I didn't have a voice any more."

'Eyes': "I get stomach cramps and my vision becomes blurred when I hear the words 'guinea pig'."

Zoe: "Those are the hormones, not the pregnancy."

'I': "It looks as if the shortsightedness was caused by the hormones."

'Disorder' can't stand the stress any longer. It gets stomach and belly cramps. Zoe recognises that. She slowly becomes aware of the situation underlying her eye disorder; that it's about her and her distress, and what happened to her.

Zoe sets up 'my'. 'My' stands in front of 'disorder' and next to 'eyes': "That's my belly, my eyes. Oh, something's coming out of me. I feel bloodless, I'm going to faint."

Zoe confirms: "I was bleeding and drove to the clinic. They told me it wasn't anything alarming and I could come back the next day. The next day I got up, haemorrhaged and lost the child. I collapsed and almost died. My husband wasn't there. When I was in hospital for the curettage, my neighbour in the ward was a woman who wanted to have an abortion and who was constantly moaning. It was too much for me. I left the clinic and was once more completely alone with everything."

'I': "Unbelievable! Now you know why your eyes were directed upwards. You couldn't look. There was a connection to the IVF treatment, pregnancy, the lost child, to your distress."

For the first time Zoe was able to perceive that she herself was in great distress. The other words from her sentence of intention identified her as her mother ('*would-like*') and indicated an early trauma of Zoe's ('*to*'). The '*contact*' was ready; Zoe has to make the decision to establish contact with herself.

In the next few weeks the truth about Zoe's past came to the surface more and more. Her mother had had two sons before her, both of whom died the day after they were born. Through the attachment to her mother, Zoe had taken on the loss trauma. She had experienced a loss trauma and existential trauma herself, and also received abusive treatment from doctors. Decisions were continually taken over her head. Zoe was alone with everything. When she was first pregnant, at 17, her mother put her on a flight to England to have an abortion. Her father wasn't told. At 21 she was pregnant again. Her husband couldn't cope with it, and her parents-in-law organised the abortion. When she was 35, Zoe only told her husband she was pregnant when she was already in the fourth month. It was at that moment that she miscarried. When she became shortsighted she began to smoke and developed multiple internal organ diseases.

Zoe became aware of her internal perpetrator-victim dynamic. Questioning the eye-related issue gave her the opportunity to access the traumas back to her early childhood. All Zoe's physical symptoms improved unmistakably. Zoe only needs her glasses now when she's driving.

Over the course of the next year Zoe wanted to access her feelings further. She had developed a close relationship with a refugee. Her husband and she looked after this refugee as if he were their own child. Zoe said she had maternal feelings she had never experienced before and she wanted to act them out. With this decision and Zoe's positive feelings, stressful resonances also came into play. The refugee, who was, in a way, adopted, was like a mirror of her own trauma experiences. His mother had left him when he was six. As an adult he sought contact with his mother and was rejected again. In addition to his life-threatening experiences of war, his own mother's rejection was the deciding factor that had made him leave his country. His life history triggered memories and feelings in Zoe from her own biography: belonging nowhere, loneliness, being alone, existential threat, rejected by the mother. She also experienced her last pregnancy when she was 40. She felt the child's passing and her own distress and life threat.

The connection with her own abortions became clearer to Zoe. Despite all the previous issues, she now feels a vitality she hasn't felt before. Another session showed her mother's intense rejection that led to an attempt to abort Zoe. Again it made sense of the lack of relationship with her parents and grandparents.

Zoe notices that she still finds it difficult to look people in the eye. She recollects her first work on her eyes, when her 'I' had its eyes directed upwards. It occurs to her that a Bible lay next to her grandparents' bed, in which she slept. All the pictures had interested her and the big, strong man – God – had from then on become her point of reference. When she was four, she had loved going to church to see this man. For others, Zoe was the strong one, and always there. She had never been able to stand up for herself.

She is now set on sensing herself, feeling herself, putting herself in first place and doing what she wants.

References

Angart L. (2004). *Vergiss deine Brille*. Munich, F.A. Herbig.
Blechschmidt E. (2012). *Ontogenese des Menschen*. Munich, Kiener.
Büchler, U. & **Becker**, K. J. (2011). *Freude am Durchblick*. Munich, Kösel.

Aurora Wolf is a singer, functional vocal coach, movement therapist and cranio-sacral osteopath. 2009-2012 she completed training in Dr Franz Ruppert's method with Birgit Assel, and followed this with further training with Franz Ruppert. Since 2011 she has worked in her practice in Aichwald near Stuttgart. www.0711-31577708.de

ANNEMARIE DENK

Chronic pain as a consequence of trauma

What is pain?

When clients talk of their 'pain' they can mean many different things: afflictions, ailments, problems, injuries, sickness, depression, grief, stress, wretchedness, misery, anguish, burden, troubles, despondency, melancholy, distress, vexation, harm, torment, worry, sadness, burden, sorrow, heartache, tribulation, agony or ache. Just looking at this list of words shows us that pain is not only a physical condition, there is an emotional side to it too. Although medicine has widened its scope in recent decades to allow a more bio-psycho-social understanding of pain, a physical cause for pain is still usually sought. The majority of Internet or newspaper articles, and even specialist literature, only shed light on the physical side of pain disorders. The psychological side often still remains hidden in the background.

Anyone who has suffered from severe pain over a prolonged period wishes to be rid of it. In Germany there are between 12 to 15 million people who seek ongoing medical support to cope with their pain. Four to five million of these would describe their symptoms as severe.

The 'International Association for the Study of Pain' (IASP) defines pain as "an unpleasant sensory and emotional experience associated with actual or potential tissue damage, or described in terms of such damage" (Sendera and Sendera, 2015). This definition stresses that pain also has an emotional component. It gives equal weight to physical pain and to pain without a physical cause.

Acute pain

Pain is a warning sign pointing out when something is dangerous and there could be a threat to our life. Acute pain is temporary and confined to a certain area. It protects us from injury, for instance when a child quickly pulls his hand away from a hotplate because of the pain, thereby preventing further burns. Acute pain prompts us to look for the cause. How important this warning system is becomes apparent when it is absent. People who do not feel pain are in great danger, because they do not feel anything when they injure themselves.

Where does chronic pain come from?

We speak of chronic pain when a constant or recurrent pain lasts from three to six months or longer. It often bears no relation to the original injury and appears in many different forms. For people with chronic pain, the pain has lost its original function; it is exaggerated, agonizing, stabbing, burning; it renders the individual helpless and makes them a victim. Most people with chronic pain have experienced years of suffering. Frequent visits to the doctor, seeking second opinions, taking medication (with side-effects) and even numerous operations have not brought any success. The pain is still there but the original illness or injury can no longer be detected. The pain has become a separate phenomenon in itself.

We now know that the regions for emotions and physical pain lie in the same area of the brain. In a study Eisenberger and Liebermann (2004) demonstrated that social rejection activates the same processes in the brain as physical pain. In a review article, Ralf Nickel, drawing on a large number of cases, proves a clear connection between traumatisation in early childhood and chronic pain in adulthood (Nickel, 2017). A hundred years ago people still believed that babies felt no pain. We now know that human beings feel pain long before birth. The nervous system develops from the ectoderm around the 17th day of pregnancy. An unborn child can feel pressure at five and a half weeks and can feel a pain stimulus via the skin, while still in the womb (Krüll, 2009). Hermann and Flor, amongst others, have shown in a study of school age children that those who experienced severe or prolonged pain as premature or term infants, during the period in which the pain processing system was still developing, would have a higher perceptual sensitivity to pain in their brain activity well beyond infancy.[53]

Pain and lovelessness

Jutta suffered for years from 'chronic pain syndrome' with pain of the cervical and lumbar spine as well as sciatic pain. When she was a child she spent five years in a children's home. When as a very young child she was left on her own she was often not given anything to eat for long periods. In one session, working with the intention method Jutta wanted to explore the cause of her pain. It became clear that her mother was beaten by Jutta's alcoholic father during her pregnancy with Jutta, and was also kicked in the belly. The person resonating with the word 'pain' experienced herself as Jutta's traumatised child part, who was extremely afraid and who drew back from the beatings and wanted to make herself as small as possible. Following the session, her mother and grandmother confirmed to Jutta that that was exactly how it had been.

Jutta was gradually able to recognise, allow and feel the fear of her early trauma experience, and this led her to experience a marked relief. She may not be completely pain-free, but she is now able to cope much better with her pain.

Since this first intention process approximately three and a half years ago, Jutta has continued to work on herself and her earlier depression has disappeared. She has been able to replace the crutches she had been using with Nordic walking sticks that she uses "just in case". She says: "I now know that I didn't get any love and today I am responsible for giving myself this love."

The theory of pain memory

The stimuli for both pain and touch reach the thalamus via neurons in the skin and muscles and are relayed by the spinal cord dorsal horn directly into the area of the brain responsible for sensitive stimuli, the somato-sensory cortex. Joachim Bauer (2002) describes a study by Niels Birbaumer and Herta Flor who carried out tests to prove the existence of pain memory. If sensitive stimuli are received, neural networks are created within this area. If an equally strong pain stimulus is received by two sets of patients, it has been shown that those with chronic pain react much more strongly than healthy test patients. These neural networks are not only formed in the cortex area, they also create interconnections to the cingulate cortex in the limbic lobe of the brain, and in the front area of the brain this pain is also emotionally assessed. So the physical pain is stored in the brain but through networks an emotional interpretation of it is stored too. An area of pain memory has been created; the physical symptoms can heal, but the networks created in the brain remain.

As a consequence a normal pain stimulus can cause an increased pain signal. These pain networks may remain silent for years, not causing any symptoms, particularly in periods of a well-balanced, happy life. But if a crisis or a psychosocial stress situation occurs, such as a separation, divorce, death of a family member or a stressful situation at work, the emotional areas of the brain begin firing. If an individual is sad and feels rejected, the pain memory can flare up again (Bauer, 2002; Egle, Hoffmann, Lehmann and Nix, 2003). This emotional stress switches onto the path that was long ago created to the cortex and is expressed as physical pain. As the original unbearable event is often split off into the unconscious, there is nothing to point to this. The individual does not know what the matter is, cannot find any connection and cannot explain the pain.

An endless search for the cause then begins, usually only looking at possible physical causes. Generally patients demand an organic reason for their pain and do not want to be dismissed as a psychosomatic or a psychological case. For the most part, doctors dispense classic medical treatment, in other words medicinal, physiotherapeutic and surgical. Only in 5% of cases is psychotherapy recommended, as a Germany-wide study with 900 pain patients has shown (Sendera and Sendera, 2015).

Risk factors leading to chronification

According to various studies in the USA, Sweden and Germany, almost 50% of chronic pain patients have experienced severe violence in their biography (Bauer, 2002). Amongst these experiences have been torture, beatings in childhood, ill-treatment, abuse, neglect, rejection, exclusion and lengthy periods of pain or stress in early life. Such traumas always leave painful traces, whether the trauma is physical or emotional. Even witnessing a trauma, when for example, a sibling is beaten, increases the activity in those areas of the brain assigned to pain, via the mirror neurons (Stelzig, 2016).

Survival strategies springing from an earlier trauma show a number of characteristics that encourage chronification. These are anxious behaviours, constant psycho-vegetative tension, a tendency to catastrophize, avoidance behaviour, long-lasting perseverance, trivialising, constantly ignoring stress limits, an inability to perceive and express feelings, passivity, self-recrimination or fatalistic thinking (Wachter and Hendrischke, 2016; Adler et al, 2017).

Patients I deal with in a pain clinic and in my practice are unable to provide an organic cause for many of these pain disorders. In about 30% of the cases no organic reason is found even after protracted investigations. They suffer from 'somatoform disorders', i.e. pain that cannot be explained physically. Some of these patients have whole-body pain and some have pain that moves around the body.

Violence and pain

From the beginning Ruth had experienced violence from her mother, both in the womb and after her birth, as far back as she could remember. The father did not stop the mother from beating the children, but demanded that they behaved and not provoke the mother.

Ruth's history of pain had begun 20 years previously, after the birth of her children, when they kept annoying her and Ruth had suppressed her impulses to hit them. She had never wanted to treat them the way she had been treated. Since then she had experienced pain in different parts of her body. First of all she had pain in her shoulder with an unknown cause. For 15 years she had severe stomach ache, again for which no cause could be found. She also complained for ten years about an unexplained pain in her right hip. Five years ago she experienced pain in her right knee and right foot, as well as her ankle. For the last two years she has had pain in her right finger. Early in 2016 she could hardly sleep at night because of pain to the right of the navel area. Over several weeks she had repeatedly felt extreme pain, with no clear cause.

As Ruth did not want to take any painkillers she looked into trauma work and came to me. In several sessions with the intention method over the course of several months, she was able to recognise what a huge impact her mother's beatings had had on her and how she had distanced herself from her self and her feelings. As she gradually allowed this to be reality and was able to feel it emotionally, her pains became less and less.

As a child, Ruth could not show her physical pain because this would have made her mother beat her again. She had no choice other than to suppress her pain so much that in the end she no longer consciously experienced it. She created survival strategies such as "dreaming herself away" and "playing dead is easier" so that she didn't feel the pain. As a child she had an accident with severe concussion when she almost died. She says that back then she would not have been sad if she really had died.

When she was 12 and broke her leg in two places she said she would have preferred not to come back into this world.

In further work with the intention method, Ruth recognised that her mother had been behind all her pain. She had been cold to her, and unpredictable and angry, and had beaten her for no reason from when she was very young, so that Ruth wanted to die rather than endure her mother's beatings any longer. When resonating for the word 'pain' I felt in my heart the pain at the icy coldness of her mother. I was close to tears. Suddenly this sensation changed, and I felt like I became the mother: I was furious with Ruth for no reason and wanted to humiliate her; I even wanted to hit her.

A few weeks later Ruth wrote to me: "This last process made me realise how strong the armour was that I had donned. Until this point I had looked at my experiences through rose-tinted glasses and had not dared to admit to myself how violent the blows were to me. I can now say: Yes, that is how this pain feels emotionally! That was and is a crucial experience for me and a great release, no longer having to hold onto this armour. I am only now becoming aware of how severe all this was for me. And this awareness, this clarity, is like a release. It feels as if metal manacles that have been binding me have now split open and been cut off. It's like a liberation. I am now myself and don't allow myself to be irritated by others who in the past have been able to upset me with their taunts. I stay in myself and am simply I." Later on, Ruth classified her pain as much lower on the scale: "I only feel a shadow, as if something was there once, but I feel almost no pain now. My quality of life has improved enormously."

In my experience, people who find an organic cause for their pain are at a disadvantage, rather than an advantage. Organically caused pain is only treated with conventional medicine, and people are therefore unlikely to look at the underlying psychological conditions. These patients insist on medical treatment, demand painkillers, are quick to accept operations and will keep hunting until they find a medical answer in the doctors' practices. I know many pain patients who, through the course of several operations to relieve the pain, have gone on to develop more serious internal diseases. However, a pain patient who has been diagnosed with an organic cause can have experienced a trauma, just like any other person. A part of him may well suspect that his unprocessed issues will be frightening, and in his effort to avoid them he will hold onto his physical pain disorder as a trauma survival strategy. However, every time he has an operation and every time he takes medicine, he might be adding to his traumatic injuries.

Why am I so stubborn?

Nicole, 54, has suffered from severe headaches since she had meningitis when she was four. These had intensified massively after a brain haemorrhage with an operation and accompanying temporo-mandibular joint pain. Nicole had tried various pain therapies. She goes to psychotherapy and practises relaxation techniques. Sometimes she feels a little better, but then it gets worse again. She doesn't want to take painkillers any more because of the massive side effects. Finally the headaches get so bad that she wants to try, with the help of a muscle relaxant[55], to loosen up the tense jaw and mouth muscles. She hopes that this will reduce the pain.

Nicole picks up the muscle relaxant from the chemist. However, as the thought of taking the medicine makes her feel unwell, she doesn't take it straightaway. At this point she comes to me for a one to one session with the intention: "*Warum bin ich so verbissen?*" "Why am I so stubborn?" The representative for 'stubborn' purses her lips and clenches her front teeth so that nothing bad can enter her mouth. This clenching in the form of "shutting her mouth" causes tension in her throat, neck and head areas after a few minutes. She feels like a little baby just a few weeks old. The representative for 'why' recognises that she is trying to spit something out. And she is appalled that she was

---

[55] Substances that bring about a reversible relaxation of the skeletal muscles.

given something to send her to sleep and silence her cries. The representative of Nicole's 'I' immediately sits down and says that she barely has any sensation of herself any more and feels as if she is "out of it".

After her birth Nicole's mother gave her to her maternal grandmother as she had to go to work. Nicole was an unwanted baby and was scarcely breastfed. Nicole's grandmother was addicted to pills. She couldn't cope with Nicole as a little baby. At that time the grandmother had been taking Valium to calm herself down. Following her experience in her constellation Nicole could well imagine that her grandmother had put Valium into her bottle so that she didn't cry so much. As a baby she had developed her survival strategy of pressing her mouth and lips together so that nothing bad came into her mouth. When Nicole realised what was happening, the muscles around the front of her mouth were increasingly able to relax and loosen up. She says that she now notices every bit of tension and can correct it. She is also happy that she now recognises that her panic when she was in an intensive care ward three years previously and, without asking, someone put a painkiller into her mouth, was connected with this early experience.

Nowadays, chronic pain is regarded as a bio-psycho-social occurrence and treated in a diversified way. The patients are familiarised with pain and stress management, psycho-education, relaxation techniques, enjoyment training, movement therapy, Feldenkrais, yoga, Qigong, and other methods that are supposed to support the patients in finding their own path out of the pain. However, Nicole's case history shows that, depending on the form of the early traumatisation, muscle relaxation processes can provoke survival strategies– for example "I have to keep my mouth shut!" – thereby increasing the pain even further. Treatments aimed solely at relaxation, without being aware of the traumatic underlying causes, can thus lead to pain symptoms increasing.

New findings about the brain and its workings show that the many pain-intensifying networks and neurons in the brain can keep altering, depending on the way the nerves and synapses are used. Pleasant images, or imagining how the neurons that are firing pain are dwindling, and using constant practice and training to distance oneself from pain, allow the brain to modulate towards a sense of wellbeing and reduced pain (Doidge, 2015). However, if an unprocessed trauma is the cause, it will continue to have an adverse effect, reducing the sense of wellbeing and not allowing calmness and equilibrium to develop. The elaborate processes of visualisation and mentalisation are then nothing more than a further trauma survival strategy.

Why do I have different pains every day?

Susanne, 57, has had various different pains since she was 17, starting with a dull pain in her left arm. When she was a child she had problems with her posture. In the years that followed she experienced tension in the cervical vertebrae with inter-vertebral disc protrusion. She has suffered all her life from spinal curvature. Susanne was the youngest child born to parents who were traumatised by war. She was a wanted child, at least by her father, although he had wanted a son. Her mother hadn't wanted any more children. Her mother was rapidly overwhelmed, lashed out and behaved in a cold manner towards her daughter. Her mother began to show signs of dementia when she was 52 and soon needed nursing care. At that time Susanne was 18 and had to help with her mother's care. Her mother seemed weak and needy after she became ill, although at the same time her unpredictable behaviour and impatience frightened Susanne. When Susanne was 33 her mother died.

Susanne had an accident when she was 20, causing a whiplash injury, which led to a worsening of her cervical vertebrae problems as well as pain in her shoulder and arm. When she was 30 she had a skiing accident with an injury to her thumb, a splintered bone and a tendon injury that healed. Afterwards she kept having mild back pains due to a deformity called lumbar scoliosis, which increased massively when she separated from her partner, a year after her mother's death. In

2002 another skiing accident caused a cruciate ligament rupture and a torn ligament. There was also meniscus damage to her left knee, and time after time pain in her right knee; in 2014 an operation to straighten the medial meniscus cartilage damage, in 2004 for the first time suspected rheumatism, in April 2015 a diagnosis of rheumatoid arthritis. Since then Susanne has consistently had severe pain in her joints as well as for years pain in her knee and back due to her existing spinal curvature, and pains in her shoulder which have in part been caused by her past falls.

Susanne has been taking cortisone for some time, and finally rheumatism medication for the severe pain, although there hasn't been a noticeable improvement. She also does rehab sport, which is important for her, but doesn't improve the pain. She also has psychotherapy.

In a trauma session working with the sentence of intention, it became apparent that Susanne had not completely come to terms with the relatively early death of her mother, and was not able emotionally to let her go. At the same time she suppressed her anger towards her mother who had only shown coldness towards her, and felt guilty because her mother was ill. In the end, this anger was directed at herself. Psychologically, Susanne felt easier after this work, but did not notice any improvement in her rheumatism issues or any decrease in pain.

There followed a further one to one session with the intention: *"Warum habe ich jeden Tag unterschiedliche Schmerzen?"* [Word for word translation: "Why have I every day different pains?"] "Why do I have different pains every day?" I am in resonance with Susanne's 'I', and I don't want to take part any more. As the 'I', I want to live and don't want to have anything to do with the dead; I don't want to dig for worms in the earth any more, I just want to live. I don't want to have anything to do with Susanne while she is still occupied with the dead and the past. I also don't want Susanne to come any closer, because all her baggage will come too. Susanne herself reacts enthusiastically towards the 'I', likes it and thinks it is good that the 'I' doesn't want anything to do with the past. Then she becomes defensive, she doesn't want to accept that the past is no longer important. At that, the 'I' moves further away from Susanne and tells her again that it does not want to have any contact with the past.

Susanne now sets me up as her 'pains'. As 'pains' I don't feel any pain. I feel I am being waited on and I like it. I feed off Susanne and her service and wish for all the gifts, including the medicines that feed me. I feel as if I fill out the whole room and I have a strong connection to Susanne whom I regard as my servant. I feel above everything, like a goddess. I occupy the whole space. Susanne recognises me in my role as 'pains' as her mother, who had let herself be waited on hand and foot, and didn't bother about anything, not even about Susanne. As 'pains' it is all about me, it is I, I, I. Susanne now feels angry towards her mother, but doesn't express her anger any further.

Now Susanne wants to discover what lies behind 'why'. I change into this position. As 'why' everything hurts everywhere, sometimes here, sometimes there; I am in pain and feel overwhelmed. Everything is too much for the 'why': it is weak and can no longer stand up. It stands between Susanne and her 'I' and finally sits down, overwhelmed, before it breaks down. It crouches by the chair, thirsty and hungry as if in a desert, and can't cope any more. 'Why' is silent, has lost its nerve, sees the beatings and no one really sees it.

Susanne now has an intense impulse to hit the 'pains', to struggle against the 'pains' (which stand for her mother), but just makes a boxing gesture. She is frightened of her anger, frightened of knocking the 'pains' over. Susanne has never dared to do that. She had to behave. Her father used to say: "Don't annoy your mother, she's ill enough".

Susanne now sets up 'have'. In this resonance I feel "What has happened to me?" I am sad; my arms hang down; I'm dejected. I am completely in the role of victim; I'm a helpless little girl and I don't know what the matter is. I am wretched and have nothing. It is only when, after a while, Susanne realises that 'have' is her as a little girl, completely alone and wretched, that feelings well up in her. She weeps. She says that she doesn't want it to be like that any more. She wants to be close to the little girl and is determined not to hang onto the past any longer.

The day after the constellation Susanne says that she woke up for the first time for many days with no pain, and that no pain developed during the day either. This completely pain-free state lasts for two further days. In the next four weeks Susanne repeatedly feels mild pain in her lower back, which disappears quickly. Since the constellation she has had no excruciating pain. The stiffness in all her joints and the pains in her knee remain much better to this day.

The aim of these four case histories is to give encouragement. It makes a great deal of sense to really look at the body's pain in relationship to its emotional origin.

References

Adler, R. H. et al (Publisher) (2017). *Psychosomatische Medizin*. Munich, Urban & Fischer.

Bauer, J. (2002). *Das Gedächtnis des Körpers*. Frankfurt/M., Eichborn.

Bauer, J. (2013). *Schmerzgrenze*. Munich, Karl Blessing.

Doidge, N. (2015). *Wie das Gehirn heilt*. Frankfurt/M., Campus Verlag.

Egle, U. T., Hoffmann, S. O., Lehmann, K. A. & Nix, W. A. (2003). *Handbuch chronischer Schmerz*. Stuttgart, Schattauer.

Eisenberger, N. I. & Liebermann, M. D. (2004). *Why rejection hurts: a common neural alarm system for physical and social pain*, in Trends in Cognitive Sciences (2004) 8, pp. 294–300.

Krüll, M. (2009). *Die Geburt ist nicht der Anfang*. Stuttgart, Klett-Cotta.

Levine, P. A. & Phillips, M. (2013). *Vom Schmerz befreit*. Munich, Kösel.

Nickel, R. (2017). *Chronischer Schmerz und frühe Traumatisierung: Wissenschaftliche Evidenz in der Behandlung sinnvoll nutzen*, in Trauma (2017) 1, pp. 6–14.

Sendera, M. & Sendera, A. (2015). *Chronischer Schmerz*. Vienna, Springer.

Stelzig, M. (2016). *Die unterschiedlichen Säulen einer individuellen Schmerztherapie*, in C. Pieh, R. Jank & A. Leitner (2016), Schmerz – eine integrative Herausforderung. Weinheim, Juventa.

Wachter, M. v. & Hendrischke, A. (2016). *Psychoedukation bei chronischen Schmerzen*. Heidelberg, Springer.

Annemarie Denk has a degree in social pedagogy, is a therapist for systemic individual, couple and family therapy. She also has health education qualifications and has completed medical studies (Ulm/Munich). In addition she has trained in hypnotherapy according to Milton Erickson, trauma therapy, and advanced training in Identity-oriented Psychotrauma Therapy with Franz Ruppert. She has spent many years working in medical practices (focusing on pain, relaxation, unfulfilled wish to have children, psycho-oncology, healing singing) and in the multimodal pain therapy of the Paracelsus Clinic in Munich. She has an independent practice working with individual consultations, groups and seminars. She also has a teaching position at the University of Applied Sciences in Munich. www.medibalance.com

MARTA THORSHEIM

Psychotrauma and skin diseases

Skin as the expression of our inward self

A person who feels well and happy has red cheeks and a rosy face. Someone who is unhappy, tired and overworked is pale and has black rings under their eyes. A person whose skin itches and feels as if it's burning usually doesn't feel well internally either. We can also tell if a person is healthy or ill by their hair. The hide or fur of an animal also gives a good indication: healthy animals have healthy skin.

The cosmetic industry provides us with any amount of creams, oils, liquids and scents to make us appear healthy and radiant. But, in the same way as a house, giving the outside a coat of paint does not alter the dilapidated condition on the inside. The way we treat our own skin reflects how much more store we set on appearance over reality. We can think of our skin as an indicator pointing to unresolved trauma.

What is psoriasis?

In my childhood older family members used the expression "the nerves are playing up" to explain the link between the psyche and skin diseases. It was a well-known phenomenon in my family that some members had 'psychological complaints' and others had 'skin diseases'. The cause of these two ailments was never questioned. They were simply accepted as 'family illnesses', which just happened to affect us. When we started to learn about DNA this was used as an explanation – it was in our genes.

In my work with Identity-oriented Psychotrauma Therapy (IoPT) I have found that the medical diagnoses received by clients and seminar participants have frequently improved or even completely disappeared, in the course of their work.[56] From that I conclude that traumas express themselves in individual physical ways and that healing requires recognition, empathy towards oneself and self-love. It is also important not to lose oneself in contact with others. As soon as an individual's healthy part begins to grow, his trauma survival structures are no longer active enough to find expression in physical illness.

For many years, Franz Ruppert has shared this knowledge with us in Oslo in his courses and seminars. When he invited me to write a chapter for this book I was delighted. I chose the subject of skin diseases because I had experience of it in my family as well as through my clients. The case history I have selected concerns a severe case of psoriasis, i.e. more than 10% of the body is affected.

'Psoriasis'[57] is the medical name given to a systemic illness that causes an imbalance in the immune system and is thus classed as an autoimmune disease. In a reference book for skin diseases I find the following information: "Many skin diseases are characterised by an increase in the immunological activity of the skin. A prescription is therefore often given for medicines that weaken the immune system, such as Cortisol, Prednisolone, Azathioprine and Ciclosporin."[58] In the last few years a range of new medicines has come onto the market with specially developed antibodies that block defined signal molecules. These are often described as biological medicines. Their price, because of side effects, is economically and in human terms very high.

Course participants and clients with chronic skin diseases have related that, despite years of using cortisone creams or tablets, light therapy and/or biological medicines, the treatments

---

[56] I am grateful to all participants who have taken part in IoPT seminars, to the students who took notes during the therapy sessions, to Grace Adelaide Andersson for making a fair copy of my hand-written notes, and to Bianca Saupe for translating the Norwegian contribution into German. You have all contributed to IoPT work in Norway – thank you.

[57] Photos of this skin disease can be found on the internet at, for example, www.psoriasis-netz.de/bilder/psoriasis-schuppenflechte

[58] https://sml.snl.no/hudsykdommer

have only managed to alleviate their symptoms temporarily. The use of creams or tablets had led to sporadic improvement or no improvement at all, or just achieved some temporary relief. Many give up and bear their pain silently – from an itching rash to abscesses all over the body, under the arms, in the vagina, in the mouth, the ears, under the feet, on the nails, on the face, the scalp, etc. They describe their suffering as painful, shameful and humiliating. Many clients are afraid of showing their skin disease openly. They hide it under clothing, creams and make-up.

Lisa: "I want me"

Lisa is a course participant in her 40s – a nurse, mother, and divorced. Sometimes her psoriasis is so much to bear that she doesn't know if she wants to go on living. Her whole body bleeds: behind the ears, under the arms and in the crotch. Blood and cream spoil her clothes. Lisa grew up with mother, father and siblings in a Christian household. An outsider would think everything was perfect.

When Lisa takes part in an IoPT seminar she first talks about her terrible nausea that began when she decided to take part in the seminar. She also relates that when she is under pressure, her skin reacts with symptoms, particularly on her forehead along the hairline, and under her arms. "I have to keep looking after myself, otherwise I have an outbreak. Recently I have put myself under a lot of stress, and I felt as if I could hardly breathe."

Lisa formulates her intention: "I want me" and writes it on the flipchart. The first representative she chooses from the group is for the word 'I'. 'I' removes all her jewellery, looks at Lisa and says: "I want to, but I don't know if I can." Lisa begins to cry; she looks at 'I' and her legs start to tremble and she says: "I am so scared!" while she and 'I' hold hands. 'I' feels nauseous. Lisa stands with her legs apart.

The process continues and 'I' comes into contact with the feeling that she is either inside a bubble, or that there's a bubble between her and Lisa; that this bubble influences how she feels and that Lisa is outside this bubble. Lisa says that something has to come out of her, and touches her crotch. 'I' looks at Lisa and says she feels panic "deep within her". Lisa now comes into contact with a feeling of retching and a conversation develops between the two of them, in which 'I' speaks of latex gloves and of something that is put deep into her throat, past the sphincter at the top of the oesophagus. Lisa sinks to the floor and cries. 'I' says: "I'm going out" and hides behind the flipchart. After a violent bout of crying, 'I' comes back. Lisa and her 'I' are in contact again. Referring to the key words 'latex gloves' that were pushed into the throat, Lisa tells of being sexually abused by her father and her brother when she was little. But 'I' looks at Lisa and says: "Yes, but there's more. We didn't get enough air."

The process continues and the two are in good contact with each other. Lisa cries occasionally and 'I' can now cope with that. She remains in contact with Lisa despite the information about the sexual abuse, the lack of air and something being pushed down the throat. Lisa herself senses that this has something to do with her own birth, and cries. She says that she recently received documents concerning her birth, in which she read that, due to differences between her blood and her mother's blood, she was separated from her mother two hours after the birth and taken to a children's ward. She was then alone in hospital for 10 days. Blood samples were taken from her temples. She doesn't know if anything more was done. When I ask if she would like to hear my understanding of the process she replies that she would.

As I see it, this process shows Lisa's pre-birth trauma (Lisa's legs tremble; the 'I' is in a bubble) and a resulting separation from her self ('bubble' between Lisa and 'I'). I also see an identification with the mother (Lisa is very afraid and stands with legs apart and her hands in her crotch, where something is supposed to come out) and a further split ('I' goes behind the flipchart). If there was a blood transfusion after the birth, Lisa's bleeding points to this early trauma. Lisa agrees with my understanding and says that this has been very enlightening for her.

The latex gloves can be an indication of the hospital staff putting a finger into Lisa's throat to free it of mucus. Lisa now understands the "Yes, but there's more. We didn't get enough air." The statement of the 'I' is a reflection of her experience immediately following the birth. Her nausea also stems from this early experience. The sexual abuse she suffered later is "the same sort of trauma" in terms of her mouth and danger of suffocation.

Lisa had worked on parts of her trauma biography in several identity constellations before, for example on being sexually traumatised by her father and her brother in her early childhood, and on the violent upbringing she experienced with her parents, and had reintegrated the split-off parts from this time. Lisa no longer needs her survival strategy as much: the strategy of being a good girl and being submissive. Her suppressed anger, which she often expressed through sarcasm and humour, was also weaker than before, after the feelings from her original trauma-tisation that had caused the anger came to light and she recognised them.

Until that moment, Lisa had never gone so clearly into resonance with her prenatal trauma, the birth trauma and the stay in hospital following her birth. She is glad that she has emotionally touched the part that had prevented her from coming into contact with a prenatal part of herself. This prenatal part clarified her own trauma in the early bonding process with her mother, whose fear of giving birth became Lisa's fear. The mother's trauma feelings had become superimposed on Lisa's 'I'.

In the closing part of this constellation Lisa told of her suppressed anger, which was primarily directed at her mother who could not look after her. She now stated clearly that this was a very appropriate anger. Her healthy 'I' now has more space and her healthy will is also growing.

A few weeks later Lisa reported that her skin disease had completely disappeared following her previous identity constel-lation. This was the first summer since she was 12, in which she had been able to go bathing in a public place. Her clothes and bed linen were no longer covered in blood from her wounds, her migraines were less frequent and weaker and her burnout syndrome had disappeared. She now had a lot of energy and it was steadily increasing.

She also said that she still developed a slight rash if she put too much pressure on herself when she was with her family. It feels right to Lisa that she had separated from her 'I' before she was born and that she instead identified with her mother's 'I'. It was important to Lisa to see that this birth experience also fitted into her trauma biography and, because it had taken place pre- and peri-natally, was anchored deep within her psyche. From this experience she now realises that the process of self-healing carves out its path without her having to do anything.

From other clients I have become aware of skin diseases that they may have borne for years, and which heal and disappear when they have worked on their trauma biography. Traumatic birth processes in particular, which were painful for the clients, and connected with feelings of disgust and early physical assaults (which could also have been medical procedures) triggered their skin inflammation. The parents' influence on the skin inflammation becomes clear when it worsens following the client's visit to their parents.

When I think about Lisa's many diagnoses, her skin disease, migraines and the professional burnout, I ask myself: Could this have been prevented if Lisa's parents had received good therapy after the stillbirth of their first child? If they had been able to work through their grief and other parts of their trauma biography before they had further children? I also ask these questions in the hope that, in the future, IoPT can contribute to prospective parents' psychological preparation for parenthood.

Marta Thorsheim is a psychotrauma therapist (IoPT) and a trainer in her own practice at the Institute for Traumawork in Oslo. She organises the International Advanced Training in IoPT conducted by Franz Ruppert. www.iopt.no

THOMAS R. RÖLL

My teeth, my trauma, my I

A little boy plays in the sandpit

He is completely absorbed in the game he's playing, when the toe of a shoe suddenly and violently kicks him right in the face. The boy screams with pain: one of his front teeth has broken off. His mother runs to the crying child and tries to comfort him. But the child can only focus on the terrible pain in his mouth. After a long walk of five kilometres to the dentist, the wound and the tooth are taken care of. Years later the tooth dies and root canal treatment is carried out.

This experience in my childhood had a decisive influence on my choice of dentistry as my profession. I have now had my own practice for 30 years and I have come to know the effect traumatisations in dental, oral and orthodontic areas can have on the whole body. Having my tooth taken out 30 years after the accident was the last possible treatment after many attempts of therapy. Afterwards I stayed in bed for a week because the after-effects in my body were so massive. During this time I recalled many traumatic experiences and the physical symptoms I had had during my life.

Many years later I suffered from severe, recurring back pain. During an imaginary journey through my body I wondered if here as well trauma might be the underlying cause. I had been involved with the constellation method for some years, and I recalled a workshop with Franz Ruppert in which I had taken part while attending a congress. The subject of the workshop was trauma constellations and it had impressed me. So, 10 years ago, I began training with this constellation method, which has since developed rapidly. It became a journey to the traumatic backgrounds of my symptoms and to myself. I now have 10 years' experience in the application of this method with many patients and clients. Constellations of the Sentence of the Intention based on Identity-oriented Psychotrauma Theory and Therapy (IoPT) have become a very effective and complementary therapy method in my dental practice.

Today this method enables me to recognise the connections between physical complaints and their underlying psychological causes, which is often the only way to ensure dental therapies are possible and effective. I am no longer surprised that through these self-encounters from 'identity trauma' to 'trauma of sexuality' (Ruppert, 2016), all forms of traumatisation can appear, entering the client's awareness one way or another via their teeth, jaw or mouth.

The dentist – simply a technician?

There is a saying that the whole person is always hanging on to each tooth. So, as dentists, we do not see isolated mouths and teeth, but people with their whole body and their personality. Thus, the dentist not only has to be proficient in dentistry and materials technology in order to treat teeth, mouth and jaw. Rather, the interaction of the teeth with the organic system and their connectivity with the whole body is of significance to the holistic dentist (Gleditsch, 1994). In addition, the dentist should also be familiar with psychological interactions, because the dentist-patient relationship is fundamentally of a psychological nature: two personalities encounter one another with their different concerns, motives and expectations and have to find a common way forward (Wühr and Koch, 2013).

One of the key requirements for successful therapy is clear communication. It is very helpful for both parties if the patient asks for work to be done that demonstrates his own understanding of his symptoms. Further suffering is frequently caused by the patient's illusory expectations as well as by the dentist's false estimation of his therapeutic opportunities (Raith and Ebenbeck, 1986; Wolowski and Demmel, 2009). This frequently results in a perpetrator-victim relationship that might have been avoided by transparent clarification of the psychological implications of the work and the dentist's understanding of the reciprocal psychological and physical interaction. The suffering is not only prolonged by this, but also frequently hugely exacerbated. This has also been demonstrated repeatedly in the special seminars that Franz Ruppert and I have held since 2012 in Ulm, where the focus is on 'problems with the teeth and trauma'.

Development of the teeth

The milk teeth and permanent teeth begin to develop approximately 40 days after fertilisation of the egg cell. In the fifth embryonic week, two dental ridges develop on the epithelial cells of the upper and lower jaw, each with 10 milk teeth buds. In the fourth embryonic month the first hard substances are formed. In the postnatal phase, the milk teeth will have erupted by the child's third year, and the roots will have developed. From about the child's sixth year the permanent teeth begin to appear and by the age of 13 the period of mixed dentition is usually concluded – we then speak of permanent dentition. Finally, between the 18th and 25th year, so-called wisdom teeth can appear, although in some cases they are absent.

Development of the teeth and jaw can be disrupted in the embryonic phase due to environmental influences, or if the mother is ill or taking medication (Leonhardt, 1981; Schroeder, 1996). In the same way, traumatisation of the unborn child by the mother, for example due to an attempted abortion, can lead later to considerable issues with the masticatory system, for instance in the form of the loss of all the teeth followed by atrophy of the jaw.

Epidemiology of 'disease' patterns

Dental patients come to the practice with the following 'disease' patterns: 10% somatic symptom disorder, 11% dental treatment phobia, 4–8% bruxism, 3–5% craniomandibular dysfunction (Kleine-Tebbe, 2009). Persistent somatoform disorders frequently occur as a result of dental treatment, for example following a tooth extraction, root canal treatment or prosthetic treatment. Psychosocial factors are often given as the cause of pain chronification, with stressful events and traumatisations being mentioned particularly frequently. Certain dental indications, such as chronic pain, clenching or grinding of the teeth, tinnitus, material intolerance and allergies, gum problems and dead teeth, can be caused or stimulated by traumatic experiences. It therefore seems crucial to me that a dentist undergoes further training to be in a position to recognise when patients are psychologically stressed, and to be able to establish a therapy concept to react appropriately to these patients. This includes, above all, in-depth information and advice prior to each therapy. In addition to specialist professional skills, successful treatment requires social and didactic skills and a great deal of empathy. Even so, it repeatedly becomes apparent that it is difficult for a dentist to understand the complexity of symptoms. The attempt to remove psychologically caused symptoms through dental treatment alone usually exacerbates the patient's condition.

Teeth and trauma

From my own personal trauma biography and my experience during 30 years of dental practice, I have observed that teeth and trauma are very closely linked. The traumatic experiences that many people have with dentists are often the consequence of a very much earlier trauma. This can be a trauma of physical or sexual violence, or 'trauma of love', or even going back to the prenatal phase as 'trauma of identity'. As a result of splitting off unbearable feelings, these traumas can appear later on in life as re-traumatising experiences during dental treatment.

Approximately every sixth patient is very fearful of going to the dentist (Wühr and Koch, 2013). Aetiologically, we frequently see early childhood stress such as traumatisations and attachment disorders as well as dysfunctional learning processes. A dental treatment phobia can develop, for instance, if an early negative experience of dental treatment leads to intense fear and avoidance behaviour when faced with further treatment.

Case history: Hannelore

When Hannelore first comes to my dental practice, she tells me that the fact that she is afraid of dentists is actually her biggest problem. A year previously she had lost a partial crown and six months previously half an incisor had broken off. She had tried several times to be treated by other dentists, but her fear had prevented her. She weeps while talking to me but remains composed and tells me that she has had traumatic experiences. The possibility of overcoming her fear with the help of my focused advice and constellation work seems to her to be the chance she has been looking for. Hannelore gains so much trust from this conversation that I am then able to look at her teeth. After explaining in detail my findings and the possible consequences of not going forward with treatment, she agrees to provisional dental treatment.

When we meet a short time later in a consultative meeting, Hannelore says that during my treatment she initially felt that she wanted to die, but that passed quickly. She then tells me the reason for her fear of dentists: when she was about 40, Hannelore was told by her mother that she (the mother) had had to marry the person who was supposedly Hannelore's father, although she loved his younger brother. She had to marry the older and first-born brother because his parents demanded it. She also had to give up her first name and her religious denomination. Ten years later, Hannelore's aunt (her father's sister), tells Hannelore that her mother became pregnant with her after being raped by her grandfather. In raping Hannelore's mother, the grandfather had wanted to show his son how to beget a son, as the mother's first child had been a girl who, in the eyes of the grandfather, was worthless. The grandfather was severely depressed and feared by all because of his quick temper and his violence. Socially, the grandfather and the grandmother were strict Protestants, but highly regarded. Her supposed father and his younger brother were regarded as weaklings in the family. Above all, Hannelore was angry with her mother because as a child Hannelore was responsible for ensuring that the grandfather did not kill himself.

When Hannelore was four years old, her mother had handed her over to her grandfather, so that she herself was no longer raped. Hannelore had become used to repeatedly being sewn up following her grandfather's sexual abuse. This was done by her father's sister, who was a gynaecologist. The worst thing for Hannelore, however, was having an abortion when she was 12 years old, after becoming pregnant by her grandfather. The abortion was carried out by her great-aunt, also a gynaecologist, together with her aunt. She was severely berated and beaten by both women because she had become pregnant. With the distress of the anaesthetic and her powerlessness came the feeling of wanting to die. She gets the same feeling of powerlessness today, and the feeling of wanting to die, when the dentist's chair is put into a reclining position.

Only when Hannelore was 13 and the grandfather was suffering from dementia, did the rape, which the whole family until then had allowed and at the same time denied, finally stop. She began to study in her early 20s. At the same time she started therapy as an outpatient, although she thought she should really have received inpatient treatment. Her further relationships with men were amicable and platonic because sexuality was no longer possible for her. She became a clergywoman but gave this profession up after a few years. Today she works as a counsellor with children and adults and is proud that, despite this trauma, she has managed to lead a seemingly normal life.

In the course of a seminar, Hannelore sets up her intention: *"Ich möchte dem massiven Gefühl der Angst und Hilflosigkeit begegnen und erfahren, wie ich besser damit umgehen kann."* [Word for word translation: "I would-like the massive feeling of fear and powerlessness to-encounter and to-find-out, how I better with-it manage can."] "I would like to encounter the massive feeling of fear and powerlessness and find out how I can cope with it better." Hannelore asks the resonator for 'powerlessness' to lie on the floor and she moves some distance away. She feels bad seeing this person lying stiff and helpless on the floor. She then sets up her 'I', who also lies down on the ground. Hannelore reacts angrily and does not want to see her 'I' being needy and a victim. However, the 'I' does not feel needy, but feels stable and with a healthy core. At the same time Hannelore's anger towards the 'I' creates a feeling of separation. In the further course of this work Hannelore is able to come closer to her 'fear' that she feels behind her anger. Finally, a profound sadness rises up within her and she begins to weep. She gently approaches her 'I' who then feels better. The 'I' tells Hannelore that it has always waited for her and is now open to her.

This new and unexpected image gives Hannelore a good feeling of being able to take further steps for herself with this form of work. She now understands how, through her traumatisations and the resulting splits, although she has survived, she has lost contact with her healthy and stable 'I' part.

Pain

Patients frequently come to the dental practice because they are in pain. It is important for the dentist to recognise different causes for the pain so that the appropriate therapy can be found. In oral medicine, according to Wühr and Koch (2013), we differentiate between nociceptive pain, neuropathic pain, psychogenetic pain and mixtures of these. In acute nociceptive pain, pain receptors in the peripheral connective tissue are irritated to such an extent that overriding centres perceive the pain. We speak of a symptomatic warning sign whereby the cause at the point of pain can be located and treated (for example by a new filling or a crown with hyperocclusion). Following treatment, the biological systems usually regenerate. With chronic nociceptive pain, the above-mentioned system is also activated. However, in this case there is not one single cause in one specific location but there are several chronic disruptive factors in different parts of the body (for instance vaccination stress, infections which have not healed completely, heavy metal stress, etc.). Over the course of the individual's life, the body's self-regulation is overloaded. Treating the painful area is then no longer sufficient but provides only symptom relief at best.

Neuropathic pain is also usually chronic. Peripheral and central parts of the nervous system that process stimuli are diseased or damaged irreversibly. Here we see, for example, neuro-dermatitis, multiple sclerosis, herpes zoster etc. Patients with chronic pain often suffer with mixed forms of the pain mechanisms described. Dentists are generally well trained in treating pain that has one definite and local cause. However, over and above that it is appropriate if dentists act professionally when the form of pain is mixed, by facilitating a co-therapy with psychologically trained therapists. Perpetrator-victim entanglements can thus be prevented and further suffering for the patient can be avoided.

'Bruxism'

This term is used to describe activation of the chewing muscles in the case of aggressive emotive behaviour patterns, by grinding and clenching the teeth. When doing this, an extremely high force is released by these muscles: measurements of 200-300kg force have been recorded in nightly teeth grinding. These forces do not occur otherwise in a person's life. They also affect neighbouring muscular and joint structures in the head, throat and neck areas as well as in the regions of shoulders, arms and back. These forces can lead to muscular and joint pain (Wühr, 2008).

Case history: Marion

Marion would like to have a constellation on "Why do I grind my teeth?" She says she feels like a replacement product of mother and father. Twins, boys, died at birth and her parents had not worked through this loss, but simply moved on and had her as a replacement child. She also has an older sister and a younger brother. She says her parents pay no attention to her as a girl – but all the more to her brother who was born after her. She has clenched and ground her teeth during the night for years, which are painful as a result. Marion believes this comes from aggression, but she doesn't know where the aggression originates.

Marion's constellation convincingly demonstrates her inner split because she didn't receive the love from her parents that she would have needed for herself and for healthy 'I'-development.

The parents did not grieve the loss of their sons or work through it. A further pregnancy functioned as a replacement for the feelings that were never expressed. But the birth of another girl, Marion, wasn't the replacement the parents were looking for. Their sadness and anger caused Marion's split.

Many years later the symptom expresses this inner split and has therefore also taken on the replacement function of not having to sense feelings. On the one hand Marion is grinding herself down between the parents and her siblings because, unconsciously, she would like to protect them from the parents. On the other hand, she identifies with and attaches herself to the mother in order somehow to find recognition and love. Thus, she grinds and wears herself down between these two sides, like her teeth in both halves of her jaw. She does not feel her profound pain, her sadness and anger, or finally her resignation. They express themselves via the symptom.

From a dental viewpoint, an occlusal splint is often the only therapeutic means. Physiotherapy and osteopathic treatment are useful additional therapies. However, these can only treat the consequences and not the causes of the pain. Sometimes further treatments follow, such as devitalising painful teeth, due to the continuing pain symptom. Such treatments indicate the dentist's helplessness and uncertainty rather than providing any health benefits. Here, if not before, it becomes clear that psychological or psychotherapeutic support is needed in order to treat such complex cases successfully.

Root infections

Inflammation of the root of the tooth is often the result of a tooth dying off due to deep caries, dental treatment (for example grinding a tooth before fitting a crown) or another trauma (a blow or fall, etc) that has an effect on the tooth. The standard traditional medical therapy is usually root canal treatment, with the aim of retaining the tooth temporarily or permanently. From a holistic perspective, such a therapy is problematic on several levels. The whole organism is gradually poisoned through toxic inflammatory products that are created by bacterial decomposition of endogenous protein frequently found within a tooth following root canal treatment.

Tinnitus and teeth

Tinnitus is the medical term for ringing and buzzing in the ears. It is often a symptom in dental patients that is not easy to treat. By definition it is a warning signal that accompanies too much physical and also psychological stress. Medically, for example, inflammation, noise stress, autoimmune diseases, virus infections, tumours, problems with the cervical vertebrae and the tooth and jaw area are seen.

Case history: Thomas

As I myself was affected by tinnitus for several weeks, I would like to relate how it came about and what helped me. The first thing I did was look at my external situation and my internal condition. I established that, professionally, I had been in a difficult situation for some time that was becoming increasingly stressful. One day the stress culminated in an argument and when I literally didn't want to hear another thing, the ringing began in my left ear. From then on, a high-pitched whistling sound with an intense feeling of pressure was the signal telling me everything was too much. I became aware that decisions had urgently to be made to alter the situation. Even though the symptom seriously affected my hearing for a time and was very unpleasant, I recognised it as a warning from my psyche and thus as help for my body.

In a first constellation, an individual session, I formulated the sentence: *"Warum habe ich diesen Druck auf meinem Ohr?"* [Word for word translation: "Why have I this pressure on my ear?"] "Why do I have this pressure on my ear?" To begin with, the representative for 'ear' said that he felt the pressure round his whole head. Everything that came from outside was too much for him and he didn't want to hear anything anymore. The symptom was therefore like relief to him. I agreed, yes, that's like my professional situation. As the constellation went on I recognised the steps I needed to take to clarify my situation. After the constellation my *'ear'* said he could no longer feel the pressure on his head. The quality of my ear symptoms also altered: the pressure reduced and the whistling sound became less intense. From my dental practice I know that an issue with the teeth is frequently the cause of tinnitus.

A further self-encounter followed shortly afterwards: my intention this time was: *"Ich möchte hören, was mein Ohr und meine Zähne sagen."* [Word for word translation: "I would-like hear, what my ear and my teeth say."] "I would like to hear what my ear and my teeth are saying." The resonator for my 'ear' appeared very fragile and weak. I hold his hands while he stands in front of me. Then he doubles over and says that he is very afraid and feels pressure on the whole of his body. Finally, he sinks to the floor while I try to hold him. I ask him while he is lying next to me in a foetal position, whether he is afraid of me. I am relieved to hear that this is not the case. Then he says that he feels as if he is in the womb and feels intense pressure and fear in his whole body. Even touching him on the back with my hand is too much for him.

From tales of my mother's I know that I was an unwanted pregnancy. My mother had strong existential fears when she was pregnant with me and didn't know how she could survive with a baby in her situation. From her I also knew that my birth had taken a very long time and was very painful for her after her waters had burst prematurely at home. After she arrived in the hospital, the midwife felt the birth was taking too long and in order to speed it up she began to press as hard as she could with her arms on my mother's abdomen, until I was born. As I appeared to be lifeless, the midwife hit me on my back until I cried.

In contact with my representative I am in tears and I feel utter despair. I realise how much strength I needed then and how much effort I had to exert in order to be born into this life in such circumstances. Finally, the representative for my 'ear', who encounters me as my split-off prenatal part, is lying relaxed next to me and falls asleep. His gentle snoring is like music to my ears, while the pressure that I have felt in my body throughout the whole process gradually diminishes. Then the resonator for my '*ear*' begins to straighten and stretch, and says that it seems as if he is waking up from a nightmare.

Meanwhile my tinnitus has also altered; I am no longer continually aware of it and it is also less intense. It has become my inner voice that tells me when things are 'too much', so that I watch out for and listen to myself. These identity constellations are an immense gift to me because through them I come more and more into contact with my identity trauma and myself. My symptoms help me to understand my survival strategies and inner splits, and to encounter them in the constellations. From the understanding that then develops I am able to experience the growth of personality parts that before now I was unable to see or live. In addition, it shows me that dental therapy, which concentrates on what is necessary, can also be very successful.

Working through my own trauma biography provides me with a realistic view of the possibilities and limits of dental therapy in daily contact with my patients, and at the same time enables me to give them good support. I see an excellent opportunity to contribute to better health and quality of life, for which everyone bears responsibility.

Glossary of terms

Aetiology: The branch of medical science that is concerned with the causes of disease.

Atrophy: Wasting away of tissue.

Craniomandibular dysfunction (CMD): Collective term for structural, functional, biochemical and psychological misregulation of the muscular or joint function of the jaw.

Epidemiology: The branch of medical science that deals with the distribution of disease in populations, and the associated variables.

Epithelium: Planar cell structures.

Indication: Generally stands for which medical measures are appropriate for a particular disease pattern.

Occlusion: Contact between the teeth in the upper and lower jaw.

Neuropathy: The cause of neuropathic pain is damage to the peripheral or central nervous system.

Nociception: The term for the perception of pain.

Somatoform disorder: The term for intense pain in a part of the body that lasts for at least six months and that cannot be sufficiently explained by any physical disorder.

References

Gleditsch, J. M. (1994). *Reflexzonen und Somatotopien als Schlüssel zu einer Gesamtschau des Menschen.* Schorndorf, Biologisch-Medizinische Verlagsgesellschaft.

Hanson, T., **Honee**, W. & **Hesse**, J. (1987). *Funktionsstörungen im Kausystem.* Heidelberg, Hüthig.

Hoffmann-Axthelm, W. (1983). *Lexikon der Zahnmedizin.* Freiburg, Quintessenz.

Hüther, G., **Korittko**, A., **Wolfrum**, G. & **Besser**, L. (2010). *Neurobiologische Grundlagen der Herausbildung Psychotrauma-bedingter Symptomatiken,* in Trauma & Gewalt (2010) 1, pp. 18–31.

Kleine-Tebbe, V. (2009). *Der Psychologische Psychotherapeut bzw. Arzt für psychosomatische Medizin und Psychotherapie als Netzwerkpartner* (Lecture in Leipzig).

Leonhardt, H. (1981). *Histologie, Zytologie und Mikroanatomie des Menschen.* Stuttgart, Thieme.

Raith, E. & **Ebenbeck**, G. (1986). *Psychologie für die zahnärztliche Praxis.* Stuttgart, Thieme.

Roissant, A. L. (1997). *Ganzheitliche Zahnheilkunde.* Heidelberg, Hüthig.

Ruppert, F. (2015). *Trauma, Fear and Love.* Steyning, Green Balloon Publishing.

Ruppert, F. (ed.) (2016). *Early Trauma.* Steyning, Green Balloon Publishing.

Ruppert, F. (2016). Lectures *Liebe, Trauma und Ich.* 3. International Congress Munich.

Schroeder, H. E. (1996). *Pathobiologie oraler Strukturen.* Basel, Karger.

Wolowski, A. & **Demmel**, H.-J. (2009). *Psychosomatische Medizin und Psychologie für Zahnmediziner.* Stuttgart, Schattauer.

Wühr, E. (2008). *Kraniofaziale Orthopädie.* Bad Kötzting, Systemische Medizin.

Wühr, E. & **Koch**, W. H. (2013). *Lehrbuch der Oralen Medizin.* Bad Kötzting, Systemische Medizin.

Thomas R Röll was born in 1958 and has been a dentist since 1990 with the focus on holistic dental medicine with his own practice in Ulm; since 2008 he has had his own practice for coaching and systemic counselling and since 2009 has completed further training and supervision in the constellation method based on attachment and trauma with Prof. Dr. Franz Ruppert. www.ganzheitliche-zahnmedizin-ulm.de

THILO BEHLA

Back pain and its causes

From death wish to staying alive

To settle one thing straight away: the pain in my back is still there. Perhaps it will be there until the end of my life. It has defined my life, and my closest social environment, for many years. The crippling severity of it almost drove me to end my life; like a parasite that sucks the life out of its host, until the host dies. However, in late 2011, something changed. I came across Franz Ruppert's trauma work and I achieved a dramatic shift in direction. It was unstoppable, from death wish to staying alive; from desperation to strength; from isolation to contact; from tiny steps to leaps; from impatience to patience. It was not a straight road without any bumps, but with sharp downward slides and exhausting climbs up the other side. At first I was scared, then hesitant, then, increasingly empathic towards myself. Now, the prospect of change is lasting. It is now half a decade since contact with my 'I' became possible, and my current now has earned the title of 'life.'

Slipped disc and external attempts at healing

In 1998, I experienced a severe slipped disc. It was so bad that I underwent an operation on the L5/S1 area of my spine. I had been loading extremely heavy chunks of granite into my car because I wanted to build a natural stone wall in my garden. If there's one thing I'm good at it's pushing my body through barriers in athletic performances. Within a very short time after the operation I was my old self again, and up for anything. Although not quite, because from then on, I was more focused on signs that my lower back was in trouble, signs that came right on cue. My reaction was to intensify my back exercises, and if I felt any pain or discomfort I would scrupulously apply imaging techniques so as to honour my physical body

Almost ten years went by like this and then suddenly, in May 2007, I experienced terrible tension in my back. It was as if I had been clamped in a vice. I identified the pain as being below the old operation scar, so I didn't connect it to my spine, and there had been no physical reason for it to occur. An MRI scan showed that there was no new slipped disc, but the feeling of stiffness didn't go away. To begin with I was able to escape the pain for an hour or two by changing my posture, going from walking to sitting or to lying down. However, this didn't help. I was filled with an increasing sense of helplessness. The overriding certainty of not being able to do anything about it ate away at me everyday, tearing apart my previously held image of myself as a person who was never ill, and who had climbed seven mountain peaks in one week's holiday.

Then began a journey of seeking outside help: rehabilitation clinics in the Weserbergland, and in the Allgäu; thermo-coagulation as an in-patient in Munich and Potsdam; a clinic for bio-kinematics in the Black Forest; injections, sling tables, acupuncture sessions and osteopathy. There were no conclusive radiological findings, but despite this surgical interventions were recommended, based on a diagnosis of what was "most likely". So, I was offered to try a new procedure called: AxiaLIF (fusing the bones of the sacrum and the 5th lumbar vertebrae with a screw). However a male nurse who worked in the place where this operation was proposed to happen turned a key for me with the simple words: "There's nothing wrong with your back. You should take a look at the psychological level."

I had paid out of my own pocket for many of the tests that I had undergone in the medical system, and because of my strong sense of order I kept track of those costs: up to 2011 it was more than €15,000! I had paid for a safety net that didn't exist. Neither the state care services, nor alternative medicines had helped me, even though many loving souls wanted to. Some very special individuals had tried to help, and catch the vase that falls to earth that was my life, but it was I who wasn't able to hold onto

this beautiful vessel. It escaped from me and shattered. The pile
of broken pieces was my landscape of misery: this wasn't why I
had come into the world.

What then followed was a tailspin into depression. I made
my condition my measuring stick with which to measure my
world. So I broke off all contact with friends, refused visits,
took sick leave from work and torpedoed my wife's enjoyment
of life, as I didn't want her to feel better than I did. In order
to protect herself, and not go down with me, she threatened
separation. I don't know now whether I was trying to raise the
'level of care,' or was actually flirting with the idea, but I did
consider taking the final path of assisted dying with Dignitas
in Switzerland ...

Searching for the problem within

I realised that looking outside for an answer had not worked, so
I was ready to try another way, this time, by looking inside. I was
given a prescription for physiotherapy, which took me to an
address for systemic family constellations in Hannover. I found
this form of therapy amazing, supplying me with undreamt of
insights into my family of origin, and my own entanglements
with it. Immediately the spasm in my lower back freed itself, like
the breaking of a delicate string on an instrument. This proved
to me that my lower back problem was not based on anything
physiological. For a few weeks after that I felt completely
healthy, then I suffered several relapses. The worst one was when
in personal contact with my mother. The subsequent sessions I
had followed Hellinger's method but did not help me, rather they
seemed manipulative and disparaging, with the facilitator
blaming me for my condition. I felt that the words I was told to
say to those representing my parents were empty; thanking them
for my conception and nourishment seemed to me to be
dishonest. It was clear to me, that this was not the way to bring
any resolutions

In chatting with a neighbour in Upper Bavaria where I lived,
we discovered that both of us had experienced constellations,

however her constellations had been at a group seminar with Franz Ruppert in Munich. She met my scepticism of constellation work by describing to me what happened in these 'trauma constellations'; it was quite different from my experience of family constellations. She explained to me that the person doing the work was always part of what was happening, they had control of the process. First of all, they formulated an intention, then they chose representatives for this intention, and that in the process there was a mixture of communication using verbal and body language between all those involved, with no 'whispered prompts' from the facilitator. A few weeks later, in November 2011, I took part in such a seminar, and at the end of the third day, I was randomly selected for a constellation. My intention was: *"Ich will meine Rückenschmerzen loswerden!"* [Word for word translation: "I want my back-pain away-become!"] "I want to be rid of the pain in my back."

What I got out of this was a snapshot of my inner psyche that was connected directly with my current psychological state. The interactions that I had with the representatives of my intention felt down-to-earth; they contained so many more possibilities than just the 'getting rid of' which I had felt in the family constellations. The intention that I set in the Identity-oriented Psychotrauma Therapy responded to requests to help me with rejection, even ridicule. As part of the process Franz Ruppert suggested setting up a representative for my back pain. This representative immediately sank to the floor and clasped my legs so that I had to drag them round the seminar room, as if they were shackles. Also suggested was to choose a representative for me as a child, and the representative withdrew in fear into the furthest corner of the room. Then we set up a representative for my mother, who rolled on the floor also suffering from back pain, and saying she felt like she was drunk. Finally we put in a representative for my father, who immediately went towards the little Thilo who withdrew even further and said he was in fear for his life.

At this point Franz Ruppert ended the constellation, and offered me his explanation: my intention was not able to solve my problem, but did illuminate the cause. The back pain came from my childhood past. My mother had been self-absorbed and could not, or would not see the abuse to me done by my father.

The bottom line was that my wish to be rid of the pain was, at that point, too great to be realised. First of all, I had to recognise that as a child I had apparently suffered a sexual traumatisation, which at the time I had been helpless to do anything about. In addition the violence that I experienced as a child led to a psychological split, and from that, my back pain began as a survival strategy to protect me, one I still hold onto today, even though the danger is objectively past. When I asked about the next step Franz Ruppert recommended a practitioner near my home: Birgit Assel in Betheln.

At my first individual session, there seemed a faint ray of light into the darkness of my past. This was accompanied by spasms of rapid heartbeat and the expressions of my mortal fear. A second session confronted me with a sense of victimisation, which I had dealt with by holding a worldview of rejection, disregard and hostility. The third session led to me registering for the next advanced trauma constellation training in Betheln.

Five years passed like this, with training and advanced training courses, study groups and day workshops where I set personal intentions, and represented for others in their intentions, all of which wove a rich cloth of increasing self-awareness. My back pain, both directly or indirectly, continually emerged in the work, and positioned itself at the centre of my intention. In small steps I began to develop from conception to teenager, and through all the twists and turns, insights and emotions began to knit together a coherent and viable foundation for myself. It resulted from my trust in the method; the skill of the constellation leader and the sincerity of the representatives, as well as from the coherence of my inner experience, because there was no actual proof: my father had died in an accident 20 years previously and my mother assiduously puts forward an image of a happy, protected childhood, of a wanted child. The following points have been disputed, whitewashed and after 'partial confessions,' once again denied:

- I was conceived because my mother was told by her parents when she was 27 that it was time she had a family;
- my conception was a formal act of creation;
- in the early stages, the pregnancy was sustained by the secret wish of both my parents that it might lead to a miscarriage;
- my mother's delusional attachment to a child she had aborted when she was 18 was mixed in with the later stages of pregnancy with me;
- due to complications, I almost didn't survive the birth;
- my unconditional love was tied to conditions: meeting the unachievable demands of my father and satisfying my mother's profound neediness;
- childish attempts to set boundaries as resistance to parental violence were met with beatings;
- as a child I was frequently left alone for half the night by my parents and when they returned I witnessed their violent arguments; and
- I almost died on several occasions on extreme skiing tours with my father during the annual winter sports weeks.

The mirror showed me a conformist, a quiescent and joyless performance body that had excellent grades, but was always in conflict with the authorities, on a narcissistic quest for recognition, and who found that being in relationships with women brought uncertainty and difficulty.

The breakthrough to clarity

Meanwhile the constellation work brought about a breakthrough. I realised a connection between trauma triggers such as the smell of sweat or "a big, black thing is coming to get me" and flight impulses that led to tachycardia or atrial fibrillation. Through the constellation work my symptoms ceased almost completely. If my heart occasionally misses a beat today, I drop down a gear, pause, and assure myself that I am not in danger. In the Identity-orientated Psychotrauma Therapy, where my 'I' and the contact with my 'I' are the central focus, I also found an increasingly gentle and more honest access to myself.

But there was still the matter of my back. The constellation work suggested the presence of an immense physical tension that built up in my body even before my birth. I tried to hide my feelings of inadequacy through a continual effort of keeping my back straight as a way to convince the outside world that I was okay. It was an enormous pressure. I began to recognise specific triggers that showed as terrible sleep disturbances, nightly whimpering that didn't fit with the adult Thilo, frequent breathlessness, and incessant itching of the anus.

I spent most of 2016 on sick leave. The persistent pains in my back almost made me chuck in my job. I used my sick leave for comprehensive diagnostics, MRI scans and X-rays, which showed the worn musculoskeletal system of a person in their early 50s with the added bonus of a disc operation. On balance, I was physically healthy, except that my sacroiliac joint was permanently locked by this continual tension that I could not consciously release. In October 2016 I again went to further training groups for IoPT therapy. I wanted to know where I was and so I formulated the intention: "*Ich will leben!*" [Word for word translation: "I want to-live!"] "I want to live! The picture was astonishing: my 'I' was turned to face me and was friendly. The representative for 'to-live' was animated and unreserved. Birgit Assel's summary: You have never been so close to your 'I'.

On 5th February 2017 I formulated the following intention: "*Ich will anerkennen, was mir passiert ist.*" [Word for word translation: "I want to-recognise, what to-me happened is."] "I want to recognise what has happened to me." Again my 'I' affectionately turned towards me. Boldly I looked at it, even if I couldn't see inside. I asked the 'what' to join us. It asked incessantly "Yeah what, what is it, what has happened to you? You know what it is! Say what it is!" 'What' got angry, walking backwards and forwards. I said: "I want to recognise that I was raped."

'What' stopped walking, closed his eyes and said: "Now you've put it into words. It fits." For a long, undisturbed, liberating time I wept; my 'I'' didn't move away from me, but stood by me, manly, adult and strong. All my symptoms fitted together, even the back pain near the coccyx. I breathed images of situations: when I lift the duvet, carefully, very slightly, for fresh oxygen; breathing deeply, when I threw back the duvet, because it is over.

I needed a week to finish writing this piece, following this constellation. My wife says I've been sleeping more peacefully since then. In a bed that offers peace and relaxation. My back is still painful, but I want to live.

Thilo Bela, was born in 1965. He works in Hannover, and lives in Lenggries. Thilo has been following Franz Ruppert's work through training programmes and workshops with Birgit Assel in Betheln since 2012.

GERLINDE FISCHEDICK

My right hip and I – the story of my rebirth

Pain from birth onwards

I was born in 1956, the youngest of three children, with a damaged hip. In those days, doctors didn't know much about hip misalignments. When I began to walk I lifted my right foot much higher than the left. I struggled to keep my balance and had to wear heavy inserts in my shoes, made of metal and covered with leather, because the orthopaedic surgeons thought my feet were the problem. It was very difficult for me, because I could only wear these raised shoes. I remember my communion, when we were supposed to wear white patent leather shoes. I couldn't find any and my black boots were coloured white.

When I was about 12, I got intense pains above my right knee. The doctors said it was a 'pulled muscle' and prescribed some ointment. After PE lessons I was often unable to walk and had to stay sitting until I could walk again. I didn't get an exemption from PE lessons. "Don't make such a fuss!" After all, it was only a 'pulled muscle'.

When I was 13, I had further problems standing up after I'd been sitting down for a while. I couldn't walk up to the board in the classroom. My knee was X-rayed again and again. There was nothing there. So in the eyes of my parents I was "moaning", and the pain was played down.

A week after Easter in 1970, I fell down the stairs and couldn't get up. My mother took me to hospital and when we were driving over the cobblestones I noticed that something on the right side of my pelvis was 'rattling'. In the hospital, the doctor asked me to lift my left leg, which was no problem, but I was unable to lift my right leg. He was a young Persian assistant doctor who had at least some idea that it could be a hip disloca-tion. The senior consultant's diagnosis was: "Your daughter will never walk again. She'll only be able to use a wheelchair." This diagnosis was kept from me. I was just told briefly that I had a 'femoral neck fracture'. For two and a half months I lay in a 'stretching bed' with weights on my feet. I couldn't move, not even sit up.

At that time there was a Professor in Mainz who had carried out two hip operations in which he had shortened the femur and implanted a right-angled plate that was screwed into the epiphysis. I underwent this operation in May 1970. As I was still growing, the doctors destroyed the growth plate in the left hip so that I wouldn't become lopsided. I have not grown from the hip since then. The operation was successful. After five months I had to learn to walk again. There was no physiotherapy in 1970. For a long time I walked with crutches. No young men courted me, and even the usual dance classes didn't happen.

Luckily I was good at swimming, and later also a deep-sea diver, which acted as physiotherapy. Through this my right hip regained flexibility. They said my hip would be good for 35,000 kilometres. After a year the angle plate was removed. The conse-quent damage was immense. I was lopsided and in time my whole skeleton grew out of shape, which led to slipped discs and permanent back pain. In addition there were migraine attacks with intense vomiting.

Family constellations and their limits

Through all the years of pain, I had no idea that I had been repeatedly traumatised. I had completely suppressed the violence and violations within my family of origin. I have to thank a girl-friend of mine who in 1998 gave me the book *Anerkennen, was ist* by Bert Hellinger and Gabriele ten Hövel (Hellinger and ten Hövel, 1996). I read the book and became aware that something in my family of origin wasn't right. With some glasses and other objects I arranged my first family constellation for myself. It immediately became apparent that my father held all the power and that my mother was not present at all. My siblings, who were 10 and 7 years older than me, were taken up with themselves. I didn't have a place in the family.

After I had separated from my ex-husband in spring 2000, an acquaintance told me about a systems therapist and mental coach near Hanover who carried out family constellations and offered three-year training courses. In 2001 I began the three-year training course with her, completing it in January 2004. Through this work, my migraine attacks improved but did not disappear. I didn't feel any pain in my hip, but I still had considerable pain in my back.

I started having doubts about family constellations in 2007 when I attended a training course with Bert Hellinger in Austria. I was asked to choose a representative for my mother (we were all doing the same), set up that representative, and then swap over, so that I was then going into my mother's experience and empathising with her, and the representative then became me. That night, following the constellation, I vomited every 15 minutes. I suffered immeasurably. I felt that something wasn't right with the Hellinger method. Despite the most intensive work, I wasn't really getting any better, there was only temporary relief. I tried to fathom why I had been so sick and suddenly I knew: Why should I be a representative for my mother and sense that she had no feelings, and none for me either? And I was supposed to forgive her? To understand Mama and pretend to myself that I can now breathe feelings into her and our relationship will therefore be intact again? That was illusory.

Getting closer through trauma constellations

While looking for another way to explore my pain, I read Symbiose und Autonomie[59] shortly after it was published. I read the book and knew that this method would help me. I have always enjoyed reading Professor Franz Ruppert's books. Books

---

[59] English version: Symbiosis & Autonomy (Ruppert, 2012).

like Berufliche Beziehungswelten (2001) and Verwirrte Seelen (2002) were substantial and at the same time easily understandable. I was able to recognise the psychological conflicts and to analyse them for myself. In the preface of his book Trauma, Bindung und Familienstellen[60] (2005) he confirmed my opinion of Hellinger. Ruppert wrote that, in a constellation in which he was a representative himself, Hellinger wanted to attribute a feeling to him that he didn't have.

Soon after reading Symbiosis and Autonomy, I was fortunate enough to attend Franz Ruppert's public trauma constellation seminar in 2010 and get to know his work myself. As I didn't know where I should start the search for my suppressed traumas, I looked first at my relationship with my mother. I did one constellation a month. When I finished one constellation, I started the next. I learnt that the traumas, of which I was still unaware, were all stored in my body. My predominant physical pains – pain in my hip together with back pain and migraine with vomiting – were all reflected in the constellations. First of all the vomiting was resolved, then the migraine attacks disappeared, but the hip and back pain stayed.

My walking got worse and worse. I would have to have a further hip operation. With the help of my orthopaedist I found a surgeon in Hanover who could tell from the 1970 X-rays that standard replacement hips could not be used on me. I limped into a CT scan and he arranged for an artificial hip joint to be made especially for me. The advantage was supposed to be the correction of my lopsided posture through putting me on two legs of equal length.

Then during a constellation I discovered that an operation would trigger an additional trauma if I didn't know which trauma was stuck in my hip. I did another constellation to find out about the trauma in my hip. I took circuitous routes. I looked at my traumatic experience as an unborn child; it turned out the unborn Gerlinde was highly traumatised and mortally afraid. I couldn't approach her.

---

[60] English version: Trauma, Bonding & Family Constellations (Ruppert, 2008).

Because of the planned operation date I had to cancel my next constellation seminar. I still hadn't understood the origin of my hip trauma. I was afraid, so I gave my partner comprehensive power of attorney, and I made my will. I even told my attorney how I wanted to be buried. He didn't want to hear that and said I should trust the doctor.

The artificial hip joint that was being made for me wasn't ready in time, so the operation had to be postponed. I immediately rang the seminar leader and asked if I could take part in the next seminar with my own constellation after all. Luckily for me, someone had cancelled. I had one last chance to discover the origin of my hip trouble. The seminar was on a Saturday and Sunday. On the Saturday I did my constellation straightaway: I wanted to look at my mortal fear as an unborn child. The representatives showed me that I would rather die than see what happened to me as an unborn child in my mother's womb. Now I understood why I had made my will. I saw clearly that I didn't want to wake up from the anaesthetic. Everybody there was shocked. The constellation leaders reacted correctly and asked me what I wanted to do. I wanted to be alone and to go away. They said I was welcome to come along on Sunday at the end of the seminar to do another constellation in a smaller group that I was familiar with. They said I should decide for myself.

I didn't say anything to my partner, although on other occasions I had told him about the insights from my constellations. The next day I drove to the seminar late in the afternoon. I observed the last constellation and the leader asked who wanted to stay on for me. All but two participants, who both had long journeys home, wanted to stay, which I found very touching. In all the previous constellations I had not been allowed to approach the unborn Gerlinde. My intention was therefore: *"Wie kann ich mich der ungeborenen traumatisierten Gerlinde nähern?"* [Word for word translation: "How can I myself the unborn traumatised Gerlinde approach"]. "How can I approach the unborn traumatised Gerlinde?"

Constellations of the intention and the original trauma

The constellation did not take place according to the later and current method of the sentence of the intention, so that while I cautiously approached myself as an unborn child, I also set up my pregnant mother, my father and my hip. I was able to approach the trembling unborn Gerlinde. She finally allowed me to be with her. Together we both watched my father's violence towards my mother's belly. My father always thought I wasn't his child. He had a short temper and was often violent. The representative for my mother tried to protect herself and suddenly cried out. Luckily, when my father punched my mother's belly, he had only caught my hip. I screamed. The silent scream finally came out of me. The unborn Gerlinde and I were able to be united and over time we both became very calm. Now I knew why I had been born with a damaged right hip.

My operation was on 21st June 2014. When I woke up in the intensive care ward I started crying. I was here. The nurse was very caring. I asked if she had been working long in the clinic. Yes, she said, 15 years on the same ward, except that it used to be a ward for newborn babies. I realised I had been reborn with a new hip. I had indeed been granted a new, pain-free life. When I went to the follow-up examination a year later, the doctor could not believe it. He was speechless: the difference in length between my legs was just four millimetres, and my crooked spine had completely recovered.

My thanks go to my partner for his love and affection, to Franz Ruppert for his insatiable investigative spirit, Birgit Assel, Detlev Blechner, Margriet Wentink and Wim Wassink, who in the wonderful surroundings of the Lower Saxony Auetal, supported by the love of Agnes and Manfred Struckmeier and Petra Grupe, all gave me their encouragement prior to the operation and are still assisting me today.

References

Hellinger, B. & **ten Hövel**, G. (1996). *Anerkennen, was ist.* Munich, Kösel.

Ruppert, F. (2001). *Berufliche Beziehungswelten.* Heidelberg, Carl-Auer-Systeme.

Ruppert, F. (2002). *Verwirrte Seelen.* Munich, Kösel.

Ruppert, F. (2008): *Trauma, Bonding & Family Constellations.* Frome, Green Balloon Publishing.

Ruppert, F. (2012). *Symbiosis & Autonomy.* Steyning, Green Balloon Publishing.

Gerlinde Fischedick lives in Hanover. She is a systems therapist, psychological counsellor, mediator and lawyer.

MARTINA WITTMANN

Chronic shoulder pain

Suffering and persistence

In the spring of 2015 I kept getting mild pains in my right shoulder that I either ignored or brushed aside, until the middle of the year. I also always had what seemed to me plausible explanations for the pains. Then the pain changed; suddenly it was always there; bearable to begin with, gentle and only occasionally intense; then intense most of the time and only occasionally bearable. I was still coping with the pain and trying to bear it. Then came the moment I adopted a posture to try and avoid the pain. My movements were hugely restricted and I was afraid that my shoulder was going to become frozen. Despite my distress I still tried to hide the pain and carry on functioning. When I talked about it I made light of the pain. I was afraid that the others wouldn't believe me; that I wasn't worth anything. I saw everything and found my own behaviour strange, but it was the only way I could function. I even blamed myself for my own incapacity and stupidity.

Unsuccessful visits to the doctor

In April 2016 I finally went to see an orthopaedist who specialised in shoulders. I had an ultrasound scan and he moved my shoulder about and came to the conclusion that there was nothing to see and nothing wrong. But he said I could try electrotherapy. He told me to come back when I felt the pain. I told him that was paradoxical because I was in pain at that time. Frustrated, I left his practice and thought that the pain was better – but that wasn't true. It was just that my anger towards the doctor at that moment was stronger than the pain. I was happy to be out of there. I went to 'electrotherapy' once. The pain was worse afterwards.

I then looked for another shoulder specialist and arranged an appointment. I thought to begin with that this doctor was more pleasant. He did the same tests as the first doctor and said that he saw some very slight calcification, but he didn't think that these could cause such pain. He recommended an operation to scrape away the calcification, and after that we'd see. I immediately knew that I didn't want that. I wanted to leave his office as quickly as possible. Now I was in a quandary. On the one hand I wanted to be helped by a doctor, to have a diagnosis and confirmation that something was wrong. On the other hand I was dissatisfied with the treatment that had been offered to me and had also had the confirmation that there was "nothing wrong" with my shoulder.

In retrospect I find it difficult to understand how long I took to think of having a constellation about these symptoms. I had been working on myself with the intention method for some time and had often formulated an intention relating to a symptom. That had always helped me. This time the possibility just didn't enter my head for a long time.

"I want to know what the shoulder pains mean"

In May 2016 I worked in my peer group with the intention: *"Ich will wissen, was die Schulterschmerzen bedeuten."* [Word for word translation: I want to-know, what the shoulder-pains mean."] "I want to know what the shoulder pains mean." First I set up my 'I' and made good and affectionate contact with it. I explained the situation to it and felt understood and supported. I then decided to set up the 'shoulder-pains'. As there were no women left in our group, I chose one of the men, and asked him to represent 'shoulder-pains' as a woman. The moment I said that, I suddenly felt it was wrong – 'shoulder-pains' was male, not female! The representative for 'shoulder-pains' also said that he felt definitely not female. He grasped my hands, held onto me and said he was feeling horny. I completely panicked. I heard the 'I' asking me whether this was my father. All I knew was that 'shoulder-pains' was male – somehow it was my father, but somehow it wasn't any actual one person, but several. I couldn't be more precise than that.

Through the question of my 'I' and my answer, I gained some momentum and was able to escape from the grasp of 'shoulder-pains' and crawled into a corner. I was tense and stiff and hardly breathing. I didn't perceive my 'I' any more, only the words of 'shoulder-pains': "I'm horny, I'm so horny." The 'shoulder-pains' wanted to come to me and my 'I' kept saying, very clearly and definitely: "No".

To begin with I only heard the words of 'shoulder-pains'. I was alone, at his mercy and incapable of taking any action. I noticed and registered that my 'I' was present and strong, but I had lost contact with it. Then I heard what my 'I' was saying and was once again more connected with it. With the contact to my 'I' I gained strength and confidence. I was able to stand up and the stiffness and panic abated slightly. The representative for 'shoulder-pains' was still there but had stopped talking. Through the contact with my 'I' I realised that the 'shoulder-pains' didn't represent one particular person, but stood for male sexual energy in general. I said this to my 'I'. It answered that it seemed the same to her, and that she was now always there for me. I felt that that was true. In contact with my 'I' the 'shoulder-pains' moved into the background. They were still there, but had no access to me and were silent.

Disappearance of the shoulder pain

From that day onward my shoulder pain had gone. This constellation showed me the depth of my injuries and splits through sexual violence. Until the age of 12, I had been subjected to sexual traumatisations by three people: my father and two men from the village where I grew up.

This was how I interpreted the dynamic of my constellation: the 'shoulder-pains' represented my tormentors' energy, not a single perpetrator. That was why my choice of a plural word was right. A part of me is still triggered when it senses, or suspects, male sexual energy. In my constellation the way I was grabbed and the predatory words of the 'shoulder-pains' made this obvious. In my daily life I encounter this energy differently and in a way that is not related to me. If, for instance, a man sweats, a part of me classifies the smell as this energy and reverts to the state at that time. This is when I split from my 'I'. It became clearly noticeable to me that I have a healthy 'I'-structure that says "No", that can distance itself, and is now in the present. And it does not fight. My focus is on myself. When I perceive my 'I', I can meet men without stress and draw the boundary I need.

In July 2014 I changed jobs and from then on I had more to do with men. Before then I had virtually only dealt with women. Through this constellation I also recognised that there are still survival mechanisms and perpetrator-loyal structures working within me that originally wanted to assign the shoulder pains differently. I am deeply moved to see how accurately my intention reflects my psyche and helps me to understand myself better.

Martina Wittmann was born in 1960 and is a nurse and teacher for the care profession. In 1998 she trained as a supervisor and in 2002 she did advanced training with Prof. Dr. Franz Ruppert. Since 2004 she has offered seminars and individual work in her own practice in Augsburg. www.traumaaufstellung-augsburg.de

JULIANE VON KRAUSE

"What has happened to my neck?"

Intense pain from childhood

Waking up in the morning with nausea and with the feeling that several people had been hitting the back of my neck with a wooden slat; severe tension and pain in my neck and throat area; headaches the whole day. Since my youth I had suffered several times a month with severe headaches, and I often had intense pain in my neck as well. Painkillers were the only thing that brought me any relief.

I decided to look into the causes of this neck pain in a constellation. An MRI scan years earlier had shown that I had suffered a slipped disc in the area of the cervical vertebrae many years beforehand. This scan had been carried out because I had suffered from dizziness following a skiing accident. Luckily, I received good osteopathic treatment and the dizziness left me. However, I could not explain the 'old slipped disc' seen by the orthopaedic surgeon.

Close to death feeling

My intention was: *"Was ist mit meinem Hals passiert?"* [Word for word translation: "What is with my neck happened?"] "What has happened to my neck?" In the individual session I asked my therapist to represent the separate words. It resulted in an extremely informative constellation: in the position of the 'what', my representative felt very ill. Everything hurt her, she felt sick and she had neck pains. As the 'is' she felt as if she was leaving her body and fainting. In the role of 'with' she felt physically unwell and dizzy. She felt as if everything was revolving and leaving the body. In the place of 'my' she felt like a little girl. Her head was pulled severely backwards and overextended, which resulted in a very uncomfortable posture. Her knee began to be painful. She said she had no orientation and did not know what the matter was. She also had a slight cough.

I recognised all the symptoms as mine: neck pain, dizziness, pain in the left knee, a cough. I found that very impressive and also alarming. I felt compassion for the little girl and all parts of me that had to suffer so.

As 'neck' the therapist said, "I feel fragmented, have to expend a lot of strength in keeping myself together so that I don't fall apart. I am very unstable and have to keep up my resistance." To begin with I couldn't make much of this statement, but I also felt compassion at that moment. When the therapist went into resonance with 'happened', she began to sway and said that she had the feeling of being whirled round and twisted. She couldn't look me in the eye. I wondered what this new information meant. When had I been whirled round?

In the position of the question mark, the therapist felt alone, abandoned and had feelings of guilt. She said: "I'm still little, I can't help it!" She thought she was wearing a cervical collar and she had a stiff neck. Into her head came the sentence: "If I hadn't held on, I'd have died." I understood: The neck muscles had to hold on otherwise I would have died! At this point I got cold: I realised how close I had been to death. Again in this role, the coughing was present. Ultimately the representative had great difficulty in breathing, and began to hyperventilate. Again, the pain in the knee. I recognised the breathing difficulty because I had experienced it several times in threatening situations.

A car accident and its consequences

In conversation with the therapist I realised what had come to light here: all my sensations, injuries and my condition during a bad car accident that I had been involved in when I was five. Our VW Beetle had been in a head-on collision with another car. My father broke his leg, my mother her arm. When the collision happened I was lying on the back seat asleep and had been whirled around on impact. In those days there were no seat belts. I was unconscious for some time. My memories of the accident start from when I woke up in the ambulance. My mother was with me. I had concussion and had to stay in hospital for a few days. I think that whiplash wasn't recognised in those days and I wasn't given a cervical collar. I had some cuts on my face that had to be stitched. They had been caused when I was thrown onto the metal ashtray in the car.

Having to stay in hospital and being separated from my parents was a shock for me. I was bewildered, couldn't sleep and didn't want to eat. I was therefore sent home after just a few days. On the first day in particular, before my mother came to visit me, I was very concerned about my father because I didn't know what had happened to him. He had been taken away in a different ambulance. My mother was able to calm me down and tell me that my father would soon be healthy again. The whole situation was all the more confusing for me because Germany was a foreign country to me then and my family had only been here on a visit for a few days.

The accident was a shock for us all. For my father, the loss of the brand new car was especially bad. He had been driving and had not given way – probably because, coming from South Africa, he was still used to driving on the left. In later conversations in the family, my father once remarked that the accident had happened because he had slept badly the night before. He blamed me for that, because I had been coughing a lot in the night. As a child I often had coughing fits. On the morning of the accident he and my mother, who had come to my defence, had had an argument. I can thus understand why, as a part of me, the question mark in the constellation felt guilty.

When I saw the parts in my constellation and experienced them internally, I realised that I almost died in this accident when I was a child. I had only just survived. Recognising this threw me into inner turmoil. I now understood what had happened to me in this car accident as a little child.

Since this constellation I have experienced a wonderful alter-ation and healing in me. For several months I have still had a slight headache in the morning, but the intense pain in the back of my neck has disappeared. The pain in my knee, too, which according to doctors is caused by arthritis, has significantly decreased. An immense improvement in my quality of life!

Juliane von Krause was born in 1958 in South Africa, and now lives in Munich. She is the director of two specialist counselling centres and sheltered housing for women threatened by violence.

CATHERINE XAVIER

Trauma and posture

Always there for others

Clients sometimes come to my psychotherapeutic practice specifically to look at their physical symptoms. They want to find the
causes behind their symptoms, and what their body is expressing. There is also the reverse process: clients work on their
psychological problems and over time a connection to their
physical symptoms becomes apparent. This was the case with
Susanne.

Susanne is in her mid-40s and has been coming to my
practice regularly for some time. She has an excellent sense of
others' moods and needs. She is very skilful in defusing a charged
atmosphere, in the family for instance, or in her workplace. Even
as a child she says she made it her job to bring harmony to the
tense family environment. She has little access to her own needs.
She is afraid her family could "break apart" if she withdraws
from her role, but she no longer wants just to step back as she
has been doing. She hasn't yet mentioned any physical ailments.
After about nine months she mentions, almost in passing, that
for years shortened tendons in her thighs and the palms of her
hands have caused her pain, and that this has improved since we
have been working together. She says she can feel that something
is happening to her shortened tendons. "Something's going on
there" she says, laughing.

"I want to live my life."

"Ich will mein Leben leben." [Word for word translation: "I want
my life to live."] This was Susanne's intention that we are
working on in an individual session. First of all she places me for
the word 'my' in the centre of the room, and as the resonator I

feel exposed and unsafe. As 'my' I need contact with her; I can only stay in the centre of the room if she is there. I have to become more stable, but it has to be with her, then I can stay standing. I have a momentary impulse to be reassured from the outside, perhaps by the parents; that I am really allowed to stand there. Susanne holds my hands and affirms that we are allowed to stand there. The contact with her is still slightly unstable, but it is there now.

Susanne then sets me up for the word 'life'. In this role I feel very small and weak. I look down at the floor. I am unable to move. I feel isolated, alone and incapable of taking any action. Susanne stands directly in front of me but at a slight distance. She looks at me sceptically: "But that's not how I see my life." I follow my impulse to sit on the floor, pull my legs up and put my head between my knees. I'm afraid of being a burden to her and being rejected. I begin to feel ashamed of myself. Finally I freeze. Susanne now remembers that as a child she had often spent the whole afternoon crouching with her doll in the hayloft, with her arms and legs bent. When she was in bed at night, she had also adopted a crouching position.

Susanne was the fourth child, born into a stressful family situation in which there was scarcely room for another child. Neither her mother nor her father was prepared for a fourth child when her mother unexpectedly became pregnant. Susanne was also the fourth girl, and her parents had hoped for a boy. Susanne learned quickly to step back in her family and try not to be a nuisance. The messages that came across were: "You're too much" and "You're the wrong sex." What became apparent about the word 'life', showed clearly how Susanne must have felt as a child and how 'life' had seemed to her. Stepping back and literally "pulling herself together" (physically as well as psychologically), was a survival strategy for her and therefore a consequence of her trauma of identity – in the same way as her flight into the role of peacemaker in the family was to justify her right to exist.

Now she puts up the word 'I' as well. As the 'I' I feel restless and as if I'm on the starting blocks: "I don't want to wait any longer, I want to act, I want action." The other two parts are too slow for me as 'I', and much too hesitant. That initially pleases Susanne, because she wants to "move on" at last.

Set up as 'want' I fluctuate between Susanne, the 'I' and the other parts. I don't know where things are heading, and with whom. Susanne says she had actually imagined that 'want' should go to 'life', but with the way 'life' is conducting itself here, she doesn't know if she does want that. Suddenly Susanne becomes quiet and then she says: "No, that can't work. I don't want a life without 'my life'. These are my childhood experiences. I can't ignore that. It's part of me and my history!

Healthy through more contact with the I

The idea of living 'her life' does not give her the longed-for vitality, but rather moves her away from herself if the unconscious underlying intention is to shake off her past. Susanne's 'I' was in survival mode and not able to 'feel' her childhood experiences. It demonstrated that Susanne is cut off from a part of herself. She recognised this through this constellation. And the more she turns towards her inner reality, and thereby finds herself, the more she can 'unfold' herself physically as well.

Susanne continues to come to me regularly and explores with the Intention Method for herself. Step by step she is increasingly successful in creating 'feeling contact' with herself and with her 'I'. That is reflected in the constellations as well as in her daily life. Among other things, she gives up her self-harming behaviours that up until now had served her as a replacement 'regulator'. She proudly tells me that she has almost given up her regular evening drink. Of course, she sometimes enjoys a glass of wine with friends, but no longer every evening. She can also now feel the exact moment when it stops doing her good. She no longer has any desire to go beyond this limit. She also only eats chocolate in small, enjoyable amounts now. She feels her body more and more, sees its signals and can stay in harmony with it.

The more she feels herself, however, the more clearly Susanne notices how members of her family ignore her needs. It is very painful for her to recognise the full extent of her familial reality. Again and again she strives to be seen by her mother and her sisters. She feels more and more that this family is not good for her, but the fear of losing her old attachment figures and being on her own is deep-seated and still affects her today. She now sees more clearly the connections between her experience with her family, her addictive behaviour patterns and her physical symptoms. She is better able to feel how she really fared as a child, and she is determined to do more work to develop herself.

Early childhood impressions are anchored deep within us, especially when they originated before we were born. Such profound therapeutic processes of change need time and the self-compassion to remain in harmony with one's own pace.

Catherine Xavier is an alternative practitioner and offers Identity-oriented Psychotrauma Therapy and the Intention Method in her own practice in Berlin, both in groups and for individual clients. www.psychotraumatherapie-berlin.de

ISABELLA GERSTGRASSER

Rheumatoid arthritis

The monster

Where is my companion, the monster? Gone! I can't believe it!
For many years it stayed with me every day, it stalked me, forced
me to cringe in embarrassment. The monster was a horrible
dragon. It was ethnic, nationalistic, anti-European, misogynistic,
xenophobic, homophobic and extremely dishonest. It was able
to eat chalk by the kilo[61] and thereby conceal its naked desire for
destruction, its criminal energy. In my hours of therapy I
struggled and fought fiercely with this beast, the perpetrator-
victim from my family of origin in physical form. Monster is
much too innocent a name for the brown scaly beast that had
tried daily to cut the ground from under my feet and snatch away
my love of life.

Victims, murderers and Nazis in my family

We didn't talk much at home, but were silent a lot. I could never
properly understand my familial reality. Interestingly, I was the
only one of six siblings who was curious and wanted to know
what had happened in the family. I wanted to find out what the
dark clouds of silence meant. As an adult, after my parents'
deaths, I really wanted to know. I did extensive research in
archives, had many conversations with acquaintances and
relations. This impulse – wanting to know what it is – was the
first significant step to finding my Self. What was difficult for me
was that my curiosity made me rather unpopular with my
relatives, but no one could stop me from learning to think more

---

[61] There is a saying in Germany that a dishonest person eats chalk like the wolf
in the fairy tale Rotkäppchen.

clearly. And so I became more daring and carried on with my research.

My grandfather, Karl, had died before I was born. Apparently he was a likeable person, friend and neighbour. But what I found out through my family research was much more complicated. He was also an official in the NSDAP (Nazi Party), and not just the harmless follower the family had made him out to be. His wife, my grandmother Gusti, died in February 1943, killed by a bullet from his service pistol. The more detailed circumstances surrounding this event have remained mysterious because no one ever wanted to talk about it. The deadly shot was fired in front of her children. My mother was one of these children: she was 11 years old at the time and my aunt was 14. My grandfather was also jointly responsible for the fact that my grandmother's brother, Pepi, and his wife Greti – both of whom were active in the resistance to the Nazi regime – were murdered by the Nazis' henchmen.

I realised that these events would also have an effect on the next generation, particularly as there was a conspiracy of silence surrounding them. Destructive family secrets are known to cast long shadows. If one's own ancestors are (co)-responsible for the violent death of family members but have never admitted to this wrong, then neither does the perpetrators' murderous energy, nor the victims' justifiable fear of being killed disappear of its own accord from the family's relationship structure. It remains present for the subsequent generations as a split-off legacy of feelings, as perpetrator-victim dynamics, as existential fear and as internalised perpetrator energy.

I have inherited a considerable part of this dynamic. On a psychological level, this presents as utter fear of destruction and blatant feelings of blame and shame. On a physical level it was my painful rheumatoid arthritis, an autoimmune disease that attacks one's own body and as a result leads to severe physical damage. I couldn't even begin to grasp what happened in me and to me. I wasn't able to access this trans-generational maelstrom of trauma that had been passed on to me. That I myself was a 'prisoner' and caught in a familial perpetrator-victim dynamic –

that idea would not have occurred to me. I just churned out my stress defence strategies like an unstoppable program of destruction. For a long time this program was my survival program. In order to survive (psychologically) in my family, I had been forced at an early age to split, to give myself up, to come to terms with obscure fears and intense emotional and physical phenomena.

From an early age I had had a special relationship with my mother's sister, my godmother, which today I would probably describe as a symbiotic love-hate relationship. The character of our family ties gave me the feeling that I had to be there for her. I was there so that she didn't have to be alone, and to give her a sense of wellbeing. My aunt was a young widow. She didn't have any children of her own, just me. If I attempted to break free of the constraints of our conflict-prone relationship, I immediately felt guilty and ashamed of my selfishness. Whatever I did, I could not break out of the prison of our relationship structure. I began to take an interest in her childhood; I talked to her a lot about the time of World War II and tried to understand why she still defended National Socialism and the Hitler period, but I didn't get very far with it.

At some point I realised that it was vital for me to free myself from the entanglements with my family of origin. I wanted to escape from it, so internally I distanced myself from my family and in particular from my aunt. My decision had a great effect on my aunt; after I ended our relationship she declined into paranoia and dementia. That, again, was difficult for me to bear because my aunt, who was now 87, had become very needy and lonely. I suffered a great deal from not being able to do anything for her. It took years until I not only thought, but also sensed and felt, that it wasn't me who was responsible for her wellbeing, but she herself. My unconditional feelings of loyalty towards her gradually decreased, while at the same time my own personal being became clearer, my true identity, the Isabella who was marked by attributions from the family, and the Isabella I really am.

My mother takes her secret with her to the grave

I'll go back to the beginning, to my earliest memories, to my mother's eyes. I was afraid of them. As a little child I probably had to suppress my own needs and feelings, especially my need for love. I remained caught in this relationship with my mother for a long time because I hoped at some point to receive the love that was not forthcoming from her. I was a child who had not received enough love and I was desperately ashamed because of it, even long after I was grown up. I thought I wasn't lovable. Although it was the grandparents and parents who didn't know what love really was, I held myself responsible for my dilemma. I quite soon turned "I am not loved" into "I am not lovable". For a long time I believed it was my own failure that I had received too little warmth, security and direction. For a long time I had hoped that if I only understood well enough what had happened to my mother, and if I forgave her for what she had kept from me, namely her love, then everything would be good between us. Then I'd feel better again. Well-meaning friends and therapists also found me to be lacking in willingness for reconciliation and forgiveness. I was ready to work on myself, so I tried forgiving. I asked my mother internally for forgiveness. It was my bad luck, and that was a very bitter disappointment for me, that despite my attempts, there was no happy end for me. Instead of peace and relief, a profound pain got hold of me. I was mercilessly confronted with the question: "Who am I really?" I felt hollow. Realising that was hard for me.

When children like me grow up and finally realise that they have grown up in a dishonest perpetrator family, they do not feel any better. Not even when they later succeed in choosing a profession and having a family. What I most longed for was to be able to be completely at peace with myself and at the same time to feel I belonged wholeheartedly to other people. But I have only succeeded occasionally in feeling what that is. My longing for natural closeness and my awkward attempts at establishing contact often ended in me running a well-disguised gauntlet. The fear of going under, of having to give up on myself, was ever-present. I sensed that something was lacking in me, something basic. Exactly what that was, I didn't know. But it had to do with me, with my suchness.

In 2002 my mother died without there having been the slightest change in our weird relationship. She was already very ill and was dying when I asked her for a clarifying conversation. It was the last chance for me to straighten things out with her. She didn't want this and refused to have this conversation. She died shortly after I had left. My siblings told me that our mother had fought against dying and had suffered an agonising death struggle.

After her death, I had a genetic test done with the help of my sisters, and found out that I have a different biological father. Clarity at last! This result was a huge relief for me because I finally had an explanation for feeling that I didn't belong with my siblings. My mother had lied to me her whole life.

It was in the year she died and I had just turned 44 that I was given the diagnosis of 'rheumatoid arthritis'. As I have already mentioned, this autoimmune disease is an extremely painful systemic disease and, according to conventional medicine, the cause has still not been identified. It is supposedly incurable.

Arthritis treatment in conventional medicine

Five different classes of medicinal products are used to treat arthritis: painkillers; non-steroid anti-rheumatics (NSAR), which are anti-inflammatory painkillers without cortisone; cortisone; so-called basic therapeutics; so-called biologicals. I have been prescribed all classes of medicinal products at different stages of the disease. Despite this, the destruction of my joints could not be arrested. The painkiller Rheutrop retard was my indispensable companion for 10 years.

When arthritis is first diagnosed, painkillers or NSARs are usually prescribed. Neither of these have much to do with healing; all they do is numb the pain of arthritis, while the latter also suppresses inflammation. Unfortunately these drugs have many side effects. Paracetamol is responsible for two-thirds of

all cases of acute liver failure caused by medicines.[62] Along with
the basic therapeutics described below, I was also prescribed
cortisone. Inflammation is suppressed more strongly by
cortisone than by NSARs. Of course cortisone does not only
affect the joint, but the whole body, although that is not
necessary. Thus side effects from cortisone also appear throughout the whole body. These side effects might be high blood
pressure, or strong pangs of hunger leading to weight gain.
When I was using cortisone I developed a 'moon face', and
people who didn't know the situation made me the debatable
compliment of saying I looked so "healthy and plump". As
cortisone suppresses inflammation by weakening the body's own
immune system, an organism treated with cortisone is more at
risk of infection.

Biologicals are brand new medicinal products developed in a
genetics laboratory. Unlike basic therapeutics, biologicals affect
specific parts of the immune system. The so-called TNF-alpha-
inhibitors, for example, disable the messenger substance of the
same name that passes on information between the immune cells.
If this treatment does not work, or is accompanied by strong side
effects, there will be further experiments, for instance with so-
called B-cell therapy. This treatment only destroys certain B-cells
of the immune system, namely those that play a key role in the
onset and continuation of arthritis. Biologicals have only been in
use for a few years and some are still in their test phase. The
long-term side effects are completely unknown at the moment,
but it is hardly realistic to suppose that there will be no consequences from long-term medicinal attacks on the organism's
highly complex regulatory and communication mechanisms. In
May 2012 I had to have an emergency operation due to massive
side effects from biological therapy, because the intern in charge
had overlooked pneumonia.

---

[62] Chantal Schlatter: *'Nebenwirkung Leberschaden'*, 'liver damage as a side
effect' in *Pharmazeutische Zeitung online*, www.pharmazeutische-zeitung-
de/index.php?id=30764

Healed, because I was in touch with myself

I was lucky enough to get to know Franz Ruppert and his work with the Intention Method at just the right moment. That was in the Chamber of Labour in Feldkirch, where he gave a lecture that changed my life. Since then I have been working on myself in individual sessions and in groups using his method, which has completely convinced me. It was through identity work with the Intention Method that I first developed an understanding of the highly complex perpetrator-victim dynamic I was caught up in. That was the turning point in my personality development. It was particularly important for me to grasp what trauma actually is, and what it had done to me. Ruppert's splitting model of the human psyche helped me understand what was behind my autoimmune disease, what caused its onset and its continuation. With the help of his theoretical concept I began to understand what was wrong with me.

For over a year now I have been completely free of complaints – I have absolutely no disease symptoms any more. But I cannot deny that it has been hard. My physical symptoms did not improve in the first two years; on the contrary, my symptoms initially became much worse with many inflamed joints and severe pain. I was close to being severely disabled and in a wheelchair. But I stuck with it, I stayed with myself, despite everything, and despite my fears. I no longer know exactly when it happened, but I suddenly noticed that healing was taking place in me and in my body.

Today is 13th November 2016. I am drinking the best cappuccino in the world. A heart-warming feeling floods through me and ignites a spark in me. A pleasant atmosphere radiates around, in the room and in me. I am sitting in the patisserie of a spa hotel, with myself as my counterpart. Where and what is home – a place, a feeling? I experience an unknown feeling of being home. Here and in myself. Suddenly it is there, the feeling I have waited so long for. I have arrived at my true self. The interior design of the patisserie allows me to look outside. Extensive glass walls usher in the familiar landscape with the almost-leafless plane trees. Everything is simultaneously outside and inside. I am experiencing the same thing within myself at this moment, with my body and my inner world. I feel complete. And absolutely right. What a feeling of happiness!

The work with the Intention Method has become dear to my heart. Today in my psychotherapeutic practice I mostly work with people who suffer from so-called 'incurable autoimmune diseases'.

Mag. Isabella Gerstgrasser has her psychology practice in Feldkirch/Vorarlberg. www.isabella-gerstgrasser.at

KATE COLLIER

Lymphoma – 'cancer'

'Cancer' and 'cancer therapies'

Thirteen years ago I had my first occurrence of 'Non-Hodgkins Lymphoma' – 'cancer' of the lymph system. My body-psyche had suppressed such a high level of stress, and so it went into a life threatening state. For a year I had nursed my husband with 'cancer', as well as looking after my children and teaching. My husband subsequently died and I was left with our 14 and 10 year old sons. My younger son, with special needs, had an emergency heart operation eight weeks after his father died.

This was followed by three more deaths in the family. Then came my brother's terminal 'cancer' which was diagnosed on the day I found my own very small lump. My doctor thought it was benign. However, when I came back from the States where my brother had died, this lump had doubled in size and another doctor also saw it as benign. I insisted on being fast-tracked – which he did – for emotional reasons. I then was told I had 'cancer'. I received the news with disbelief and dissociation and got on as best I could with looking after my children and working. I had little time to think about myself.

Then after having radiotherapy I thought my 'cancer' was gone. And when it returned three years later at Stage 3 and was life threatening, I was strongly advised six months of chemotherapy treatment. I remember thinking, "if I don't take this treatment I will orphan my children". My reaction was that it was not about me; in fact I wasn't emotional about it at all. I was frozen; I felt isolated and alone. I felt unsupported without my husband and concerned about how the children would handle the news. And yet it was my fierce independence and inability to know or say my needs that fed my isolation.

I was living and working in a special needs community with my son in the USA at that time and a long way from home. My treatment was highly medicalised of course. I had four brightly coloured chemical cocktails in the drips above me and felt the shock and repulsion as they rushed up my veins and as I sucked ice to stop being sick. I remember a friend shaving my hair, crying for me as it fell to the floor, the chemo hats to keep the cold winter air out, and I remember the cold touch of a succession of body scans. The steroids sent me into a disembodied state and I was drained of energy as the effects of the treatment accumulated.

Fortunately I was well nourished with organic food, healing therapies and support from those around me in the community. Above all, I was positive, sustained by a spiritual practice – partly another form of survival ritual. I was looking straight at my mortality and managing to feel okay.

It is only now in identity therapy that I see how dissociated, split and disembodied I was, and always had been. In other words I had the pathology for 'cancer': my identity was in others' emotions; my survival patterning was to suppress my own emotions and be happy for them.

Trauma and identity constellations

When I started following Franz Ruppert's method, called trauma constellations then (Ruppert, 2016), I began to see my earliest traumas and the way my survival mechanisms affected my illness, and how my so-called 'cancer' was the ultimate survival strategy.

In self-encounters with different intentions, my implicit body memory and the resonance of others allowed me to see for the first time the layers of trauma that had been there from the very start of my life. I was born with jaundice and I saw the fragile, traumatised baby that wasn't seen by the medics and nearly died, and the survival parts that were disconnected, isolated and hyper vigilant. I felt myself plucked from my mother in the emergency. The resonance of the representatives showed lots of bright lights and a fight for my life. I was alone, isolated and without the warmth of my mother. In those days babies were put in a ward apart from their mothers and taken for feeding every four hours. So I split because of the existential trauma from the cultural and medical practice of the time creating for me a trauma of love.

I often see with my clients, when exploring pre-birth trauma, an unfriendly, unsafe womb and I realise that if a woman holds the fear and mistrust of trauma, her womb is like an object to her, disembodied and external to her – and so for the baby growing inside her. So I began to wonder about my own in utero life. I set up an intention to sense how it was for me in the womb. I wanted to separate what was mine from my mother's to understand the entanglement.

In the womb one representative reported it was cold with no sense of feeling of where to attach, I was unwanted, my mother was exhausted and the only way I could make that life-death connection with my mother was to not want myself, to give up on myself. The representative for my *'want'* was hanging on by a thread. What I saw in this encounter was how I had given up on myself in order to be able to attach to my mother. I saw everything I held about myself explained: a feeling that I had no true place in the world, was not wanted by others and that I had to apologise for being here, for living. I felt a lot of shame around my very existence, enhanced by being at the bottom of a sibling pecking order. The inner turbulence and anxiety were compensated for by an exterior social confidence and smile on my face.

So I survived by taking on my mother's identity, feeling the emotions of my parents and siblings at the expense of my own, and, as one representative reported, actually feeling alive by perpetrating against myself. In this way I lost my identity in a family where true, honest emotions of love, sadness and pain were covered by a 'happy, fun' survival ideology. Such a pathology for 'cancer' was created from the start in my survival mechanisms – suppression of my emotions and needs and constant vigilance and care of the emotions of others. An automatic regard for the emotional needs of others, while ignoring your own, is a major factor for chronic "illness" (Maté, 2003).

With the pain and grief during these processes, I experienced greater embodiment, a warming up of my body and thawing of my emotions. I became interested in how medical intervention in adulthood triggers our very earliest traumas and survival patterning, and how recovery is about seeing, feeling, sensing and re-embodying ourselves.

Traumatisations through the medical system

I also see a parallel between the way we lose our identity in the medical system when we are adults and our earliest experiences of identity trauma at birth, and in our attachment with mother and father. When we enter a hospital, we are a number, called 'a patient' and tagged – at a hospital birth we have a number, are called 'a baby' and tagged. We lose something of who we are from the very start in life. When we are diagnosed we are labelled with the identity of the 'illness'.

I was sensitive to being labelled 'a cancer patient'. Inside I refused to take on the identification. Partly this was healthy and partly my survival way of not wanting to be a victim and vulnerable. But I *was* a victim and the consultant was in authority – I was depending on him to keep me alive.

The unconscious, victim-perpetrator dynamic with the consultant, though kind and of good intention, was not so different from my authoritative but well-meaning father who took his role, duty and responsibility seriously. Even the way we experience medics as cold and withdrawn can trigger our earliest bonding trauma. In their own survival system, they are hiding behind the symptoms and treatment plans and asking you to comply with fear of the consequences. This has parallels with the parent-child dynamic and fear of being excluded by not accepting the norms of the family.

I have clients who have experienced medical procedures as similar to physical assault or rape, often having been witnessed by students and medics in physically intimate positions, exposed to their detached eyes and the cold touch of surgical equipment. The client may have been conscious or under anaesthesia but this memory is held in the body. We may also be traumatised by medical intervention because we carry unresolved trauma from previous medical treatment done to ourselves or others – in my case I entered the same oncology unit I had been to with my late husband during his treatment. My love and identity traumas were retriggered by medical intervention and my survival pathology responded in exactly the way it always had.

Knowing more clearly who I am

For years after my 'cancer' treatment I felt fear, panic and anxiety not only that it would return but that I'd die in another way – fear therefore to live. As I got in touch with primal feelings of pain, anger, sadness, and shame and saw what my trauma was, and what was not mine, the healthy part of who I am felt clearer, stronger, more compassionate with myself and more connected. One day I woke up realising that the fear of 'cancer' recurring had gone, and my anxiety around 'illness' no longer had a hold on me. Instead I have a greater understanding and a more authentically present sense of who I am. So I could say the Intention method has helped me to recover from illness and medical intervention but, in fact, it has helped me truly meet myself for the first time.

References

Maté, G. (2003). *When the body says No. Exploring the stress-disease connection.* Hoboken/New Jersey: John Wiley & Sons.
Ruppert, F. (ed.) (2016). *Early Trauma.* Steyning, Green Balloon Publishing.

Kate Collier was a teacher from 1973 to 2007 in UK, Africa and the USA. She became a Body Therapist from 1996, Qualified as a Therapeutic Counsellor and Systemic Constellations Facilitator in 2010. She engaged IoPT Supervision / Training 2013–2016. Kate now has her own practice in Brighton, UK working with IoPT and EFT in individual, workshops and online sessions. www.katecollier.net fkatecollier@yahoo.co.uk

NADJA PALOMBO

Sleep disorders and psychotrauma

The function of sleep

Sleep is a natural phenomenon and is essential to human life. It is not a passive state but passes through the brain in rhythmic cycles. A person spends about 3,000 hours a year, and about a third of their life asleep. An adult's sleep requirements varies from individual to individual and lies between four and nine hours, with an average of six to seven hours. If a person sleeps for fewer than four hours or more than nine hours on a permanent basis, this correlates with an increased risk of, for example, heart disease or diabetes, impaired performance and poor concentration, depression, weakening of the immune system and increased susceptibility to infection (Pape, Kurtz and Silbernagl, 2014).

During sleep the body's temperature drops, as does the amount of energy required to keep the body's vital functions going, and so the heart rate and respiratory frequency slow down. Today we assume that the phases of sleep and physical relaxation also play an important role in our ability to learn and our memory capacity. Sleep activates the immune system and helps to regulate the metabolism. The body's inactivity during sleep creates optimal conditions for the process of cell renewal. Insufficient cell renewal encourages premature deterioration and aging.[63]

Individual sleep cycles can be analysed in a sleep laboratory. Detailed measurements are taken of brain activity, muscular

---

[63] www.prosomno.de

tension, eye movement, heart and respiratory rates as well as physical movement. There are five different stages of sleep: Stages 1–4 are non-REM sleep, stage 5 is REM sleep (REM is rapid eye movement).

Falling asleep and light sleep (stages 1–2) account for 55–60% of the whole period of sleep. Stages 3 and 4 are termed deep sleep (15–20%). Stage 5, REM sleep, also called active sleep, is characterised by intense dreaming and an increase in heart and respiratory activity and cerebral blood flow. In a healthy person, sleep begins with shallow sleep (stages 1–2), followed by a period of deep sleep (stages 3–4) and REM sleep. As a rule there are four to six such cycles per night.

If people are woken up during a period of REM sleep, 80% of them say they have been dreaming. During REM sleep, our brain makes our skeletal muscles extremely limp so that we don't actually carry out all the movements we are dreaming. That is why in some nightmares we feel we have to run away but we can't; we're unable to move. Sleepwalking, therefore, doesn't happen during REM sleep but during phases of deep sleep.

While deep sleep is accredited with the task of physical regeneration, REM sleep seems to be necessary for psychological recovery. In summary, we can say that the five stages of sleep have to appear in their proper order to ensure that sleep is restful and restorative. Brief periods of wakefulness are completely natural in this process.

Sleep disorders

Sleep disorders are distinguishable by their symptoms as well as their causes. On a symptomatic level, we can broadly differentiate four forms of sleep disorders or sleep-wake disorders:[64]

---

[64] www.schlafgestoert.de

Form of disorder	Symptoms
Failure to fall asleep and/or inability to stay asleep (insomnia)	Difficulty falling asleep; frequent waking up in the night; difficulty going back to sleep; waking up too early in the morning; the feeling of not really sleeping deeply; not refreshing and too little sleep
Disorders with increased sleepiness during the day (hypersomnia)	Problems staying awake during the day; involuntary falling asleep or dozing during the day; being permanently sleepy despite sufficient length of time asleep
Disruption of the sleep-wake rhythm	Problems going to sleep at 'normal' times; instead, those affected go to bed significantly earlier or later, but then as a rule have no problem sleeping (can be caused by shift work, medicines or substance abuse)
Disorders/abnormalities/ disruptions occurring during sleep (parasomnia)	Abnormalities in sleep, e.g. sleepwalking, sleep-related breathing disorders (temporary suspension of breathing), nightmares, nocturnal groaning, restless legs syndrome, sleep-related eating disorders, nocturnal bedwetting or talking, teeth-grinding during sleep

Sleep disorders often occur during stressful situations (if one cannot switch off) or through unfavourable sleeping habits. The reason for sleep disorders can be, for example, chronic pain, hormonal diseases, gastrointestinal disorder, multiple sclerosis, etc. Sleep disorders often appear as a side effect of medications. These include, for example, antibiotics, certain anti-depressants, blood-pressure medications, asthma medications, cortisone, thyroid hormones, medication for dementia, antihistamines (for allergies), and chemotherapy. Similarly, drugs such as alcohol, caffeine, nicotine, cannabis, heroin, cocaine and ecstasy can cause sleep disorders.

People with sleep disorders complain most frequently about difficulty in falling asleep, followed by disruptions in staying asleep and waking up too early in the morning. There is frequently a combination of several sleep disorders. About 15% of the population in industrialised nations suffer from chronic sleep disorders. A further 20% complain of occasional problems going to sleep or staying awake. The percentage can be much higher in certain population groups (for example shift workers, 50% of whom are affected by sleep disorders). Sleep disorders, headaches and backaches are the most frequent psychosomatic complaints. In the age group 65 years and above, 40% complain about not getting enough sleep or about problems to do with sleep. Men and women are equally affected in the age group up to 40 years; thereafter, the proportion of women to men affected increases to 3:2.

Acute sleep disorders often vanish when the cause (such as acute stress at work) disappears. However sometimes some sleep disorders take on a life of their own after a few weeks, then the original cause doesn't play a role any more and the sleep disorder becomes chronic. This is true of two-thirds of the patients with severe sleep disorders that may have been ongoing for anywhere between one to five years, with 40% of those concerned suffering from a chronic sleep disorder for more than five years. In outpatient clinics for sleep medicine, patients with sleep disorders report that the sleep disruption has already been going on for an average of 12 to 14 years.

Sedation of children – an alarming trend

At this point I would like to point out a dangerous trend: parents are sedating their children with soporifics. Infants and toddlers rarely sleep through the night; some cry and scream the whole night. Parents then want to be able to sleep through the night; they are exhausted and have insufficient strength to manage, and then may become aggressive. In the past some parents used to dip the child's dummy in beer or wine to calm a child down. Today frequently overtired parents make use of what they think are harmless soporifics for fretful children. Parents seek advice and understanding on internet forums. One popular 'sleep mixture' is Sedaplus, which is available in chemists without a prescription. The active substance Doxylamin used to be an ingredient in anti-allergic medication and one of its side effects is to make the person drowsy. The same soporific side effect is used in cough mixtures and cold remedies or medication for nausea. These medicines are also approved for small children in a weak dose. "As their sedative effect is commonly known, we can assume that these products are also used to calm down or sedate."[65]

Soporifics disrupt the natural rhythm of sleep: the children sleep too deeply, impeding the nocturnal phases of dreaming and learning, and their breathing is too shallow. This can lead to organ damage and respiratory arrest. As these 'sleeping aids' are available over the counter, there are no figures or statistics concerning their use. Parents who take their overdosed children to paediatricians are often too ashamed to admit to this practice. Estimates assume that at least two out of 10 children are given soporifics in some form. The actual figure might be far higher.

---

[65] Hannsjörg W. Seyberth: '*Rezeptfreie Antihistaminika bergen Risiken für Kleinkinder*' 'Prescription-free antihistamines put little children at risk', in: *Deutsches Ärzteblatt* German Medical Journal (2012) 109, H.37, S. A 1822.

Psychotrauma as the cause of sleep disorders

Many people who have experienced a psychotrauma also suffer from sleep disorders such as nightmares or difficulty falling asleep or staying asleep.

As a small boy Egon and his parents experienced expulsion from East Prussia. He had psychotherapy for several years but still suffers from nightmares today. He says: "I have often been woken up by my own screams. I wasn't able to talk to people around me any more. And when something was said, I still wasn't helped. It's a vicious cycle: not able to sleep, not able to rest, exhaustion, becoming ill, weakening of the immune system. Pills are no help with that."

Traumatised people are at pains to suppress their trauma experiences. They attempt to split off all the feelings that have anything to do with the trauma. This mechanism also has to be continued in their sleep. This is a paradox, because we actually need the sleep phases to switch off our control mechanisms. Thus, people with sleep disorders encounter problems as early as the first two phases of sleep. They are unable to switch off because they are afraid of losing control. In the light sleep phase – which is after all about 50% of our sleep time – their stressful thoughts and feelings continue.

Case history: Heike

Heike says that for many years she has had nightmares several times a week. In her dreams she trembles, is afraid, can't defend herself and feels frozen. She wakes from her nightmares with a profound feeling of desperation. In her dreams she tries to scream, which for years she was unable to do. This only changed when she began to work through her nightmares. The muted scream was finally vocalised, after many years – a part was able to express itself audibly with a loud, long-drawn-out "NOOO!" not just internally but externally as well.

In one of her first constellations Heike said that, as a child, she was alone in the evening, almost on a daily basis, and watched television until late at night. She remembers falling asleep in front of the television and being woken after a while by scenes in horror films. Her intention was: "What trauma is reflected in my night-mares?"

A representative in her constellation said that the horror in the films was nothing compared to the horror she had to endure. It also became evident that it wasn't one single traumatic event, but an ever-present danger that caused Heike great distress. Another piece of information was that it had to do with violence and that Heike was alone in those situations without any help from her mother or anyone else. So it wasn't a case of it being a one-off event that was regularly re-enacted in her nightmares, as Heike had thought. Her nightmares were the symptom for her ongoing childhood experiences of being alone and in great distress. After this constellation her screams during her nightmares were not so frequent and not as loud. She also felt the nightmares were less threatening.

Heike was always very afraid of going to bed. She regularly looked under the bed and even today she sleeps with her bedside light switched on. She set up several further intentions with the following wording: "What happened to me as a child?", "What violence have I seen and what have I experienced myself?", "What precisely happened to me that I am so afraid of?"

The results of these further constellations showed that her mother had attempted to abort Heike and had tried to commit suicide while pregnant with Heike. In the constellations Heike could plainly feel that she wasn't protected in any way. This made her extremely afraid of relinquishing control during sleep. Heike then remembered that she was often rudely awakened out of a deep sleep in the middle of the night by her father shouting and punching her mother. As a child she sometimes got up at five o'clock in the morning so as to enjoy some peace and quiet. Usually by this time, things had calmed down in the family and her parents were asleep. But sometimes the peace was deceptive and after a 'ceasefire' her father's terrorising would start again. She wept while she was talking about it and it took a long time before she was able to calm down. "Those were the very bad days, when he even robbed us of those few hours to recover from the horror the previous night. He simply kept on with his beatings."

Heike explained that she felt she could only sleep reasonably well if she was in a room with someone she trusted. Then she felt as if she could let go. Her previous partner had been someone like that. He had also confirmed to her that she trembled shortly after falling asleep, that her whole body was tense and she had whimpered quietly.

Heike's next intention was: *"Ich möchte fühlen, wovor ich Angst habe."* [Word for word translation: "I would-like to-feel, whereof I fear have."] "I would like to feel what I am afraid of." In the constellation, the representative of the word 'whereof' embodied the father's aggression. The word 'fear' stood for the connection to her mother. The representative of 'fear' said: "It's not that bad!" Heike had heard this sentence again and again from her mother in an attempt to calm her down. In her relationship with her mother Heike also came into contact with her mother's trauma feelings, in other words with the violence that her mother had experienced, as well as with her mother's survival strategy of playing down her experiences. In the constellation Heike had made a significant physical experience for herself: "Tension is created by threat; release is created by good contact."

In the conversation following this constellation, Heike became aware that there is a part inside her that prefers any form of contact with her mother to emptiness and loneliness. The bond between Heike and her mother still exists today through the common feeling of helplessness and being a victim.

For Heike, sleeplessness is the result of violence and abandonment. As a child she was entirely at the mercy of continual violence from her father. Staying awake, therefore, is her attempt to avoid being subjected to threatening attacks. Although she knows that the actual danger has passed, her protective mechanism is still active. The second thing Heike experienced was being abandoned, associated with the feeling of loneliness. The mother could only make light of Heike's father's violence, because she was also helplessly exposed to it. As a consequence, Heike was alone with the horror she experienced and had to split off all the feelings that engendered fear.

Heike's sleep remains her yardstick, determining what degree of trauma feelings she can allow and tolerate. On the other hand new sleep problems appear, whether it be falling asleep or staying asleep, whenever she is overstressed in her life. Heike's level of suffering has become significantly lower and her quality of sleep has improved, and she continues to work on understanding her traumatisations, and fitting them into her life and thereby coming more into resonance with the healthy parts within her.

Conclusions

The following insights are based on Heike's example. Sleep disorders are frequently a consequence of

- insufficient parental care,
- emotional abandonment,
- hostility towards the child,
- sexual attacks which took place in the night.

A trauma is often re-enacted during sleep in the form of a nightmare. In many cases, sleeplessness can be seen as a survival mechanism of the psyche, to try to stay awake, because the perpetrators came at night.

In my experience, sleep disorders are frequently more than an isolated symptom. They have a history and causes that often reach back into childhood. It is worth getting to the bottom of them by trying to establish a link between symptom and cause. Then the memories, the feeling and perception within will return into connection and harmony. What we need is healing relationships.

Egon, whose history I have touched upon, expressed it in this way: "What helps me is if people take my feelings seriously, and I have a perspective it's worth living for. I don't need any theories or medicines, but people who believe in me, who feel with me and encourage me."

References

Pape, H.-C., Kurtz, A. & Silbernagl, S. (2014): *Physiologie*. Stuttgart, Thieme

Nadja Palombo was born in 1965. She has had her own practice since 2003 at the South German Institute for Logotherapy and Existential Analysis in Fürstenfeldbruck. She is also an alternative practitioner for psychotherapy, graduate social pedagogue, and supervisor, having completed an advanced training in logotherapy and existential analysis, systemic therapy and traumatherapy with Franz Ruppert. www.nadja-palombo.de

BETTINA SCHMALNAUER

Childhood diseases, parents and trauma

Children in distress

Babies brought to my practice are often babies who cry a great deal. They may have digestive problems, problems with sleeping or skin rashes. In the case of toddlers, it is often a matter of difficulties in their relationship with other children, fears, wetting or soiling themselves, infectious illnesses or frequently a high temperature. Children of school age may be bothered by schoolwork and exam fears, as well as bullying, and exhibit nightmares, grinding their teeth, frequent stomach-, ear- or headaches, severe coughs or allergies.

Recognising and finding out the causes of these childhood messages is the basis of my work. A child or a baby is not yet able verbally to express how he feels. If conventional medicine does not achieve the desired healing, many concerned parents today turn to other methods. I work with the BodyTalkSystem© with babies and children, while I have had good experiences with the Intention Method in one-on-one work with children of 12 years or older. Depending on their personal maturity, adolescents from the age of 16 upwards can also work in group sessions with the Intention Method. The best results can be achieved if the parents are also prepared to look at their own childhood issues.

Luckily enough, the distress of babies who cry, who don't want to sleep or drink is today, as a rule, taken seriously. Most mothers and fathers no longer want to toughen up their children by letting them cry. My questions to the mothers prior to a session are chiefly about the course of the pregnancy and how both mother and child experienced the birth. It is always fascinating how clearly and precisely the babies 'tell' me their experiences, using all methods at their disposal: their facial expressions, gestures, body language and their crying. They tell of their mortal fear during the pregnancy and the birth process, for example if the birth was induced because it wasn't progressing and they experienced stress and shock, or if they became stuck in the birth canal, or if they had to survive a Caesarean section.

Children at kindergarten and their parents

At kindergarten age, children sense exactly how their parents are feeling, and express this unconsciously but clearly, especially if the parents have split off their feelings and memories. If parents come with their children, I see it as my duty to speak for the children and to translate what they are trying to express. It is often the only way to gain the mother's attention.

Laura is four years old. She had suffered repeatedly from infectious illnesses, and frequently had a high temperature, a cold, inflammation of the ears and above all an exhausting and persistent dry cough. At night she often gets into 'Mummy's bed', and has difficulty falling asleep and sleeping through the night. Her mother, Sabine, comes with her to my practice. I ask her about her daughter's complaints. These are explained to me while the little one waits on the couch. Then the mother talks incessantly and in detail about her mother-in-law. I take the liberty of pointing that out to her. She looks at me, shocked – she hadn't even noticed. In our further work together, Sabine, Laura, her brother David, who is three years older, and the father, Gerhard, all come to my practice. Laura's cough and her infections quickly improve. As Sabine and Gerhard are willing to work with the Intention Method, their trauma biographies become apparent.

Gerhard's parents are both alcoholics and his sister is frequently in a psychiatric ward. As a child, Gerhard was often left alone, had to endure his parents' arguments and as a result was very withdrawn. He appears very introverted and his body language indicates many beatings. Unfortunately he also seeks refuge in alcohol. Sabine has often spent nights looking for him, particularly when she was pregnant with David. She didn't know what state he'd be in when she found him. At home, Gerhard often shouts at the children, who are already scared of him. As the wellbeing of his children is also important to him, he is prepared to look at everything.

Through Sabine's constellations of the intention, we discover that in her childhood she suffered from a weak mother and a silent father. The conflicts between her parents were not dealt with, but were always in the air. When she was in puberty, her father insulted her by calling her "incapable and too stupid" with regard to schoolwork. All this went so far that, as an adolescent, Sabine was thinking of committing suicide, and developed 'bulimia'. In holidays she spent with her grandparents, an uncle sexually abused her. Over a period of three years, Sabine was able to look at all this in individual and group sessions. Afterwards she felt very much better.

Since then, Gerhard's and Sabine's children have developed well and are physically healthy.

Schoolchildren who wet themselves

The parents who come to my practice are usually those who make a serious and credible effort to be good parents. Sometimes they even want to do "everything for the child" better than their own parents did. These are often families where everything should really be good. Often the parents have worked a lot to provide well for the family, but there has not been time for relationships and emotional care. This is where the parents are challenged to look closely at their own childhood. "How were you at the age your child is now?" I often learn of traumatic events when I put this question to the parents.

Schoolchildren wetting themselves is a common problem that is very much a taboo. Statistically it affects more boys than girls. I also have children coming to my practice who soil themselves. The sense of shame here is even greater, as is the reluctance to ask for help. It is not only the parents who are embarrassed; the child is also deeply ashamed in front of his parents. In these cases I have often observed that the child goes by the maxim: hold everything in during the day, and take off the pressure at night and "cry downwards". Working with these children, I aim to talk to them at eye level, to create a trusting relationship and let them understand my honest intention to help them. The subject of wetting and soiling demands a great deal of intuition and tact. Not infrequently, I cannot even talk about it directly.

Ilona comes with her son Florian, because he's "so restless and fidgety", but above all because of his 'nightly problem': he wets his bed almost every night. When Ilona sets up her intention: "Why am I an anxious, negative person?" the final words in her sentence make her think of a miscarriage. This was some time ago, but even so, Ilona immediately bursts into tears. Many unwept tears and things unspoken now come out of her. After this process she is visibly relieved and seems more alive and 'more present'.

Fritz, Florian's father, is a tall, well-built man and successful at work. His intention is "Why am I inwardly restless and why do I submit to social pressure?" In his constellation his mother's belief comes to light: that everything has to look good on the surface. Working through his intention frees him and relieves him visibly of his inward pressure.

"Florian can now let himself go and relax, which was difficult for him until now. He appears relaxed and liberated. We have noticed a considerable improvement", his father writes to me later.

Absent parents, absent friends

Leonie is now 12 years old and has been coming to me with her mother, Sandra, since her first year at primary school. They are both concerned about what's happening at school. Her best friend from primary school is plotting against her, passing her mistakes off as Leonie's and making out that Leonie's achievements and ideas are her own. In class, Leonie is always excluded and she is hardly ever invited to parties. I explain the Intention Method in the individual setting to mother and daughter. Leonie is quickly convinced and willing. Sandra doesn't yet have the courage to do her own work.

Leonie's intention "I want to have the courage to say something and not worry what the others think of me", reveals the following: because of her parents' guesthouse, Leonie was frequently left on her own as a little child. Mother and father worked a lot and although the flat was on the first floor of the guest house, Leonie often has to occupy herself, and go to bed alone, while both her parents are busy downstairs. Her search for an accepting person she has transferred to her friends. If it doesn't work with her parents, then perhaps with friends! So don't say anything that could annoy them or chase them away.

So the original rejection was from her parents, who had also grown up with self-employed parents who had only worked for their own business. The good of the firm was always put ahead of anything else. Sandra often hears from Leonie: "You always leave me on my own!" Until now Sandra has put forward counter-arguments and justified her actions. I encourage Leonie to tell her mother truthfully how she feels and what she needs. I recommend to her mother that she listens to, sees and accepts the needs of her child. During the work it occurs to Leonie that she could look for other girls, and boys too, as friends and forget about the ones who don't want her. Several occur to her straight-away.

I am very pleased to hear later from Leonie and Sandra that everything has turned out well. Emboldened by her daughter, Sandra later comes to one-on-one sessions in which she looks at her own issue – being left alone by her mother – and frees herself from her mother's dominance.

When parents' trauma feelings end up with the children

Vera has been coming to me for six months. Her 13-year old daughter, Anabel, sometimes has fits of screaming, outbursts of rage and the problem of not being able to sleep on her own. She is a very anxious child and can only go to sleep when her Mummy is there. She also suffers from violent stomach-aches as soon as bedtime approaches. They've tried hot water bottles, but up until now nothing has helped, and the doctor hasn't been able to find anything either.

Encouraged by her mother, Anabel is willing to try intention work in the individual setting: "Why do I sleep with Mummy and Daddy?" Anabel chooses a cushion for each word. All the cushions are at about the same height, except for the 'I' which lies a long way back under the table. I notice that the girl falls into a trauma paralysis straightaway: she sits motionless on her chair and stares towards the 'sleep', which is lying on the table above the 'I'. Gently I try to reach the girl. It takes what seems like an eternity. Finally she is able to tell me that she is anxious about her parents. She is afraid of losing them. She can't explain it; it is simply 'a feeling'.

As I have already worked with Anabel's parents, I understand that well: her mother was sexually traumatised by her grandfather when she was a little girl, and her grandmother didn't want to know about it. She even locked Vera in the cellar when she couldn't stop crying at night. Anabel's father's mother was diagnosed at a relatively young age with 'cancer' and the boy was completely alone with his fears and worries.

I can only reach Anabel with a great deal of sensitivity. I can now offer to go into the role of 'I' in her intention. My feelings and images are there: disoriented, alone, the parents are both rushed, and always very busy and stressed. So if I want something from my parents, I am forced to get involved in their stress. With sadness in her eyes, Anabel confirms my description. Strengthened by her agreement, I, in the role, go so far as to want to say that to her parents. Healthy anger arises in me: "I need a

Mummy! I don't want to have this permanent stress any more! I want my Mummy to look after me. I want her to be there for me! I want to be seen and loved and not to have to look after Mummy and Daddy myself!" I make these demands indignantly as Anabel's 'I'. Anabel sadly agrees with me. We decide that Bettina – in other words, I as myself – should say that to her mother. Anabel agrees with that and hope flickers in her eyes. "That's a matter for grown-ups" is how we summarise it.

As I am bound by professional confidentiality and can only speak to the parents about our work if the children expressly ask me to, I again ask Anabel in my role as her advisor if she really agrees with the course of action we discussed. "Please, you talk to Mummy", Anabel answers, anxiously and unsettled.

Her mother Vera is taken aback by my remarks about the work with her daughter, but also grateful. It is significant that Vera had had an individual session with me in the morning before Anabel, and her intention had been "Why does Anabel sleep with me?" It was quickly revealed in this work that Vera's preoccupation with Anabel was a distraction from her own traumas. It is important for her to look at these. In the role as 'me' I am, to begin with, very unhappy and sad. In the further process with Vera, however, I am really indignant about the rage I've swallowed down. I don't want to stay silent any longer; everything must be brought into the open! Vera has tears in her eyes and the lump in her throat actually hurts her.

Again in the role as her advisor, I explain to Vera that it makes no sense wanting to speak to her mother. Her mother has split off her perpetrator self, and will not want to listen. However, there were now several people who believed her and would help her. She should turn to them.

Vera's feedback after four weeks: "Anabel is going to a new school which is more suitable. That was her own wish, which we quickly and happily sorted out for her. We've also now bought our dream holiday home on a lake. Anabel immediately wanted to sleep in her own room in the holiday home. She generally goes to sleep more easily now and her stomach-ache has gone! She is no longer afraid!"

The trauma knowledge of Franz Ruppert has enriched and deepened my work with parents and children and made it highly effective. I have accompanied many parents for several years. I have often known the children since they were babies. It is a great pleasure for me to see how well many parents and children have developed. I am particularly pleased about the parents' willingness to try something for the sake of their children, that they might otherwise not have dared to: to look at the trauma in their own childhood. In retrospect, it was always worth it!

Bettina Schmalnauer was born in 1970 and is the mother of three children. In 2011 she completed advanced training with Prof. Ruppert. She is self-employed as graduate Life- and Social Counsellor in her own practice since 2008 with the BodyTalkSystem© and Gordon family training. Certified coach with the Intention Method according to Franz Ruppert in the individual setting and in groups. Her practice is in Ohlsdorf near Gmunden (Upper Austria). www.gesundheitswerkstatt.co.at

ELLEN KERSTEN

Who am I in my body and in my sexuality as a woman?

Body and sexuality

Many women are deeply uncertain about their sexuality and their body. They usually look for the cause of their difficulties in current events or relationships. However, these are frequently not the primary cause, but the re-enactment of previous experiences. A non-existent or derogatory reference to their own body and their own sexuality is usually the result of traumatising experiences in childhood. Through such experiences, the relationship to oneself and one's own body is lost, which often already happened in the womb (Ruppert, 2014). From then on parents, partners, superiors, doctors or therapists become the focus of one's own life.

What does my body feel like? Where do I like touching myself? Where do I like to be touched? What do I smell like? How do I look at my body and myself? Do I like what I see? What does my vagina look like? What excites me? Many adult women don't really know. Often they can only vaguely recognise their own needs. They identify with the sexuality of their partners and what excites them, but access to their own body and sexuality is often blocked. Many women accept that as being unchangeable.

The more stable our contact with ourselves, the more likely we are to experience sexual intimacy with our partner. We only reach our full potential to enjoy intensive sexual experiences when we know and feel who we are. The sexual therapist David Schnarch puts it like this: "Differentiating is the ability to be myself when I am close to people who mean a lot to me. Real togetherness requires a clear dividing line between us at an emotional level." (Schnarch, 2006, p.66) That means that even when I am in a relationship with others, I remain my own point of reference. If I merge with my partner and his feelings, and give up my own identity in favour of the relationship, my own sexual desire disappears. If I don't recognise myself, I don't recognise my own sexuality. Meaningful intimate sexuality is not based on innate physiological reflexes. They need their time to become fully developed.

Vital, sensual sexuality takes place within and with our body, a body that first and foremost we find attractive ourselves. But why do we often feel so strange in our own body? Why do we often reject it harshly and condemn it? Why do we want to have a different body, one we think is perfect? Why do we always compare ourselves with other women – rate them, judge them and compete with them?

Doing this we no longer see and feel ourselves as a whole organism, but reduce ourselves down to, for example, our legs – supposedly too fat; our backside – too wide; our breasts – too small or too big. This fixation on individual parts of our body has something self-tormenting about it. At the same time these thoughts are accompanied by feelings of extreme helplessness and powerlessness. The self-abasement is expressed, for instance, like this: "If only I were a bit slimmer, my relationship would be much happier". Or "If my breasts were larger I'd feel more like a woman". Our own body is perceived as the offender that is preventing us from achieving our personal desires and goals.

Diets and, increasingly, cosmetic surgery, are frequently an attempt to win back control and power over our own body. In 2015 in Germany 43,287 aesthetic plastic surgery operations were carried out (12% of those on men). The most frequent operation was breast enlargement, followed by liposuction.[66]

---

[66] www.vdaepc.de

Sexual traumatisation and its consequences

A lack of relationship to one's own body can have many causes. However, sexual traumatisation appears so frequently in women's trauma biographies that it's important for me to go into this possible cause in more detail. Sexual violence is a boundary violation and means every sexual act that is carried out on or in front of a person either against their will, or which this person, due to their physical or verbal inferiority, is unable to consent to knowingly (Bange and Deegener, 1996). It is violence if an older person uses their position of power, or the ignorance, trust or dependence of a girl (or boy), to satisfy their own sexual desires. This can happen with physical contact, but also hands-off, for example through the showing of pornographic images. Sexual traumatisation is always an act of violence. There is a very wide spectrum of activities and degrees of severity that violate the boundaries. What is critical is how the person experienced the boundary violations themselves.

The closer the relationship between victim and perpetrator, and the more frequently the assaults happen, the more severe the consequences of sexual violence will be. Perpetrators almost always deny the act, and the child is generally dependent on her relationship with the perpetrator. In order to stay in a relationship with him, she cannot recognise him as a perpetrator. This leads to intense confusion in the child, out of which she can only gradually find her way in adulthood.[67] A perpetrator will usually form a 'special' relationship with his victim, which he then takes advantage of.

The long-term consequences depend to a great extent on whether the child receives emotional support and comfort following the sexual exploitation, and whether she is believed. The World Health Organisation (WHO) calculates there are a million children in Germany who have experienced or are experiencing sexual violence.[68] The number is probably very much higher.

---

[67] www.vincent-regensburg.de

[68] www.hilfeportal-missbrauch.de

A typical characteristic is for concrete images and memories to be completely absent. Denial and secrecy are integral in sexual traumatisation. As a rule a child becomes sexually traumatised because she has previously experienced a 'trauma of identity' and a 'trauma of love' (Ruppert, 2012). The sexual traumatisation rocks the child's trust in the world down to the very roots of her existence.

A child's healthy development requires the protection of her parents. If the mother herself is traumatised, she misuses the child as replacement for her own lack of identity and to fulfil her own needs. The child herself therefore has no nurturing and warming contact; she suffers from endless loneliness. From the depths of despair and existential distress, the child clings onto any straw offered to her. The slightest hint of attention is sufficient. She does not have the option to say No. In her emotionally starved state she is unable to differentiate between 'good' and 'bad' contact, and so she is easy prey for the perpetrator.

The perpetrator regards the child's body as his (or her) property. It's all about *his* (or her) needs, not those of the child. Even his own child is abused to satisfy his wants. For example a father only adores and spoils his daughter because he needs her as comfort in his own despair. The father is absolutely convinced that he is only doing himself and his daughter good in his worship of her. The daughter regards the entangled relationship with her father as normal. She senses that her father needs her and that she is important to him, but it is impossible for her to know that this is not about her, but about her father.

Sexual traumatisation is accompanied by extreme feelings of fear, powerlessness, helplessness, shame and disgust. The body freezes and the unbearable feelings are frozen. The child has to leave her own body, and a profound inner split is the result. The child's own 'I' and her own wanting have to be abandoned. The child is completely at the mercy of the overpowering perpetrator, and any resistance is impossible, or would make the situation worse. The perpetrator often threatens even more violence, which increases the feeling of powerlessness. What happens in such a child is hard to comprehend in its impact and drama. The child is not the subject but the object of the perpetrator; the child has to submit to the perpetrator's will. In her hopeless situation, she has to bond with the perpetrator and so cannot see him as a perpetrator. It is impossible for her to separate and distance herself from the perpetrator. The victim will experience the perpetrator's needs as if they were her own and she reacts automatically, with no will of her own. Her feelings are split by the experience. Out of mortal fear and because she is completely at the mercy of the perpetrator, the child can only behave in such a way that it looks as if she is going along with it willingly, otherwise it would make the situation worse. The child's body may respond involuntarily to the perpetrator's touch with desire and a moist vagina. The child is very confused. The victim feels ashamed and guilty instead of the perpetrator, and her need for contact adds to her feelings of shame and guilt.

The consequences are extremely serious. Many women are only sexually stimulated when they fantasise about scenes of violence, and later sexual desire is often coupled with suffering pain. The pain may even be experienced as a relief. The woman's own body comes to be regarded as the source of feelings of profound powerlessness, fear and uncertainty. Consequently, such a survival strategy makes sense: "I am only safe when I am not in my body!" From then on, the woman experiences her body as foreign, to the point of fighting with it as an enemy. When having sex, some women take flight into inner imaginary worlds. For example, they fantasise about 'Mr Right' who does everything for her and anticipates her every wish. They don't feel their own body but just go along with everything and fake their sexual desire both to their partner and themselves.

Exchanging sex for emotional and material security is a typical relationship pattern in sexually traumatised women. The relationship is more like a partnership of convenience. The woman pays with sex for the security that the man offers (house, money, social standing, relationship status). At the same time she may try to avoid sexual contact, and sexuality becomes split off in such a way that, even in a relationship over many years, it is seen as foreign to her and not belonging to her identity. The woman then does not experience herself as a sexual being.

Sexually traumatised women try in many different ways to exercise control over their partner or their children. Such women often have exploitative relationships based on dependence that get stuck in a perpetrator-victim dynamic. They cannot access an identity of their own that gives them stability, and continually ask others: "Am I OK the way I am?" "Am I doing everything right?" They are dependent on the opinion of those they look to for support and security. They do not satisfy their own needs or take decisions – everything is left to their partner or other people who are close to them. They are therefore unable to become emotionally mature. Emotionally, they remain a little girl inside the body of an adult woman.

Sexually traumatised women may often unconsciously send strong sexual messages to men. They want to have contact and to be noticed. At the same time they are afraid of aggression and want to flee. They continually avoid a relationship among equals. This behaviour is also an attempt to gain control over the situation in the past that violated their boundaries. They either have no relationship or jump into bed with anyone. They may feel good when they are able to dominate men or when they are paid for sex. There is nearly always a background of sexual traumatisation when women prostitute themselves. They thus re-enact their own trauma again and again.

They may expend a lot of energy in preventing the memories of the terrible experiences and the suppressed feelings from rising to the surface: vital energy that then is unavailable for other aims in life. They will create denial mechanisms that are supposed to protect them from being emotionally overwhelmed. However, these may increasingly lead to a loss of connection with reality, and suppressing the truth becomes a survival strategy. It can go so far that they find themselves permanently in a fog of confusion; feelings such as panic, pain and disgust are completely split off. The person's own body, with all the terrible things that happened to it, is seen as unimportant, it is devalued and despised. The split-off feelings then lead a life of their own, and the result is a permanent state of tension. And then suddenly, with no explanation or association, feelings of panic or disgust will appear. Life becomes more and more insecure and unpredictable because the person's own inner security and stability are not present.

Frequent physical symptoms are:

- inflammation of the vagina, fungal infections, cystitis, period pains,
- dry vagina and pain during sexual intercourse,
- migraines,
- skin diseases and allergies,
- sleep disorders,
- autoimmune diseases,
- refusing to eat (so-called anorexia) or eating too much.

Behavioural problems that appear are:

- obsession with cleaning, being a workaholic or a shopaholic,
- abuse of medication, alcohol and drugs,
- self-harming, such as cutting, or scratching the skin until it bleeds,
- sex addiction, compulsive promiscuous behaviour, prostitution, sadomasochism,
- not experiencing orgasm, compulsive masturbation or the loss of all sexual desire and feeling of numbness in the pelvic area,
- excessive 'wanting to feel oneself', for example by extreme sport,
- compulsive rituals, such as compulsive washing.

Diagnoses such as 'borderline personality disorder', 'depression', 'psychosis' or 'anxiety disorder', can also be added as attributions by psychiatrists.

Body awareness is profoundly disturbed by sexual traumatisation. One's own body is radically rejected and experienced as a heavy burden. Such people believe themselves to be caught inside their own body, which they would prefer to be rid of. In cases of 'anorexia' the body is supposed to be prevented from maturing and growing up. The female shape attracts men and is therefore seen as dangerous. The less substance one's own body has, the less sexual needs it will have. The wish to vanish physically by starving oneself is an ultimate survival strategy. There is a huge longing for an intact, flawless and pure body, basically for sheer nothingness. If there is not a complete reversal, the starvation can end in death.

Self-harming is a reaction to the deep rejection of one's own body. The body that has brought so much suffering into one's life has to be tortured. The body is experienced as the enemy and treated as such.

Helena – a self-development report

"I am only now, at the age of 47, gradually realising the magnitude and extent of my terrible childhood with the subsequent consequences for my life today. Both my parents are alcoholics. And always have been. My mother was 'not present'. She lived in her own world as a result of her traumas. I tried so hard to reach her and save her. I didn't succeed. I was there for my mother, not her for me. I was also there for my sad grandmother, who lost a child in the war. I was there for my father. His mother died before I was born. I was his replacement mother. Everybody always said I was a 'wished-for' child. Yes, a child who was there for their wishes! I was so lonely that I read all the books in the library. In the world of books I had a place. Not in reality. No one saw *me*.

"Until my uncle came. I was so desperate in my loneliness and lack of contact. And he wanted me. I had so hoped for that. At last, someone who is kind to me. In my neediness I had no option, I couldn't sense that even he wanted to use me for his own wants. His sexual wants. It happened in my grandmother's house. Again and again. From when I was six until I was ten, until we moved away. My uncle had an afternoon nap and I was supposed to come to him. Sit on his lap. Take his penis into my mouth. Swallow his sperm. Let him feel me between my legs. And always smile. He said that I wanted it too. That it was nice. But I was mortally afraid, but only inside. My body had reacted with the play-dead reflex. I could not let him see my fear. He threatened me with violence if I said anything to anyone. The quicker he came, the more quickly my ordeal was over.

"For decades afterwards I wept bitterly during sexual inter-course. No wonder: today I know that I had sex as an adult woman with the body of a little girl. My body's outward sexual characteristics had developed. Not my sexuality. That was fixed at the age of a six-year old girl. Since then I survived as if inside an icy prison cell where time stood still.

"Before and during my period I was in an unbearable state of nebulous confusion. During my period I felt really ill. With aching limbs, mood swings, migraine. My period was strangely uncoupled from my body. My period was like a dominator that demanded my submission. That was how it felt to me. It also had something to do with the fact that there was a discharge of blood. On the one hand that was a relief, on the other hand stressful. Today I connect this with the uncle's ejaculation. The situation was very stressful, but the ejaculation was a relief. That was the moment he let me go.

"I suffered repeatedly from inflammation of the vagina. With a sensual itch. It was only the burning pain and agonising itch that allowed me to sense my genitals. I continually scratched at my skin until it ran with blood and I had a strangely satisfied feeling that came from the burning pain. I also rubbed my eyes compulsively until they emitted a slimy liquid that I sensed as being foreign. Today I know: all this was a re-enactment of the oral abuse. I continually and obsessively pulled out my hair to remove inner tension.

"I have had recurring panic attacks since I was 14. A fear of death. Overwhelming mortal fear and over-excitation. The trigger has always been seeing corpses and dead bodies. The difference is important. Corpses will be buried; dead bodies can live on. The panic attacks were always accompanied by obsessive thoughts: I lie there, dead, and at the same time I observe myself from the outside. This condition kept recurring and lasted for months at a time. I wanted to understand it! When I was 17 I started having therapy. I sought answers about life after death from priests. From psychologists, psychiatrists, astrologists and alternative practitioners. I was martyred, tortured and driven. My parents said I was mad. I always paid for my therapies myself.

"As a child I had had to pay with my body in order to have contact with a man. Therefore I thought that men could give my body back to me. I believed that for years, and didn't notice how dependent I made myself with this expectation. On the one hand I am mortally afraid of all men and at the same time they are supposed to be my saviours. It took many years of therapy for me to understand that this wouldn't work. I am the only person who can reclaim my body for myself. Only I can approach my body again if I no longer have to destroy it as my enemy nor keep it at a distance for fear of further assaults.

"I can't throw food away. I always have to keep very large reserves of food, shower gel and other things for daily use in my flat. Not throwing food away and at the same time having to keep a large amount of food causes me great anxiety and stress. Food and things that I need daily and can touch are my substitute for my body. That's why it feels so existential to me if I have to throw away food that has gone bad. I no longer condemn myself or put myself down for the obsessive behaviour now that I can clearly attribute it to the sexual traumatisation. It has resulted from that, and the little girl had no option other than to make use of this survival strategy. Simply attributing it calms me down and allows me to escape from the destructive cycle: "I am bad and worthless because I can't manage to stop this behaviour." Today I have empathy and understanding with myself and no longer put myself down. I feel the change that's happening and can give myself all the time I need to work through the process.

"I was only able to feel myself through extremes, such as eating too much, scratching my skin until it bled, etc. At the same time I was also super-sensitive to external stimuli such as heat, cold, loud noises, crowds of people, etc. I was always in protective and shielding mode and even so I felt I was light years away from my own body. Food and I had a very ambivalent relationship with each other. As a little girl and in the many years afterwards I would actually have preferred just to be able to vanish away. The only way I could survive was to crawl away into my innermost being and barricade myself there. Being there by not being there. To flee so far away that not even I sensed that I existed. I only existed broken up, disintegrated into lots of little pieces, without a body.

"At the same time I wanted nothing more in the world except to live! To be there. Alive. Whole. With everything, what and who I am and what makes me me. In my body. The more I wanted to disappear, the more food took over my wanting to exist. My whole day was focused on food. Hunger was hunger for life. I kept putting on more weight, more existence in my body. I became fatter and heavier, weighed almost 120 kilos. I was 37 years old and was hardly able to move, I was so heavy.

"Then a girlfriend of mine died. I was standing in the funeral parlour to say farewell to her. I looked at her dead body and suddenly felt myself falling into a bottomless pit. Looking at her dead body had catapulted me from one moment to the next into the traumatising situation from back then. Extreme panic attacks, heart palpitations, an extremely high pulse rate, massive over-excitation – these were my companions from then on. The agonising feeling of being a stranger amongst strangers, uncoupled from any life, grew and grew. I was unable to have any human contact. It was as if I was in a spaceship. Detached from all life, broken up, totally alone. I was completely helpless, like being caught up in a maelstrom. The more I tried to cling to something or someone, the worse the panic became. What had held me externally up until now had been blown away, my children, my husband, my girlfriends, my food. What was left was a void without any support. It was a complete loss of control. Functioning in a lifeless survival-existence had ceased.

"I was almost at the point of voluntarily admitting myself to a psychiatric ward and taking psychotropic medication. I didn't do either. And for that I am today endlessly grateful. Because underneath all this horror and terror that was raging inside me, I felt the tiny seedling, me. I felt this hint of support within me. Felt the thing that is me, who I really am. I felt more and more that I am my own salvation. From within me and not dependent on other people. That was *the* turning point in my life. Since then my reference point is increasingly *me*. I orientate myself around me. I connect with what I am. I detach myself from what I am not. It is a process to be developed step by step. I am here. I want to be here! More and more. Becoming increasingly whole. Identity therapy is a significant part of this.

"For a long time I refused to believe what I had experienced as a child. It was a constellation that first brought me the necessary clarity to be able to say 'Yes' to it. My intention at this constellation was: "I want to perceive the reason for my mortal fear".

"By that time I knew that my parents used to have parties that involved a lot of alcohol. I was about two or three years old. In other constellations it had become apparent that these parties were like sex orgies and that I, as a little girl, was in the middle of them. Until then there had only been vague physical perceptions that I had experienced boundary transgressions during these sex orgies.

"The representative for my 'I' was very sympathetic towards me from the beginning and in a good contact with me. 'I': "We are right. We haven't done anything wrong". This sentence greatly relieved me. I sensed how responsible and culpable I otherwise felt for absolutely everything. For 'reason' I chose several men as representatives. They felt as if they were drunk or stoned. The representative for 'perceive' couldn't then open her eyes, felt so threatened from outside that she had to withdraw into the innermost part of her body. I began to cry. I felt myself in my body, felt the boundary of my skin and the outside, the men, simultaneously. This outside is 'too near, too big, too much'. Through sensing that these men were too near, too big and too many, I was more present in my body. With my own truth I suddenly felt completely calm and relieved. I felt much closer to myself. In the presence of 'perceive' I was able to sense my body and the truth of the sexual trauma.

"I no longer doubt my sexual trauma. I can recognise it as my trauma experience. I can now progress, I can grow, devote time to other things. I am no longer caught up in that. I am arriving in my own life.

"There used to be total chaos within me. Like an orchestra without a conductor. Every part thought it was calling the tune. Now a conductor is there. I am there. And the pieces of music are becoming more harmonious, more in tune with each other, more connected. I feel that I am maturing, developing, becoming grown up. For this process of mine I have needed a considerable portion of trust, hope and persistence. There have been and still are many exhausting lean periods. But I am not becoming bogged down any more for a long time in unpleasant conditions. Today, my inner regulation works much more quickly. There is an unprecedented stability within me. My life has become so much more positive in recent years that I am sometimes amazed at myself. I realise today how exhausting it was to be there, by not being there. My weight has reduced considerably. The recurring inflammations of the vagina have ceased completely. My period now feels a part of me and not the other way round. The complaints during my period are much less intense. I feel inwardly and outwardly much more secure. My sleep is more relaxed and deeper. I live much more mindfully and consciously. I am developing more and more empathy and love for myself. I discriminate between contacts that are good for me and ones that aren't. I can now feel that exactly. I no longer give myself up for the sake of a relationship. I am more important to myself than the relationship, whoever it is with. I feel my boundaries again. I am beginning to become friends with my body. When I have sex I can stay inside my body. Can feel my desire and myself. Can join with another person and disengage again. Without disintegrating myself. I am discovering my I, self-determined, with my own will, my feelings, in my body, with my sexuality. That is absolutely the greatest happiness for me."

References

Bange, D. & **Deegener**, G. (1996). *Sexueller Missbrauch an Kindern.* Weinheim, Beltz.

Lindner, L. (2011). *Splitterfasernackt.* Munich, Droemer.

Northrup, Ch. (1998). *Frauenkörper, Frauenweisheit.* Munich, Zabert Sandmann.

Röhr, H-P. (2015). *Ich traue meiner Wahrnehmung.* Ostfildern, Patmos.

Ruppert, F. (2011). *Splits in the Soul: Integrating Traumatic Experiences.* Steyning, Green Balloon Publishing.

Ruppert, F. (2012). *Symbiosis and Autonomy.* Steyning, Green Balloon Publishing.

Ruppert, F. (2015). *Trauma, Fear and Love.* Steyning, Green Balloon Publishing.

Ruppert, F. (ed.) (2016). *Early Trauma.* Steyning, Green Balloon Publishing.

Schnarch, D. (2006). *Die Psychologie sexueller Leidenschaft.* Stuttgart, Klett-Cotta.

Ellen Kersten was born in 1969. She is an alternative practitioner since 1995, and she offers open and set groups in Identity-oriented Psychotrauma Therapy as well as individual constellations. www.naturheilpraxis-kersten.de

DIANA LUCIA VASILE

Cervical cancer and becoming a mother

Two years of individual psychotherapy

Rebecca, 27, came to therapy due to general feelings of sadness, physical pain and relational difficulties that were couple and work-related. The symptoms that troubled her were irritability that produced conflicts in relationships and with herself, excessive work (two jobs), nightmares, emotional confusion, and work-related confusion.

Rebecca was the third daughter in her family, the youngest living child. During her entire childhood her father was an alcoholic, constantly neglecting his daughters' activities. The mother was depressed, overwhelmed by house chores and children's needs. They both had low-paid jobs and therefore financial difficulties. When Rebecca started her psychotherapy, the mother and the daughters were struggling with caring for their suffering father.

Rebecca's therapeutic goals were to become more relaxed, to improve her relationship with her partner, to be clear about who she was and what her life was all about. She was considering marrying the man she had been with for more than seven years, and having children.

Exploring her life story and focusing on her feelings, intentions and resources, using self-observation, mirroring, self-reflection, and dream analysis, Rebecca got in contact with her traumatic feelings and their consequences:

- Physical and emotional numbness: confused feelings for her partner, absence of symptoms when sick. For example, around the age of 26, she suffered a renal colic and even though she was severely bleeding she did not feel anything. She only went to the hospital emergency room after she noticed the blood on the floor when she was working overtime. The doctors confirmed that she had been in real danger of dying due to late presentation at hospital;

- Avoidance of pleasurable moments and activities: small amount of time for relaxation and friends;
- Avoidance of peaceful moments: compulsive work and activism;
- Avoidance of medical doctors to check out her health and medical difficulties;
- Intrusive symptoms: emotional pain, nightmares, flash-backs, sadness, anger, pain;
- Dysfunctional cognitions: "I can cope with heavy workloads", "Relationships are difficult", "I have to take care of my parents, even if it is a tremendous effort and causes me losses".

Twenty-two sessions in 18 months of individual psychotherapy helped Rebecca become more aware of her needs and survival strategies. Thus, she used her personal and social resources to make important changes in her life:

- quitting her most stressful job, and focusing on her own business,
- new life-style: healthy food, sleep and relaxation time, sport and leisure activities,
- deciding to marry her partner,
- setting objectives for herself and her relationship with her partner, not for her parents, thanks to the clarity she received through her relationships within the family that were "making her ill".

Rebecca decided to take a break from psychotherapy and enjoy her changes, right after her wedding.

Group therapy and Identity Constellations

Two years later she phoned me, absolutely terrified: she had been diagnosed with genital problems, severe 'Human Papilloma Virus alteration' of the genital area. Seven gynaecologists had told her about the danger of developing cervical cancer within two years. On top of everything, Rebecca found out that she could not conceive.

The following therapy session focused on reducing the intensity of her feelings, regaining self-confidence in her ongoing process of healing, and emphasising the connection between body and psyche, that obviously needed to be reconsidered. Thus, Rebecca started the second part of her psychotherapy, focusing on taking her trauma seriously: the experience of splitting from her body and needs. Rebecca made two major decisions:

- to be the person responsible for believing in and stimulating her healthy structures: the only person who can heal her physical illness and generate her vital energy and fertility, and
- to be responsible for the treatment, a personal one, with natural nutrition with only fresh vegetables and fruits, no sugar, no meat, self-prepared food according to her own needs, longer sleep and relaxation time, meditation, essential oils and remedies as the main medical treatment, trauma-psychotherapy oriented towards facing traumatic feelings and identifying a profound victim-perpetrator dynamic as a survival strategy produced by her early traumas.

Rebecca then attended group therapy using Franz Ruppert's Intention Method and doing Identity-Constellations. In the course of two further years, she slowly but steadily improved her medical condition. She was healed, even though gynaecologists did not support her decision to refuse drugs and surgical interventions.

Three group processes were the most significant for Rebecca, as she focused on her infertility. For the first one, her intention was: "I would like to free myself and my husband from what blocks us from conceiving". After the constellation she wrote to me:

- "My blockage was not about my relationship, but about a deep depression and deep anxiety related to my own life experiences". This helped Rebecca look more closely at her own trauma and not at her marital relationship.
- She re-discovered and re-connected to her 'I': "There was a moment, when I stood face to face with my 'I', embraced ... I felt how everything and everybody around me faded. It was my deepest dive inside myself, though at first it was with a lot of fear, pain, effort ... I received her body warmth and her breathing helped me breathe easily, naturally. Slowly, I began to feel every little part of my body, an extremely pleasant experience ... as if something was coming back to life. I felt the strength to support myself ... nothing complicated ... very hard to put that feeling into words ... it was very new to me. Since then, I have not felt alone any more. I have preserved this protective sensation, as if nothing bad can happen to me or put my life in danger. This feeling was so welcome – considering that in the last two years I was tormented by the fear of a serious deadly illness, the threat of cervical cancer that about seven professional doctors had exposed me to."
- The desire to have a child was a survival strategy: to take care of her childhood wounds. Rebecca created an illusion that taking care of her own child would bring her peace, because she did not know what her own wounds were. She identified two deep beliefs: "to be a child is awful", "pregnancy and giving birth are very painful experiences". Rebecca realised that the pain was real, but that it came from her real childhood experiences that had generated the wounds in her genital system.

Rebecca's second intention, "I wish to be able to continue my life with peace, joy and freedom along with my husband and our child", brought two most important clarifications:

- "The representative for 'my life' showed me very clearly that she needed breaks in order to breathe ... I saw her as being very close to dying." – Rebecca faced her split off traumatic reactions: loss of vital energy and giving up. A few days later, Rebecca felt exhausted, "as if I had lost the ability to fight". She gave up an aggressive attitude towards her body and herself – not taking her body's needs and sensations seriously.
- "I also learned that silence, joy and freedom are survival strategies, not healthy ones. This helped me greatly ... the information and the attitude that I received from the representative of the word 'life': she told me to be patient ... when tired, to enjoy the fact that I am breathing, when sad, to let the sadness be."

Rebecca realised her survival mechanisms, obtained clarity about her deep feelings of fear, pain and life-threatening loss of vital energy due to the aggression towards her basic needs for body contact, eye contact, maternal care and protection. This aggression resulted from an abortion attempt by her mother while she was in the womb, neglect and then, through the survival mechanisms of denying the traumatic feelings, generating maladaptive thoughts, feelings and actions. A month after this process, Rebecca found out that she was naturally pregnant.

Becoming a mother

As her third intention, when Rebecca was 18 weeks pregnant, she formulated: "I want to live (see and feel) how I can be a healthy mother for my child". These are some of her insights:

- "The fears toward my child were confused with my mother's feelings about me, while she was pregnant with me. She wanted and intended to abort me. At that time, my father came out of prison, having been convicted for a crime he had not committed, but he had wanted to save a close relative. So I realised that my existence began with survival, not with relaxation and peace. Now I realise that all my life I had tried to please my parents, to make them proud of me, not because I exist, but because I fulfil their needs. This took a huge effort, a feeling of constant tiredness, few moments of superficial relaxation and incomplete satisfaction in everything I achieved."

- "To be a healthy mother means to take care of me all the time! This ensures a good and permanent contact with my baby."
- "There is still confusion between good and aggressive contact."

Rebecca understood that a healthy mother is a clear mother who does not obey her child simply because the child looks at her with a tender look – a look that Rebecca did not receive when looking into her own mother's eyes. A healthy mother also perceives and protects her own strength. Rebecca gave birth to a healthy baby girl. They are now both developing a constructive relationship.

Diana Lucia Vasile, PhD, is a Logos Consultant in Bucharest, Romania. She is a Psychotherapist, Clinical Psychologist, Supervisor, President of the Institute for the Trauma Study and Treatment and Associate Professor of the Hyperion University in Bucharest diana.vasile@istt.ro www.istt.ro

STEPHAN KONRAD NIEDERWIESER

The male body, sex and trauma

Sexual traumatisation

Prior to 2010 in Germany, when the sexual violence perpetrated on a massive scale against boys at boarding schools and in choirs became known, the word 'abuse' was usually thought to refer to girls. Today experts believe that about 10 to 15% of all men have experienced sexual violence in their childhood or adolescence (Schlingmann 2016, p.1).

Celebrities often raise awareness of the issue; the author and critic Fritz J. Raddatz revealed in an interview with the *Süddeutsche Zeitung* that, at the age of 11, he had been forced by his father to have sex with him and his step-mother. We can ask ourselves whether that influenced his decision to end his life by suicide. The interview was originally published with the title *"There were too many wounds"*.[69]

When we talk of perpetrators of abuse, we usually think of men. They are considered transgressors, aggressive and violent. The fact that women and mothers are also able to commit acts of violence against children is scarcely making its way into society's consciousness. The former pimp, Andreas Marquardt, went public with his ordeal: for years his mother had forced him to have sexual intercourse with her. His autobiography *Härte* was made into a film and was released in cinemas in 2015.

Tauwetter, Berlin's counselling centre for men who have suffered sexual violence, assumes that 25% of all acts of violence against boys are carried out by women. If we check with the

---

[69] http://sz-magazin.sueddeutsche.de/texte/anzeigen/41802/Es-gab-zu-viele-Verwundungen

Commissioner for Child Sexual Abuse, we find right at the beginning of the expert's report "Figures on the Frequency of Sexual Abuse" the sentence: "It is almost impossible to give precise figures on the frequency of sexual victimisation of children and adolescents in Germany due to the available data".[70] Differences in the numbers arise because researchers base their data on different criteria. Is the term 'violence' confined to putting pebbles or shards of glass under the foreskin, or is it used for burn injuries or penetration? Last but not least, memories are deceptive, particularly in the case of trauma. Above all victims are often only questioned, and that has several drawbacks: For example Andreas Kloiber, in one of the few studies that have ever been carried out in Germany on sexual abuse against men. He says that men tend to re-interpret their victim experiences, concluding: "In most surveys ... the majority of test subjects rated their experiences of sexual abuse as meaningless or even positive for their later development". (Kloiber 2002, p.25). However it seems that at the same time many of those questioned suffered from alcoholism, drug abuse, were unemployed or psychologically badly affected.

In cases of sexual violence we often only think of lust as one-sided, of penetration or other acts that lead to a climax in at least one of the participants. However, there are many other forms of sexual violence. For example in the course of constellations, different parts of clients remember that, while being washed their genitals were treated roughly because the mother regarded the child as dirty. To cause a traumatisation it may be sufficient that the mother just wrinkles her nose or hesitates when cleaning the baby, or if she smiles into the baby's face but emotionally freezes at the sight of his genitals.

Children identify with the treatment they receive. They develop their self-image based on what they are met with. If they are treated with love, they think they are lovable. If a little boy,

---

[70] https://beauftragter-missbrauch.de/fileadmin/Content/pdf/
Pressemitteilungen/Expertise_Häufigkeitsangaben.pdf, taken from website on 1.12.2016

as a baby or toddler, experiences disgust in his mother, or if she rejects his sexuality, he will conclude that something is wrong with him. At this early stage of development he cannot possibly understand that his mother is afraid of all male genitals, or has had bad experiences with men, and that her rejection, hesitation or fear have nothing to do with him personally. Sabine Bode writes: "Women who were raped as children and never experienced support and comfort are [. . .] in most cases poison for their sons." (Bode 2014, p.215).

The organ that is connected with the mother's trauma is unconsciously rejected just as are the unbearable feelings that cannot be integrated. The unconscious rejection of the organ is the best protection from being reminded of the trauma. Men whose psyche is traumatised then look for self-accusations along the lines of: "It's all my penis's fault," "If only I didn't get erections," or "If only my lust wasn't so great".

Genital mutilation

The circumcision of little boys has all the makings of a traumatising experience: at the mercy of someone, helpless, powerless, something is happening against their will. Sometimes many people witness the process – which increases particularly the feelings of shame and humiliation. Just imagine this situation as an adult: surrounded by strangers, having your penis operated on in full view of others, while suppressing any protest or natural impulse to resist, and all possibly with no anaesthetic.

A man of Jewish heritage told me that at his little brother's circumcision he began to hit out at the gathered community. Even as an adult he couldn't speak about this experience without flying into a rage. Until then he hadn't even considered that his own circumcision might have been traumatising for him.

When entering the gender in the register of births, there used to be just two possibilities: 'male' or 'female'. Newborn babies who were not conclusively male or female had to be 'corrected'. In 2012 the German Ethics Council called for this legislation to be reconsidered. The Council said the obligation to define the gender was: "an unjustifiable interference in personal rights and the right to equal treatment". As of November 2013, if the baby's gender is not totally conclusive, the entry in the register of births can be left blank. This is no trivial matter as, depending on the statistics, we are talking about up to 4 in 100 newborn babies. One prominent example was the sex therapist Tiger Devore. He has so far had 20 genital operations, two of which were full penis reconstructions. According to him, all operations up to age 19 were unnecessary.

In the case of David Reimer (born in 1965 in Canada), circumcision at the age of six months caused irreparable damage to his penis. On the advice of the sexologist John Money, his parents decided to bring David up as a girl. He was castrated, the testicles 'corrected' to form the lips of the vulva, his sex organs 'adjusted'. From the age of 12, David, now called Brenda, was given female sex hormones. At the age of 15, Brenda discovered that 'she' had been born as a boy, and underwent treatment to reverse the reassignment with a double mastectomy, testosterone injections and a phalloplasty operation. David got married when he was 25, and adopted children. When he was 38 he committed suicide. According to his mother, David would still be alive "if he had not been the victim of that 'catastrophic experiment' that had caused him so much suffering."[71]

Emotional violence

In Germany approximately 1,300 expectant mothers per year blank out their pregnancies. 270 children are only detected because the woman suddenly goes into labour.[72] Although the child has been supplied with nourishment and oxygen during the pregnancy, he has been emotionally ignored for nine months, which for the child is similar to solitary confinement. The 'Still

---

[71] https://de.wikipedia.org/wiki/David_Reimer
[72] https://www.welt.de/gesundheit/article154460998/Wenn-Frauen-ihre-Schwangerschaft-nicht-bemerken.html

Face Experiment' gives some idea of the effect of two minutes of no contact on babies.[73]

Our bonding system allows us in situations of distress to seek protection from our attachment figure, but if they look impassively, or are in some way the cause of our distress, our natural impulses are compromised. The person who should be protecting us becomes the danger. Our biological systems, which as a rule support each other, suddenly begin to fight each other – the bonding impulse and the fight-and-flight impulse. Afterwards closeness cannot be experienced without fear; there is no love without violence, and no contact with one's own body without pain. Touch is experienced as threatening, being noticed is shameful.

If a boy grows up in an environment in which men are thought of as perpetrators, there is no possibility of him developing a healthy image of himself as a male being. He might then try to suppress his aggression. One solution might be to behave in a particularly endearing way: gentle, tender, emotional, helpful, approachable, careful, undemanding, domestic, or similar. 'Male' features such as energy, single-mindedness and assertiveness might then fall by the wayside.

'Sexual functional disorders' and 'illnesses'

It becomes clear that functional disorders such as so-called 'erectile dysfunction' ('impotence'), 'ejaculatio praecox' (premature ejaculation) or 'anorgasmia' (inability to achieve orgasm), can be survival strategies when we consider the function these 'disorders' have.

For his whole life, Mr D. had experienced sex as a way to relax. For the last two years however this had not worked. He tries Viagra – but then feels he is deceiving his partner. In a constellation he cannot differentiate between his lover and his mother. In the following therapy sessions further significant problems come to light: he never felt he was wanted; he was not allowed to show his need for intimacy and he had 'learnt' to manage on his own. At the same time, he had remained deeply

---

[73] https://www.youtube.com/watch?v=apzXGEbZht0

dependent on the receptivity of his respective counterpart, so that it was almost impossible for him to experience his own will, let alone follow it. These issues ruled his everyday life to such an extent that he had cut himself off from his physical sensations. He was really scared of experiencing himself in his own body. He called himself a "head with legs".

Many steps were necessary before Mr D. was able to transform his automated sexuality into a satisfying and nurturing experience: security in his own body, in order to be able to experience himself at all. Recognising and questioning the shame about his mother's rejection, allowing his need for intimacy, being held and cuddled, instead of being fixated on penetration. Learning to formulate his needs and accepting the frustration of rejection without having to withdraw. Trusting that his counterpart really saw him, and of course recognising his fear of his own will and being able to rise above it. Last but not least, he repeatedly encountered the pain of rejection; that he was never seen by his mother, which for a long time he thought was his own failure. At the same time it became increasingly clear to him that his former sexuality was only an outlet with which he tried to regulate his chronically overexcited nervous system. His real needs were intimacy and contact.

For Mr D. the path to healthy sexuality was lengthy. This example shows how complex this basic human function is, that we normally assume will work itself out of its own accord. Symptoms in this area are often just the tip of the iceberg. If we restrict ourselves to investigating the function of the organs, conduction systems and hormones, we do not do justice to the multidimensional complexity of the human organism.

Physical violence

Another very common survival strategy is to reinterpret the suppressed traumatic experience by giving it an erotic charge. The pornography industry lives from a customer base that uses rape scenes for sexual satisfaction. In this, the mixture of sexuality and violence is limitless.

When talking about violence and sexuality we ought to mention sadomasochism (SM). In the television report "Farewell to a double life"[74] a man called Walther, husband and father, describes his path to SM. While he is standing at his father's grave he hints at the reason he is unable to separate violence from love. In the same programme, a dominatrix, who earns her living with SM, says that in her experience this form of sexuality is usually a re-enactment of violent experiences in childhood.

An example from my practice is the following: Young Mr J. wanted to discover his true sexuality with the help of a constellation. As a child he had experienced a great deal of violence. As an adult he believed he would enjoy it if strong, muscular men 'used' him as a slave. His true sexuality proved to be a longing for tender, loving touch and being noticed. Sexuality in an adult sense was completely foreign to his representative parts in a constellation; they were only interested in being able to have physical contact, intimacy and warmth that they could decide on for themselves.

"Mother, sex, object – a popular movement raises the mature woman to an icon of lust" was a title in *Die Zeit* newspaper in May 2015. It described the increasing desire for MILFs (Mom I'd Love to Fuck ...) and DILFs (Dad ...).[75] Perhaps this is just a further sexual variety, however the constellations of Mr H. showed that hidden behind his preference for much older women there lay sexual abuse by his own mother. The erotic charge helped him to hide the pain of his experience.

However, we need to exercise caution: to conclude from the above that all sexual preferences that are different to the missionary position have their origin in traumatic experiences that have not been processed, would be a simplification with

---

[74] 'Abschied vom Doppelleben' broadcast on 6th November 2014 in the ORF (Austrian national television) series 'Am Schauplatz'.

[75] Christian Fuchs: 'Mutter, Sex, Objekt – Eine Bewegung aus dem Volk erhebt die reife Frau zu einer Ikone der Lust', in: *DIE ZEIT*, 19, from 7 May 2015, http://www.zeit.de/2015/19/milf-gesellschaft-mutter-frauen-sex.

which one might upset and shame people. We also fall short if we reduce sexual symptoms to sexual traumas alone and overlook the complex contexts in which they happen.

Sex as trauma survival mechanisms

Shame-based attempts at coping are born from core beliefs such as "There's something wrong with me", "I don't deserve …", "It's the fault of my penis (body/gender)". In the same way we can develop strategies that are based on pride, for instance hyper sexuality: a different partner every night, or, even better, several in succession, or even at the same time. This definitely does not fall into the realm of myths, but is 'normal' for some men. The problem with this trauma survival structure is that in our society men earn recognition for 'virility'. It is therefore difficult for most hyperactive men to question their 'virility' and to recognise it as a trauma survival mechanism.

Buying sex is a further strategy of avoiding feeling the trauma of rejection. By forcing someone (as a rule, someone who is dependent on the money paid) to put their body at my disposal, I can avoid the risk of being reminded of my original trauma.

A further pride-based strategy can be to become a porn actor. Instead of being devalued, debased or feeling wrong about one's own sex, sexual organs, need for sexuality or for sexuality itself, one receives recognition in the porn industry. Today that is simpler than ever because there are internet portals on which one can upload self-made pornographic films. Many people even achieve fame in this way, and they believe they are validating themselves by these means.

Trying to attain physical perfection is also a strategy to make one's body, to which one has no positive relationship, 'lovable': cosmetics, gym, hormone injections, operations, etc. all help to oppose the feelings of self-debasement and "It's all my body's fault". To mention just one statistic: with 2,800 penis enlargements a year, Germany is the world leader.[76] "The motivation

---

[76] 'Wunderwerk Penis': *3sat.*
http://www.3sat.de/mediathek/?mode-play&obj=58453

behind trying to optimise oneself is in my opinion not only 'beauty' or 'slimming mania', but inferiority complexes, or fear of failure." (Ahlers 2015, p.191)

To avoid having to confront the violence suffered, an individual can 'level off' their own suffering by perpetrating violence in their own environment, by using other people for sex instead of entering into a loving relationship with them that would inspire both partners equally. They may become an exhibitionist, a rapist, a pimp. They may traffic adults and children, beat them, force them to perform acts they would never willingly perform – or kill them during or for sex. People are reduced to goods to be traded, money to be earned. The previously mentioned pimp, Andreas Marquardt, "took out his anger on women. As a pimp he despised his whores. They were simply objects of lust, there to make him a profit. 'I wasn't able to have a normal conversation with women'".[77]

A person can equally well become a perpetrator against himself. In my practice I support men who masturbate compulsively, are addicted to porn and/or sex, or who have knowingly infected themselves with contagious diseases. Bill Clegg describes this obsessive maelstrom in his autobiography (Clegg 2011). At the age of 30, the successful New York literary agent spent $70,000 and ruined his life within a few weeks with crack. The cause of this obsessive activity is often a chronically unregulated nervous system. Depending on other self-calming methods that can be found, the person's need to have orgasms will subside to a greater or lesser extent.

Self-harming behaviour puts a strain on any partnership, by emotional imbalance, neglect and lies. Professional work also can suffer as a result, because while at work, the person is only thinking of sex, browsing pornographic pages on the internet, or desperately looking for a sex partner on dating portals. Money is squandered, the rent isn't paid – many such lives end in complete ruin. A biographical novel about the exceptional and legendary

---

[77] *SPIEGEL ONLINE*, http://www.spiegel.de/panorama/gesellschaft/sexueller-missbrauch-durch-frauen-verkehrte-lust-a-788332.html

dancer, Rudolf Nureyev, describes how he would leave the theatre even during a short break in his performance, to have sex. He died in 1993 from the complications of AIDS (McCann 2005).

Until our trauma is integrated, the likelihood is very high that we will re-enact it again and again, in other words that we will seek a partner or situation in which we can re-live what has not been completed.

A young man came to me in distress following a Tantra workshop. The participants were asked to disclose their most secret erotic fantasies. His was to be more or less attacked, caressed and sexually stimulated, before being dropped suddenly again. That is exactly what was enacted with him in the course of the weekend, with no warning. He dissociated and for days afterwards he wasn't present in himself. In his constellation it was revealed that his sexual fantasy was not a fabrication but a reflection of his early childhood experience: to be picked up and put down according to the adults' needs, not his. He had been given up for adoption immediately after his birth.

The sexual therapist Esther Perel says: "Tell me how you were loved as a child and I will tell you how you make love as an adult".[78]

Processing trauma

In an ideal case, symptoms linked to male sexuality can be traced back to a concrete traumatising experience, and then shifted from the inside to the outside. Now symptoms can be attributed to an experience and the consequences can then disappear.

As in the case of Mr R., who came to my practice with recurring chronic inflammation of the urethra. Conventional medicine and homeopathic treatment had not been able to resolve the problem. However in a constellation it became clear that, from the very beginning, his mother had confused him with

---

[78] http://www.estherperel.com/tell-me-how-you-were-loved-and-i-will-tell-you-how-you-make-love

the perpetrator whose victim she had been. Over the course of many sessions he found more and more of himself and cleared up his complex confusion of identity, and the infection disappeared.

This path is stony and does not necessarily lead to the required goal. Seeing repeatedly how badly one was treated often increases the shame in having experienced something like that, in being an off-spring from such parents.

Trauma not only causes us injury and renders us powerless. It also causes "a permanent shake-up of self- and world-under-standing" (Fischer and Riedesser, 1999, 79). This shake-up is caused by the fact that we remain identified with the traumatising experiences and derive distortions of identity that result in limiting views about ourselves. However, these beliefs are not cognitive decisions that we achieve by weighing up pros and cons. At a trauma level, beliefs are autonomous reactions, physical, emotional and mental, that shape our daily experience. They shape our "habits of perception and the automatic process by which we, without thinking, lend a meaning to our experiences" (Kurtz 2002, p.36).

Once installed, these distortions of identity function as filters, interpreting reality. Through them we experience our relationships and our work, and feel our world. These unconscious models, stored in our body's implicit memory, direct our thinking, feeling and actions. They make us behave in a certain way with others and ourselves, and they shape our concepts of, and fantasies about sexuality. We are so convinced by them that we believe them to be the truth. We find it difficult to accept anything outside them as true. They make us feel unloved, too much, not enough, a nuisance, invisible and anything else, although we have long ago – often decades ago – outgrown the traumatic situation.

Because identifications, distortions of identity and beliefs are not consciously felt, we cannot stop them with affirmations, meditation or conscious behavioural modifications. Giving them up is difficult. "Who am I if I give up my survival mechanisms?" a client asked me recently. By questioning one's own identity, which is held to be true, one indeed enters an emotional vacuum, which causes anxiety in many people. This has to be cushioned therapeutically.

Constellations are one method by which these distortions can be lifted into our consciousness. If they are consciously felt, they can undergo correction through the current experience in the constellation. But there are several obstacles on the way.

Auto aggression

As soon as we feel threatened, our nervous system switches into fight or flight mode, which on an emotional level can be perceived as anger – but is often confused with fear. But if we thought fight or flight might decrease our chances of survival, we would have suppressed our natural aggression impulse. From then on we were fighting ourselves. This internal perpetrator-victim dynamic frequently becomes visible in constellations.

In the trauma situation our own anger is coupled with fear of losing our attachment relationship. Because these personality parts did not develop further, this fear usually continues into adulthood. If this becomes visible in a constellation, it is important to keep the client in his experience and at the same time point out the possibilities that are available to him as an adult today. Only when he has the option to commit to himself instead will he be able to give up identification with the attachment persons.

The shame and guilt barrier

Not infrequently distortions of identity are hidden behind a protective shield of shame. We haven't managed to cope with a situation. We think we are inferior, a loser. Then come the self-accusations: "If only I'd tried harder", "If I weren't this or that, I'd have received the love".

Shame is considered to be a feeling. Looked at more closely, though, it is an autonomous reaction. When it has been triggered, the neck gives way, the shoulders fall forwards, the chest narrows, everything constricts. The person breaks contact and looks away. An ashamed person would not even notice that his counterpart is sympathetic to him and the correcting experience cannot be integrated – a vicious cycle that is very clearly visible in constellations.

The ashamed person wants to hide. In the worst case, shame triggers the impulse to disappear completely. In 2010 the fate of 18-year-old Tyler was in the media. His room-mate secretly filmed him kissing a boy and tweeted: "My room-mate is gay!" As proof he added the video. As a consequence Tyler took his own life.[79]

Shame "determines how people live their lives", says Prof. Dr. Stephen Porges. "On a physical level, shame triggers responses that are very similar to a threat to life ... When people are ashamed, they lose their ability to act according to their will."[80]

John Bradshaw formulates shame as a 'toxic state of being': "Once shame is transformed into an identity, it becomes toxic and dehumanising ... [it] is unbearable and must be covered up, necessitating a false self ... As soon as one takes on a false self one ceases to exist psychologically". (Bradshaw, 2005, p. xvii) "Shame is highly correlated with addiction, depression, violence, aggression, bullying, suicide, and eating disorders", adds Brené Brown, Research Professor of Social Work at Houston University.[81]

Janina Fisher, student of the trauma expert Bessel van der Kolk, made a statement that corresponds with my own experience in practice: "The persistence of shame reactions, even years after trauma treatment, is an obstacle to the complete resolution of trauma"[82], because shame prevents those affected from communicating what they have experienced. There is a further

---

[79] Ulrike Meyer-Timpe: 'Vor allen bloßgestellt' in: *DIE ZEIT*, 50, 1 December 2016, http://www.zeit.de/2016/50/ausstellung-scham-deutsches-hygienemuseum-dresden

[80] https://nextlevelpractitioneer.nicabm.co (Week37, Day 1).

[81] Brené Brown: 'Listening to Shame' (TedTalk), https://www.ted.com/talks/brene_brown_listening_to_shame?

[82] https://www.youtube.com/watch?v=bYR7BAQDq6U&list=PLfSzB01WfIJL_19TiLbH-pxIKcGYWezYA

vicious cycle: most people are ashamed of their shame. Not infrequently they even despise themselves for it and berate or hate themselves: "There you go again, withdrawing. Don't be so sensitive! How much more therapy do you want to do? You're hopeless!" However, if the trauma is brought to light in an unprotected setting, or incorrectly addressed, it can even increase the shame reaction.

It is a similar case with feelings of guilt: when, with victims of sexual violence, one explores their associated feelings, one often encounters guilt. Unlike girls, boys are unable to hide their sexual arousal; their body shows it. And that is precisely what perpetrators use to convince them that their victim is enjoying it and wants it. Thus victims of sexual abuse often feel guilty of experiencing lust in such a situation. Sometimes they are even convinced that they have provoked the abuse themselves. If male perpetrators abuse heterosexual boys, the boys often fear that they are homosexual.

According to Gahleitner victims who are subjected to sexual violence by their mother fall into a double bind: "If [the victim] has experienced positive feelings in the abuse situation, then it wasn't regarded as abuse; if that wasn't the case, [the victim] is stigmatised as abnormal or homosexual because sex doesn't give him any pleasure". (Gahleitner 2005, p.70) It doesn't matter what a boy feels, he's going to lose.

After I had given a talk on sexuality and shame, Mr N. set up his intention: "I want to come into contact with my shame". The representative for his 'I' immediately casts his eyes downwards and freezes. Mr N. tries to encourage him, to assure him of his affection and understanding, and because nothing seems to help, he finally wants to embrace him. But his 'I' recoils from him. A moment of anger flashes across Mr N's face. He quickly suggests asking another part to come into the constellation, but I advise him against it because it is clear that he is already standing facing his shame, but is unaware of it.

I ask Mr N how he perceives his 'I'. "Rejecting", he answers. I mirror him my impression: "Your 'I' doesn't want to be embraced, but wants to be seen, with all his feelings". I advise him to take a step backwards and to find what feels like a healthy distance. His 'I' heaves a sigh. I make Mr N. aware of the dynamic: not seeing oneself causes freezing and resistance. Giving oneself space, showing understanding for one's own needs, creates trust.

When that gets through to him, Mr N. puts his hand on his heart. I ask him what he experiences under his hand. He answers: "A deep pain". I ask him whether he is able to give this pain space and he begins to weep. He remembers how he had to pretend as a child, how he had gone along with it when someone wanted to be close to him, how he was not allowed to be who he was, and how he had been ashamed of not being lovable.

I mirror to him that today he is doing to himself what was done to him as a child. That reaches Mr N. in the form of a further wave of pain. His 'I' raises his head. The more Mr N. understands that he has closed his heart off from himself, the more his 'I' is released from his frozen state. In a process that takes a good half hour, he cautiously moves his arms, becomes less stiff in his hips, can finally take small steps. Finally the 'I' opens his eyes and looks at Mr N. The internal process of shame towards self-acceptance becomes visible externally.

Two months later Mr N. emails me: "I was very pleased to be accompanied by you in my process of becoming I. You really helped me with it. I can still see the constellation in my mind's eye and I am very grateful for the development that came out of it. I want to thank you and share my joy about it with you".

References

Ahlers, C. J. (2015). *Himmel auf Erden und Hölle im Kopf.* Munich, Goldmann.

Bode, S. (2014). *Kriegsenkel.* Stuttgart, Klett-Cotta.

Bradshaw, J. (2005). *Healing the Shame That Binds You.* Deerfield Beach, FL/USA, Health Communications, Inc.

Clegg, B. (2011): *Porträt eines Süchtigen als junger Mann.* Frankfurt/M., S. Fischer.

Fischer, G. & **Riedesser**, P. (1999). *Lehrbuch der Psychotraumatologie.* Stuttgart, UTB.

Gahleitner, S.-B. (2005). *Sexuelle Gewalt und Geschlecht*. Gießen, Psychosozial.

Homes, A. M. (2004). *Von der Mutter missbraucht*. Norderstedt, Books on Demand.

Kloiber, A. (2002). *Sexueller Missbrauch an Jungen*. Kröning, Roland Asanger.

Kurtz, R. (2002). *Hakomi*. Munich, Kösel.

McCann, C. (2005). *Der Tänzer*. Reinbek, Rowohlt.

Schlingmann, T. (2016). *Mythen und Fakten*, in Deutsche Kinderhilfe (2016), Praxisleitfaden Kinderschutz.

Stephan Konrad Niederwieser was born in 1962 and has been an alternative practitioner since 1989, he also practices Hakomi and NARM [NeuroAffective Relational Model]. He is the author of 28 books, which have been translated into English, Polish, Czech and several other languages. Ten of these are books on sex advice. Stephan Konrad Niederwieser lives and works in his own practice in Berlin. www.stephan-niederwieser.de

ANDREA TIETZ

The menopause – opportunity for a change in perspective

The menopause and psychotrauma

"During that time I would have separated myself from me, if I could have," a girlfriend said recently when I was telling her about my research into the menopause. Many women have already split from themselves much earlier. Some symptoms of the menopause only arise as a result of this early separation from their 'I', and at the same time the symptoms of the menopause often contain the necessary information for healing. I gained this experience and knowledge by accompanying many women in my practice.

It is striking that there is comparatively little specialist literature on the topic of the menopause, or advice based on studies. Women often say spontaneously: "Me? I haven't started that yet!" It still seems to be a taboo to talk openly about the subject. This may also have something to do with the fact that ageing is decried in our youth-oriented society. There are of course studies and guides on hormone replacement therapy, but these do not explain how the psychological stress develops. Women are usually alone with that, and so far we women have only been able to make unsatisfactory attempts at explaining why we often become 'contrary' during the menopause.

In my 25 years as an alternative practitioner I have not really been convinced by the possibilities of healing menopausal complaints with naturopathic means. For years I have worked psychosomatically. The Intention Method developed by Franz Ruppert simplifies the process for discovering early psychotraumas, and also for healing them. I have therefore asked myself how menopausal complaints and psychotrauma are connected and what effects the menopause has on the identity development of women willingly going through the menopause and those reluctantly going through it.

With Franz Ruppert's constellation method (Ruppert 2014) we can explain:

- why an early adjustment in childhood can be necessary;
- how the splitting-off of traumatic experiences affects our contact with our own 'I', our will and our own impulses;
- how the journey into a satisfactory 'third phase of life' can be pioneered through such findings.

The older we are, the greater our need is to accept ourselves as 'I'. The feeling we have of never being good enough, the quest for self-optimisation in order to please others, the effort we make to comply with the image others have of us, becomes less strong. On the contrary, the longing grows in many women to be able to say of oneself: "I know who I am and what I want to live for."

Even though these issues are equally important for everyone, in this article I am dealing with the female menopause and its effect on the development of the identity of those women willingly going through the menopause. I facilitate women's groups on the topic of the menopause and during them I provide information and facts about the menopause. Findings from brain research, attachment theory and developmental psychology form the foundation for my practical work.

Women suffer in different ways

In connection with the menopause, conventional medicine talks of 'climacteric syndrome', a typical combination of symptoms brought about by changes in the hormonal balance. There are many different menopausal complaints: nightly panic attacks, heart palpitations, night sweats and hot flushes, feeling overwhelmed, general anxiety, reduced ability to perform, loss of libido, weight gain, partnership problems, depressive symptoms, perhaps for example due to an unfulfilled wish to have children. Questions about the meaning of one's life return.

Almost all women I know experience the above symptoms, but they tend to focus on one particular symptom: they suffer particularly from the loss of the ability to define themselves as they used to. Women say things such as: "I never used to be afraid!", "But I always used to be slim!", "I never had a problem with sex!", "I never blushed!", or "I always had more energy than others!"

Why do women suffer in such different ways? In order to be able to answer this question we have to look for a reference to these specific symptoms in the biography of each individual woman. In other words, it will be possible to find a solution or healing if we look more closely at this 'hated' symptom.

Symptoms as signposts

In therapy we often see that precisely the mentioned condition (for example: "But I've always been strong!") has been in fact the woman's survival part, and the survival part also points us towards its origin – a traumatisation. In the current 'challenging' phase of life as an adult menopausal woman, the compensatory forces that, until now, through the survival part, have helped to keep the trauma at bay, no longer work. Instead the symptom is now perceived as an 'illness'.

The events that traumatise a woman in the early years of childhood, and/or any influences from the parents' or grand-parents' generation, lead to the child programming herself to adapt in order to be part of the community, the family – an essential programming for the children's survival. Trauma comes not only from experiences of war, accidents or natural disasters. Constant disparagement, lack of attention, and extreme neglect as a child can all be traumatising if the child is unable to cope with the situation in a healthy manner. The psyche tries to find a solution to prevent the child feeling overburdened. And the 'solution' is frequently psychological splitting as a trauma survival strategy.

As an example, during the menopause Gisela suffered increasingly from panic attacks and feeling overwhelmed. Her wish was "to function as I did before". That seemed like an instruction to me to help strengthen her survival parts – one of the most frequent forms of intention of my menopausal clients. The most important goal of therapy is to recognise that their survival part is not a 'resource' that will encourage healing, but that this old childhood behaviour pattern is no longer beneficial in this form today. Holding on to it prevents development. There can only be creative ability and healing if the survival part's rigid behavioural routines are changed.

The menopause is not an illness

I consciously use the word 'suffering' instead of talking of 'symptoms'. The term 'symptom' is generally used to refer to pathological changes. The menopause is not an illness – although subjectively it often feels as if it is. Professional 'menopause rating scales' contain questions about physical complaints such as hot flushes, urinary problems or muscle pain. The complaints associated with the drop in hormones also contain distinctive features that can be attributed to the person's psychological state. Sleep disorders, irritability, depressive moods or anxiety are also seen in conventional medicine as factors that affect the quality of life.

Conventional medicine is also aware of the subjective perception of symptoms. A study by Prof. Dr. Kerstin Weidner, Psychologist at the University Clinic in Dresden, confirms this. She has investigated the validity of the 'menopause rating scale'. In summary she says: "According to scientific literature, complaints that occur in the menopause should not be attributed prematurely to hormonal causes alone."

This confirms my conclusion: that there is a strong connection between menopausal complaints and the psyche. We generally assume that one third of women have a normal menopause, one third have moderate symptoms and one third have pronounced menopausal syndrome.[83] Current studies on the consequences of transgenerational trauma have established, for this group, a trail of earlier traumatisation in the brain, which is verifiable with imaging procedures.[84] Reinforcing factors for this particularly badly affected third of women are the menopausal (usually from the age of 45 or 50) strong fluctuations in the hormonal cycle as well as a steady reduction in the production of sexual hormones. The drop in oestrogen levels in particular leads to increased irritability (Riecher-Rössler, Kuhl and Bitzer, 2006). A psychological state, which until then was 'manageable', increases to become a psychological stress. According to the vulnerability/stress model, the stress limit is then exceeded. Usually this supplies the motivation to deal with the suppressed and yet stressful background of their present distress. In connection with the menopause then, a 'symptom' is more of a health-guide, not a sign of illness.

The menopause as a chance for personal growth

I interpret the menopause – just like other 'weakening' situations – as a period of transition, like the time after a severe illness or a bereavement, a period in which upheaval causes the gradual lessening of the strength necessary to maintain the survival programs from childhood. The menopause does not generate new symptoms – it reveals issues that have existed for a long time. This reinterprets the menopause as a time of profound opportunities for development. And that completely changes the perspective. The focus, then, is on the possibility for growth – not on loss or depletion, which is how this time is usually described.

---

[83] Feministisches FrauenGesundheitsZentrum e.V. (Publisher) (2012): Wechseljahre – Praktische Begleitung für diese Lebensphase [Menopause – Practical guidance during this phase of life].

[84] Bundesgesundheitsblatt Gesundheitsforschung Gesundheitsschutz (2016) 59(10), p. 1255–1261; doi: 10.1007/s00103-016-2436-2.

- Women can begin to recognise how they are being controlled by trauma coping strategies.
- They can begin to understand and feel the stress they are generating, instead of controlling it.
- Women can begin to understand their childhood survival programs as emergency solutions, and to replace them with new and useful abilities.

In the women's group 'Menopause – an illness?' we do a lot of work with the sentence of the Intention method, seeking our own identity. In this way women can often drop their external orientation and/or stop allowing themselves to be directed and defined by it. The women discover why they are suffering under certain conditions. They share experiences. This strengthens social acceptance. Women treat themselves more kindly and gain new zest for life. In one-to-one work with women and in this 'women's menopause group', I have experienced how, through working on their physical suffering and psychological intentions, women are able to accept the process of change through ageing, and also seize the opportunity to develop a healthy 'I' and sense of stability.

In group work and in one-to-one sessions, women pursue the causes of their subjective suffering. Questions arise from physical and psychological symptoms, such as: "Who am I really?", "What self-conceptions have I adopted?", "Can I really make decisions freely, or do I have to continue to react with acquired automated responses?" Here are a few examples, which are representative of the many women who have opened themselves up to encounter their own inner parts. Not 'stories', but approaches to their own female biographies connected with strong emotions. Women recognise their early splits, recall painful experiences and finally rediscover healthy, helpful parts of themselves that were left behind long ago.

I'll tell you about Heike, who is grieving because she has been unable to start a family; about Christa, whose sexuality suffers from massive changes of the mucosa; about Katja who has been experiencing profound loneliness since her daughter left home, and who is searching for energy for herself; and about Gisela who would like to know why her belly is so fat.

Gisela: "Why is my belly so fat?"

Gisela was born in 1962, has an adult son and has been part of the menopause women's group from the beginning. Gisela is a lively, independent woman who seems very self-confident. To begin with she sits there laughing about the planned intention "Why is my belly so fat?" I ask her whether she has any idea what that might have something to do with. Gisela's mood changes abruptly. She talks in a choked voice and through her tears, about panic attacks at being alone, from excessive demands that in the worst case lead to her fainting. Her father was a verbal and physical tyrant. She was constantly afraid of him, but didn't show it. "On the contrary." But today, despite her stressful childhood experiences, she wanted first of all to work on why her belly keeps growing.

First of all Gisela chooses a representative from the women's group for the word 'belly'. They hold hands and 'belly' immediately says: "I have a feeling of fullness in my own belly and a tension that has to hold onto everything." Gisela confirms this perception. One after another, she sets up representatives for the other words in her sentence. The 'why' says that she is almost fainting from fear and panic. The 'is' confirms what the 'why' has said and emphasises that it isn't over yet – it still *is*. She describes how she is on guard and has to sound out the surroundings in order to track down possible dangers.

Gisela can go along with all the statements and classifies the information: "Yes, this fear and panic is always there, especially when I'm alone. I feel that I push everything into my belly and hold it there." Now she sets up the word 'my', which looks afraid and says she is still very little. She withdraws from everything – even hiding herself. When Gisela asks her why she's doing that, 'my' replies: "You can't look after me – you don't want me". Gisela confirms this information. She recognises the 'my' as a traumatised child part and also recognises its distress. But she has more contempt for the supposed weakness than empathy for her self. Gisela ends the day's work at this point with the realisation that the fears have assumed their places in her belly. She decides to approach her vulnerability and sensibility.

As a child, Gisela had learnt to 'swallow down' her fear. Feelings or, worse, 'weaknesses', triggered her terrorising father. Gisela had had to develop a sort of foresight to protect herself as far as possible from her father's attacks. Even today she says: "I have to finish my work and I have to have everything planned in advance" – which is a survival strategy that is very important for her – otherwise she would not be able to bear the turmoil and fear.

Through the encounter with her survival part, Gisela was able to understand herself much better. In further constellations she slowly approached her scared, traumatised child part. She came into contact with an ability that, back then, she had had to split off: being able to look after herself by addressing injuries instead of "cramming feelings into my belly". Instead of automated reactions, Gisela can now react more flexibly to life. In other words she can structure her plans well, and does not have to plan ahead in a panic. She has become softer and can show her feelings better. Her belly is sometimes fatter, sometimes thinner – but other things have become more important to her.

At that time Gisela was living in a state of internal threat – a consequence of her childhood psychotrauma. She reacted with her survival patterns to circumstances that resembled the stressful situations of her past. In brain physiology this reaction can be attributed to the amygdala, the task of which is to evaluate risks in situations. Immediate reactions are initiated even before conscious actions are carried out, and we feel how the memory of the trauma is stored in the body. In constellation work, the unconscious can become conscious, and we can stop looking at life through a 'trauma scanner'.

Katja: "How can I find the way to my strength?"

Katja, 54, is separated and has an 18-year-old daughter. She is a lively, exuberant person who is frequently chosen as a representative because of her evident empathy. This time it's important for her to have her own constellation. In tears she tells us that her adult daughter has gone travelling and when she comes back she's planning to move out, but that's not why she's crying. On the contrary, after her daughter's departure she felt strong and self-confident and plunged herself intensively into planning her further career as a coach and team trainer. Then suddenly and inexplicably her energy collapsed, which shocked her and made her despair.

Her intention was: "How do I find a way to regain my strength so that I don't feel so abandoned?" Katja's sentence contains the word 'I' twice. She begins with the first 'I', who immediately appears self-confident and strong. The next word Katja sets up is 'strength'. She chooses a participant whose behaviour outside the group is independent and steady. 'Strength' immediately appears vulnerable and defiant and draws back from the 'I' with the words: "I'm not available to you like that any more". 'I' reacts in a disparaging and pugnacious manner.

Katja now sets up the 'how'. The representative shows solidarity with the 'I' and tries to convince 'strength' to join them. Katja feels connected to both of them and doesn't understand why 'strength' doesn't want to be touched by her or by the two other parts. She now chooses the second 'I' in her sentence. The representative doesn't want to be in contact with anyone, she feels alone and deserted. We recognise a child part of Katja in this 'I'. Now 'strength' is interested and moves towards the child part. She feels that she wants to "use her strength for the child 'I' and not for the removal of this abandoned child 'I'".

Katja recognises that in this constellation the first 'I' is a survival-'I' that has used its strength to avoid feeling abandoned, and wants to continue doing this. Katja knows that, as the third and unwanted child, she was neglected and she tried not to be a nuisance to her parents. She says: "I used my strength to make it easier for others". She ends the constellation when she can not only see but also feel that she no longer has to waste her strength on such a survival strategy. As her daughter grew up and left, Katja's own, split-off feelings of abandonment were triggered.

In a follow-up conversation a few months later she tells me that now, in the menopause and ageing, she has become reluctant to make it easy for others. She experiences that as positive: "It's over!"

Christa: "I want to be able to have sex again"

Christa was born in 1956, lives alone and doesn't have children. She came to my practice in 2014 following a three-year odyssey through gynaecological practices in different towns. She is now 58, slim, smart and in despair. Her husband left her six years previously for 'someone younger'. Christa was already suffering from menopausal complaints – depressive moods, hot flushes, sleep disorders. Due to 'operational cost-saving reasons' she lost her full-time secretarial job. She had her last period four years previously and shortly afterwards she complained about discomfort in the genital area. At the same time she began a relationship with a man a little older than her. Burning and dryness of the vaginal mucosa meant that shared sexuality became agony for her. To begin with, she kept her problem to herself because she was afraid her partner would leave her if there were any difficulties in having sex. At this time, Christa lived in Munich and she went to gynaecologists seeking help. She was given differing answers and different remedies. She tried to stay available sexually by using anti-fungal drugs, oestrogen creams and even antibiotics, which in her impatience she sometimes used at the same time. After a year her new partner left her. She assumes that her mucosa problem was the reason.

Christa moved to Berlin. Again she visited different gynaecologists and through an acquaintance she came to my practice. She said that she was now open to alternative methods, after the last gynaecologist had said to her that she would have to "live with the pain and just grit her teeth when she was having sex". First of all we worked on her problems with naturopathy before I suggested, in 2015, that we could look into a possible psychological background. Christa didn't want to do this work in the group so we arranged a one-to-one session.

Christa is an only child – 'her father's star' as he always called her. Her parents met after the Second World War when, according to her mother, "you were lucky to get hold of a healthy man". After her parents had been married for six years she was born in 1956 in the Ruhr area. Christa didn't know anything about the circumstances of her conception or her mother's pregnancy. In her opinion, her parents' marriage was 'difficult'. Her mother frequently had depressive episodes. The father left the family when Christa was 12. Her mother was then 40, had no vocational training and earned some extra money on top of her support payments in the catering trade. Her mother "kept bringing different men home", who also somehow paid their way, but never stayed long. She had no contact with her father any more. Her mother died 10 years ago.

Christa doesn't have a relationship at the moment. She is still unemployed and survives on very little money. She is afraid of "never getting a man again" and remaining unemployable. Her intention for the constellation is: "I want to be able to have sex again".

I make myself available to her as a representative in the one-to-one setting along with some felt floor-markers, which are characterised by their shape as female (circular) or male (square), to represent her words. She first chooses a round floor-marker for her 'I'. She stands opposite this marker and says that "first of all I can't do anything with it". Then she stands on it and says that she feels as if she is shrinking. After that she chooses a marker for 'sex' – "because this is what it's about" – and decides on a square marker. She places it next to the 'I' and at my suggestion she stands on it. She describes her feelings as a mixture of powerful and superior. Then she stands on her 'I' again and immediately begins to weep. When I ask her what is happening she says that, now that 'sex' is lying next to it, she feels a great loneliness and longing. That reminds her of the evenings alone at home when her mother was working.

Christa leaves the marker and then stands with one leg on 'I' and the other on 'sex'. She describes her plan to "bring the two together". As she stands there with straddled legs, she notices that she feels "somehow torn". She turns down my suggestion of setting up further elements from her intention with the words: "I think I already know what it's about – I've actually known it for some time".

Christa tells me her interpretation: "I have quite often not wanted to sleep with a man – not even with my husband. I would have preferred to leave it at the tenderness stage before – the closeness would have been enough for me." Christa's child-'I' longed for attention. Sexuality would of course not have been able to fulfil her child need for love. The image of her constellation – one leg here, one leg there – showed the split from her actual (suppressed) wish for intimacy. Christa's depressive mother was not able to give her the necessary closeness and presence. Turning to her father was the alternative – even if closeness to him was connected with splitting off her child needs and early sexuality.

Christa was satisfied with the result of this work and happy to have "talked about" her intermittent aversion to sexual intercourse and her inner turmoil about it. She decided she wouldn't try and heal her complaints with regard to "functioning during sex", but "simply wanting to heal herself".

The healing process is ongoing. Christa is no longer looking for a relationship at any cost. Her mucous membrane is slowly recovering, and she has moved back to Munich.

Heike: "Why can't I start a family of my own?"

Heike, 45, is in a relationship and doesn't have any children. She is a tall, slim woman with an alert mind, and is self-employed as a coach and lecturer. She talks about her desire to start a family but, following an operation on her ovaries, in-vitro fertilisation is her only chance to have children. After several unsuccessful attempts, she and her partner have come to terms with a life without children of their own. In the past, Heike has always had cats and she wants to have a cat again. She realises there are difficulties involved, because she lives on the sixth floor and is at work a lot. All this makes her sad and leads to her intention: "Why can't I start a family of my own?"

Heike first chooses a representative for her 'I'. The 'I' spontaneously says: "There's nothing wrong with me. I'm adult and I'm there for you". Now Heike chooses 'family'. The representative is sad and says: "I finally want to develop". The 'why' that Heike now sets up in the constellation seems approachable and affectionate: "I want to give you a lot, I'm around you, I'm enveloping you". Heike sees a connection with a womb – her mother's womb. When she mentions this, the 'why' says: "Yes, but I can't protect you – you should be there for me!"

Heike recognises traits of her mother in these sentences. She says it was her mother's 'marketing': I am the good, all-enveloping mother. But Heike knows that she was only 'right' if she wanted what her mother wanted. The 'why' then alters her behaviour and mutates from the enveloping mother to the smothering mother. She holds onto Heike tightly and says: "You're here for me – why should anyone else be important to you?!" Heike takes a step backwards and distances herself from the 'why'. She is visibly pale and upset, but also understanding what is happening. At this point she ends the constellation. Heike's sentence of intention was a wish for understanding, and she is satisfied with her insights.

Heike has seen and felt that a part of her is still under the influence of the 'smothering mother'. In order to maintain vital contact with the mother, this part subordinated itself as a child to the mother's desire for 'non-separation'. Heike's autonomy could not develop – her own plans for a family were thwarted by her mother's neediness. The 'I' in this constellation has shown a part of Heike that is already sufficiently grown up to lead an independent life. Heike has taken the opportunity several times to deal with her mother issues. Through her growing contact with herself she is now able to encounter her mother without self-abandonment.

Summary

The 'menopause-women' are always aware that it is the healthy parts that have brought them together. Contact within the group is described as 'sisterly-supportive'. The group grows through empathy for each other; it promotes better perception of the women's own female body. In this way, traumatising social experiences can also heal. Suppressed memories appear and lose their threatening nature through the orientation in the present. They can be disengaged.

The women learn which overwhelming circumstances from the past still trigger anxiety. That makes those things visible that have fixed us in old behavioural patterns. But it is not only the level of suffering, but curiosity and confidence too, which make the transition into this new phase of life easier. The women recognise their own competence; they see the abilities they have acquired in their life. That helps the women approaching the menopause 'willingly' to have a close look at the advantages and freedoms of becoming older. Through their constellations they experience understanding for themselves and affirmative self-acceptance.

References

Riecher-Rössler, A., **Kuh**, H. & **Bitzer**, J. (2006). *Psychische Störungen in Zeiten hormoneller Umstellung bei Frauen*, in Neuropsychiatrie (2006) 20(3), pp. 155–165.

Ruppert, F. (2016). *Early Trauma: Pregnancy, Birth and the First Years of Life*. Steyning, Green Balloon Publishing.

Weidner, K. & **Becermann**, M. (2016). *Beschwerden in dem Wechseljahren: Nicht nur eine Frage der hormonellen Situation*, in Deutsches Ärzteblatt (2016) 46, pp. A2101–A2106.

Andrea Tietz was born in 1959, and has worked as an alternative practitioner in Berlin since 1994. She is married, and is a mother and grandmother. www.core-evolving.de

CHRISTINA FREUND

Sport, the body and trauma

Sport as an over-exploitation of one's body

Sport is physical activity that we engage in for pleasure, to strengthen our body or competitively. According to the original meaning of the word, sport serves as a diversion, pleasure, amusement and play – exciting pleasure that comes from movements of the body.[85]

At school sport was my favourite lesson. I always loved to move, to be outside in all weathers, playing football and skiing. Later running became my passion, until it started to cause me suffering; I always had to run my distance, even if I was in pain. My pleasure in movement and physical expression became a compulsion: I had to run – until a sudden back operation stopped me and I couldn't run any more.

Unfortunately, my progression – from moving my body for sheer pleasure to it becoming a self-harming behaviour that damaged my body – is widespread. In the world of sport – and by no means only in competitive sports, but also in leisure and health sports – remarkable phenomena can be observed:

- putting oneself into life-threatening situations voluntarily and unnecessarily;
- disregarding the body's warning signals and thereby injuring oneself;
- doing training despite injuries, and making them worse;
- experiencing physical pain as pleasure;
- taking performance-enhancing substances and thereby permanently damaging the body.

---

[85] www.duden.de/rechtschreibung/Sport#Bedeutung1a

Why do athletes damage their bodies until they can no longer do the sport? On 3rd November 2016 there was a report in the *Süddeutsche Zeitung* about the end of the career of a 27-year-old, highly-talented cyclist: He was "an example of how a carefree attitude, the suppression of pain and an almost pathological ambition can turn an athlete bursting with strength into a decrepit young man". In this article he comments in retrospect: "I should have listened to my internal signals more, and never set out on the Tour". In the previous year alone he had had six bad falls, each time onto his head, but had carried on, and had only been stopped by a stomach bug.

Pressure to perform, doping, sports addiction, excessive demands and a mania for optimising the body testify to a fight for distance and times, for kilograms and muscles. Ultimately it is often a merciless struggle against one's own body that revealed itself to me in several conversations with doctors, physiotherapists and athletes. There is no meaningful data on the resulting damage to the athletes[86], but in the light of the approximately 23 million German nationals who regularly engage in sport, in other words several times a month, the number of people who damage themselves through sport is probably very high.

Sport injuries and sport science

Sport injuries are events that happen during sport. We have to differentiate between macro-traumatic injuries (massive external forces, accidents) and micro-traumatic injuries (protracted, recurring, often underlying strains and sport-related damage) (Würth, 2014). In what follows I will only deal with micro-traumatic injuries that result from chronic over-exertion, because these are avoidable. From a sports-scientific viewpoint, these injuries occur when movements continue despite physical warning signals. The body sends pain signals, which the athletes do not notice or do not interpret correctly.

---

[86] https://edoc.ub.uni-muenchen.de/8682/1/Seither_Berenike.pdf

Tim, 41, came to several individual sessions to explore his compulsive perfectionism. One day he rang me up to cancel an appointment: Because of a stress fracture in his foot he couldn't get up the stairs. He had exceeded his training schedule. Tim is a perfectionist, an enthusiastic runner who wants to improve his marathon time and trains according to a specially formulated schedule. When I asked, he said that before setting out, he had clearly felt that he should probably not run, but he ignored the feeling.

Why don't athletes take pain signals seriously or notice them properly? In their search for answers, sports scientists are increasingly looking at the athletes' psyche. Professor Sabine Würth summarises the existing explanations of sports injuries as follows (ibid, p.40–64):

- Action-psychological approaches: Injuries are caused by mistakes in the movement sequence. Personality characteristics such as willingness to take risks, fear, and lack of concentration and coordination lead to athletes deviating from normal movement patterns, thereby injuring themselves.
- Stress-theoretical approaches: Injuries are caused by stress management mechanisms. Athletes have different personality characteristics and are driven by stressors such as performance pressure. The interaction between stressors, personality characteristics and stress management mechanisms leads to injuries.

Würth notes that neither of these basic theoretical concepts go far enough in explaining the injuries; they view injuries predominantly as something that takes place largely within a person: injuries occur due to personal demands, performance pressure and personal characteristics. However, athletes not only make comparisons with themselves, but also with others. They see their achievements in relation to other people. That is why Würth places the relational aspect at the centre of her research. Using three empirical studies, she examined the influence of personality characteristics, such as "willingness to exert effort or exhaust oneself completely", and of social reference norms, such as "performance motivation and performance behaviour" on injuries. This shows that:

- it is mainly the willingness to exhaust oneself completely that often leads to injuries, due to hoped-for and/or perceived social recognition;
- over-adaptation to codes of conduct and values inherent in sport, identification as an athlete and the desire for appreciation and social recognition leads to injuries, unfavourable treatment of injuries, doping and eating disorders.

Accordingly, the need to be recognised and appreciated, to belong to the world of sport with its special code of values and conduct, and to have an identity e.g. as a football player, are stronger than the need for protection and the integrity of one's own body. These needs lead to one's own body being stressed past healthy limits, to pain signals being ignored or incorrectly perceived, and to injuries and damage. But why are some athletes so over-adapted and exceptionally willing to perform? Why is Tim such a perfectionist that he exceeds his training schedule and ignores all pain signals? Sport science has not yet asked these questions, which are important to me. That is why there are no studies in this regard.

I will therefore restrict myself to the individual biographies of athletes whom I accompany in my practical work with the intention method on the basis of identity-oriented psychotraumatology (IoPT).

Leo: "Playing football to save my life"

Leo, 31, injured his left knee very badly when he was 26 while playing football, without any external interference. He suffered an unhappy triad of injuries – a combination of a tear in the anterior cruciate ligament, inner meniscus and inner ligament.

How can the ligaments tear without any form of external interference? From a medical point of view it is very probable that Leo's knee was already damaged with micro-injuries through his excessive football playing. With such an impairment and continuing to put undiminished strain on the knee, it is likely that the ligaments will tear. When I question him, Leo says he did not feel anything beforehand that might have suggested an injury, but he also says that he had felt little or nothing at all at this time.

Leo comes to my seminar to look into a possible psychological background to his knee injury. His intention is: "Why have I completely destroyed my knee?" In his work Leo reveals himself from the beginning in a traumatised part: He weeps, his whole body trembles, he can hardly string two words together and can only write with difficulty. He starts with the word 'I'. Leo's 'I' feels uncompromisingly neutral, even uninvolved, as if it were none of his business. His 'knee' is very different: it desperately tries to come into contact first with the 'I' and then with Leo himself. It is not successful until it goes over to Leo, shakes him and shouts at him: "We're playing football for our lives! Don't you realise that?" At that Leo breaks down and only stands up again after a long while. "But I don't want to sacrifice my knee." When I ask him why he is playing football for his life, he shakes his head. He doesn't know. He started playing football when he was 11. First of all he played on his own, then with friends, then in a club, for hours every day after school, and the whole day long in the holidays.

Next Leo sets up the word 'destroyed'. This representative feels a life-threatening rejection, almost panic attacks. "You want to kill me! That's outrageous!" Leo freezes visibly. After a while he turns to his 'knee': "I am beginning to understand you. You don't have to fight any more. I don't know how, but I'll find another way." After that Leo ends his constellation.

In the next therapeutic process, Leo was able to further clarify this work: Leo's mother became pregnant unintentionally when she was 17. After he was born, Leo repeatedly spent several weeks at a time with his grandmother. The relationship between mother and grandmother was tense and prone to conflict. As an illegitimate 'child of shame', Leo was subject to massive rejection, to the point where his grandmother even tried to smother him with a cushion over his face. For years, Leo woke up in the night, paralysed and frozen with mortal fear, except for his left leg, which twitched uncontrollably. These panic attacks only stopped when Leo achieved clarity for himself about the attempted murder. In another constellation he wanted to know why the word 'destroyed' had shouted: "You want to kill me!"

Leo's unconscious memories and his work with the sentence of intention suggest that his knee injury could be a late physical consequence of his early childhood traumas. This remarkable connection between psychotrauma and subsequent sport injuries is new territory in the world of sport: so far, no research has been carried out on unresolved trauma experiences as a cause of sport injuries. Scientific research on the psychological consequences of injuries has only been available for a few years. According to this, serious injuries can traumatise athletes.

But how can a split-off trauma which happened a long time ago, be the cause of sport injuries? In Leo's traumatising environment, his psyche was evidently unable to develop in a healthy way. This is evidenced by the fact that Leo was unable to grasp the reality of his knee and act accordingly. He didn't feel any pain signals and went on playing. Correspondingly Leo's 'I' in the constellation described above was a survival I. He was playing football for his life. Football allowed him to bear his mother's and his grandmother's rejection and hostility. When he was running, taking shots at goal, or tackling, he was able to reduce the tense trauma energy stored in his body, so that he could live on for a brief while. However, this trauma energy repeatedly built up in his childhood through his continued contact with perpetrators, and in adulthood through his contact with his internalised perpetrator. Through football, Leo also gained access to his body, but that was exactly what had evoked the split childhood trauma experiences.

We can thus say that Leo repeatedly played against the threat of being killed, and fought against the perpetrator energies of his mother and his grandmother, in vain since Leo was a prisoner of the damaging re-enactment of his trauma. As a result, Leo could not stop playing football. He went on playing for his life, until almost all the ligaments in his knee tore – the 'unhappy triad' – literally an unhappy threesome (Leo – mother – grandmother). With this newly acquired understanding about his childhood and his self-destructive survival mechanisms, Leo gave up playing football. He doesn't want to do any more damage to his knee and is looking for other healthier ways of getting fun out of movement.

People are not always successful in transforming their survival parts into healthy structures.

Ina: Arthritis in both knees and ankles

Ina, 24, comes to an individual session because she has arthritis in both knees and ankles. The severe pain has stopped her from doing any form of sport and she is hardly able to move without pain. When I ask her what it means to her, not being able to do any sport, Ina begins to cry bitterly. Sport has always been her favourite thing. She cannot imagine life without running, cycling, skiing, and climbing.

For three years, Ina has been receiving excessive amounts of conventional medical and alternative treatments, but with no lasting success; the pain always returns. One of the doctors treating her speculates that her pain could have a psychological cause, and so she has come to me following his advice. She says that although she wants to understand why she is continually in pain, she also wants to do sport again. Her intention therefore is: "I want to do sport again".

Ina begins her work by standing on the floor-marker for 'again': "That is my mother. I've incorporated this part of her. But I have no problem standing there. I'm really angry with myself there." The next word she chooses is 'sport': "My knees are cooler here; they're usually so warm because they're inflamed. It's calming me down standing here. I'm becoming calmer here." After that she chooses 'want': "I don't get anything. This one feels empty. It feels like absolutely nothing.

It's neutral." On the word 'to-do' Ina's knees give way visibly: "It's pulling me downwards. It's like a lost perspective – hopelessness and desperation; like I've felt recently without sport." Finally Ina stands on her 'I': "What is that? I? No idea... 'You're bad and spoilt! You'll pay for your happiness!' That's how my mother used to curse me, for as long as I can remember, whenever I was happy."

Ina's mother had longed for a boy. After giving birth, when she saw that her child was a girl, she began to shriek loudly and curse the newborn child. She was quickly admitted to a psychiatric clinic. Even today, she cannot bear the fact that she has a happy, lively and agile daughter. She reviles and curses Ina repeatedly, prophesying her death and that she will go to hell. Her mother is only able to treat Ina normally when Ina is ill or physically injured. As a result, Ina's childhood and adolescence were dominated by illness, accidents and sport injuries. In between there were phases in which Ina was healthy, when she was outside a lot and played many different sports successfully and with great enjoyment. Since moving away from home it has become worse. Ina can now hardly move because of the inflammation.

Ina was already traumatised and lost her identity in the womb, through the fundamental rejection by her mother of her gender. According to the theory of the trauma biography, as described in the introductory chapter of Franz Ruppert's book, Early Trauma (Ruppert, 2016), this 'trauma of identity' leads to a 'trauma of love'. The mother can only tolerate Ina when Ina is ill or injured. As a result, Ina's psyche cannot develop in a healthy way, and she does not recognise her own distress and the desperation of the mercilessly rejected child that she was. On the contrary she sees her 'arthritis' as an enemy to be fought against. Her 'I' is identified with the destructive 'mother-energy', and so in Ina's body a terrible perpetrator-victim dynamic is raging (Ruppert, 2016). In order to survive and endure her mother's destructive energy, she permanently damages her body, thereby carrying on her mother's destructive work herself as an adult. In the process of her trauma biography Ina has become a perpetrator against herself. A few weeks after this work Ina wrote in an email: "No, there is no distress behind the inflammation. It is my enemy. It has to go. I have to fight against it. Then I'll be able to do sport again. Then I'll have conquered my mother."

Ina has apparently not found a path out of her self-damaging behaviour towards herself into a healthy life. For her, the fight against her body and its needs is still the only way to live with the reality of her prenatal traumatic experiences.

Manu: Periostitis in both shins

Manu, aged 47, wants to find out who she really is with the help of the intention method: "Who am I without my survival parts 'competitive athlete' and 'manager'?" She ended her career as an alpine skier as a consequence of periostitis (shin splints) in both shins. Despite all the treatment, her legs still hurt today. After the end of her skiing career, Manu put all her energy and strength into her professional career. After a few individual and group sessions, I asked her to summarise her findings to date regarding "her identity and the injury to her legs":

"When my legs refused to ski even one more turn, I thought I would die. How could my body do that to me? That was the first time in all my years of competitive sport that I even tried to talk to it ... or, more precisely, scream hysterically at it. I had consistently ignored its screams in all that time, and they had been loud and often. My body had been signalling endless exhaustion and frustration, and finally with increasing pain in the periosteum, but I couldn't afford to listen to it. My happiness, yes, even my life, depended on staying in the ski team, to continue to be part of it, at any cost. The team was somehow my family, where would I go without it? How could I bear not going to competitions any more, no longer being seen and not belonging anywhere?

"But it was not a family in which one could experience stability or security. It was a group in which I had to fight, and in which the trainer told me that I should become more selfish because otherwise I wouldn't get anywhere in individual sport.

How big was my disappointment when the familiar, cheerful childhood sports group, with whom I had had such great enjoyment of going on courses, being silly, and simply enjoying nature, turned into an elite of individual contestants, and 'sport' no longer stood for freedom and joy in movement, but ended up becoming a struggle for survival.

"Anger, sadness and grimness governed my final years in competitive sport. My movements, which had been light-footed and joyful, suddenly became hard and jerky. The fear of not being good enough and losing my place meant that I could hardly sleep at night, and a leaden tiredness blighted my day. At that time a part of me wanted to give up. Being in the public eye felt flat, and even occasional successes couldn't preserve the illusion that I had what I wanted.

"Today I know that I was searching desperately for love and recognition, and wished so much to have everything I had missed in my own family. And it was precisely this disappointment that repeated itself in sport ad infinitum, until my body called a halt to it. And it did that thoroughly, because the ski run 27 years ago was my last."

As an unborn child, Manu experienced existential rejection. Although her mother hadn't thought consciously of abortion, or made any attempt to carry one out, the womb was still a threatening place for Manu. For her mother, the pregnancy was overwhelming, because of a trauma she herself had experienced. As Manu's work repeatedly showed, from the very beginning it was Manu's determined will to live that allowed her to survive the time in her mother's womb. With her will and her child's unconditional love after her birth Manu tried to convince her mother to see and love her. But despite all her efforts, her mother remained ambivalent towards her daughter – trapped in her own unresolved trauma experiences. Manu's 'trauma of identity' led directly to a 'trauma of love'.

Manu transferred this struggle for survival against rejection and for recognition and love, into competitive sport. There she met with the destructive energy she had first experienced in the womb (it has to be 'I' or 'You'), in the competitive struggle for places in the squad. And, just as she had as a child, she reacted with her strong will to survive and her childlike search for love and recognition. She didn't manage it. She wasn't loved or recognised there either. This hopeless task led to the constant re-enactment of her original identity trauma – until her shins became permanently inflamed.

Even today, Manu finds it almost impossible to do any sport. But it doesn't have to stay that way. What opportunities might open up for her in sport if she can end her survival struggle? If she continues her search for her healthy 'I'-parts? And looks after them and nurtures them? I wonder.

On the move with a healthy 'I'

In summary, the insights of sports science described earlier can be found in many examples from my practical work with the intention method; people who do sport may injure and damage themselves when their psyche is not in touch with the reality of their body; when they do not know by feeling that their body needs a break or that it is injured; or when they feel the warning signals but don't pay them enough attention. Sports science sees personality traits as the cause of injuries. In my opinion that is a mistake with far-reaching consequences because these are only symptoms, attributions or 'masks'. But the question is: what is hidden behind these athletes' masks?

The case histories indicate that the causes of these serious failures of the psyche can lie in very early experiences of trauma. The 'trauma of identity' fundamentally disrupts the development of the psyche with its special functions, particularly of the 'I' and the will. If people's identities are traumatised very early in their life they develop illusory identities that consist of identification and attribution: "I am an athlete. I want to be successful, loved and recognised". Thus athletes do not perceive the reality of their body and behave accordingly, which can be very damaging. As a result, we cannot prevent self-harm and self-injury in sport at the level of symptoms as sports science suggests. An athlete I know describes it like this:

"An 'I' who practises competitive sports cannot be a healthy 'I'. Because the aim here is to make the body as fit as possible for a certain period of time. And in doing that, signals received from the body are simply a nuisance and have to be blanked out. Some [people] can partially develop a healthy 'I' when their career is over, but many cannot."

So if we succeed in overcoming existing survival structures and strengthening healthy 'I'-structures, we can engage in sport healthily and with enjoyment: "It would be best if I could find the child in me who had so much fun from movement", once again in the words of the above athlete.

References

Ruppert, F. (2016). *Early Trauma: Pregnancy, Birth and the First Years of Life*. Steyning, Green Balloon Publishing.

Ruppert, F. (2014). *Trauma, Fear & Love: On the Path to Healthy Autonomy, How Constellations can be Helpful*. Steyning, Green Balloon Publishing.

Schmid, M. (2016) *Gegen die Wand*, in: *Süddeutsche Zeitung* vom 3.11.2016.

Würth, S. (2014): *Verausgabungsbereitschaft und Overconformity im Kontext von Verletzungen im Sport (=Spektrum Bewegungswissenschaft, Bd. 8)*. Aachen: Meyer & Meyer.

Christina Freund, born 1974 has a degree in social pedagogy, completed social work studies at the University of Applied Sciences, Munich, and advanced training in psychotraumatology and trauma counselling with Lutz-Ulrich Besser (2006–2008). Subsequently she completed an advanced training in 'Trauma, Bonding and Family Constellations' with Franz Ruppert in 2008, and since 2009 has offered group seminars with the method of self-encounter. Since 2012 she has had a private, independent trauma counselling, and a lectureship at the University of Applied Sciences, Munich. www.christinafreund-selbstbegegnungen.de

Green Balloon Publishing

By Franz Ruppert:

Trauma, Bonding & Family Constellations: *Understanding and healing injuries of the soul* (2008)

Splits in the Soul: *Integrating traumatic experiences* (2011)

Symbiosis & Autonomy: *Symbiotic trauma and love beyond entanglement* (2012)

Trauma, Fear and Love: *How the Constellation of the Intention Supports Healthy Autonomy* (2014)

Early Trauma: *Pregnancy, Birth and First Years of Life* (2016)

By Vivian Broughton:

In the Presence of Many: *Reflections on Constellations emphasising the individual context* (2010)

The Heart of Things: *Understanding trauma – working with constellations* (2013)

becoming your true self: *a handbook for the journey from trauma to healthy autonomy* (2014)

---

www.greenballoonbooks.co.uk
info@greenballoonbooks.co.uk

42 Goring Road, Steyning, West Sussex, BN44 3GF, UK.
Tel: +44 (0) 1903 814489 – info@greenballoonbooks.co.uk

www.ingramcontent.com/pod-product-compliance
Lightning Source LLC
Chambersburg PA
CBHW020654270326
41928CB00005B/113